Praise for

Transition Strategie
Adolescents & Young Adults

D1324567

"Communication plays a substantial role in anyone's involvement with friends, family, neighbors, and coworkers. Too often, communication strategies are an afterthought, especially as students leave school and migrate into the world of adults. This book is not simply critical reading for educators and families, but also for staff throughout the adult system, and especially for those charged with employment. Alternative and augmentative communication is vital to understanding complex behavior, to understanding anyone's vocational themes and desires, to designing instructional strategies, and for increasing worksite integration. The authors transcend most books focused on this age group by addressing the whole person, and by moving transition planning away from simple compliance and paperwork to the impacts of real-life outcomes."

—**Cary Griffin and Dave Hammis**
Senior Partners
Griffin-Hammis Associates

"As you know, effective transition planning requires that transition teams help students with disabilities identify goals for their adult lives and then plan the supports and services that can help them achieve those goals. It's not always easy: Students' goals may not be the same as the goals that adults have for them; the necessary supports or services may not be available; or the student's needs might be so diverse that they are beyond the expertise of the planning team. Students who use AAC who are planning for their transition to adult life may fit into this category: Not only do their transition teams need to address the typical supports and services, they also must address their diverse AAC needs in all transition domains. This book helps transition stakeholders who find themselves struggling to understand the needs of adolescents and young adults who use AAC as they plan for their transition to adult life. The book uses concrete examples, case studies, and step-by-step instruction to provide the kind of guidance that transition teams need to help them tailor their individualized transition planning for students and young adults who use AAC. Thanks to Drs. McNaughton and Beukelman for preparing this book to help educators, parents, transition specialists, and other transition stakeholders assist students with disabilities meet their dreams for a transition to a preferred adult lifestyle!"

—**Colleen A. Thoma, Ph.D.**
Director, Doctoral Programs
Virginia Commonwealth University School of Education
Richmond

"I am delighted to see this addition to the AAC Series. This text fills an important gap in the literature between school-based services and those provided in the adult community. It provides a wealth of practical information about a wide range of topics vital to service providers and their adolescent clients with complex communication needs."

—**Kathryn M. Yorkston, Ph.D.**
Professor and Head, Division of Speech Pathology
Department of Rehabilitation Medicine
University of Washington, Seattle

"McNaughton and Beukelman have compiled a much-needed book addressing individuals too long neglected in the secondary transition literature: youth and young adults using AAC support who experience some of the lowest employment, literacy, and community participation rates of people with disabilities. This edited book is packed with up-to-date research, lively case examples, and down-to-earth 'how to' strategies covering a gamut of everyday life from literacy to sexuality. Both in-school and postschool outcomes are addressed by contributing authors who are experts in their areas. This is a must-have book for parents, teachers, caregivers, support providers, and AAC users themselves."

—Carolyn Hughes, Ph.D.
Professor of Special Education
Vanderbilt University

"This comprehensive text covers virtually all aspects of the often-complex process of transition to adult life for young people who use augmentative and alternative communication. It is an outstanding resource for anyone who is in a position to assist these individuals effectively prepare for and navigate this transition."

—Richard Luecking, Ed.D.
President, TransCen, Inc.
Rockville, Maryland

Series Editors:
David R. Beukelman
Joe Reichle

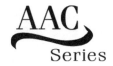

Transition Strategies for Adolescents & Young Adults Who Use AAC

Also in the *Augmentative and Alternative Communication Series:*

Autism Spectrum Disorders and AAC
edited by Pat Mirenda, Ph.D.,
and Teresa Iacono, Ph.D.

*Practically Speaking: Language, Literacy,
and Academic Development for Students with AAC Needs*
edited by Gloria Soto, Ph.D.,
and Carole Zangari, Ph.D., CCC-SLP

*Communicative Competence for Individuals Who
Use AAC: From Research to Effective Practice*
edited by Janice C. Light, Ph.D.,
David R. Beukelman, Ph.D.,
and Joe Reichle, Ph.D.

*Exemplary Practices for Beginning
Communicators: Implications for AAC*
edited by Joe Reichle, Ph.D.,
David R. Beukelman, Ph.D.,
and Janice C. Light, Ph.D.

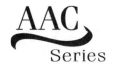
Series

Transition Strategies for Adolescents & Young Adults Who Use AAC

edited by

David B. McNaughton, Ph.D.
The Pennsylvania State University
University Park, Pennsylvania

and

David R. Beukelman, Ph.D.
University of Nebraska
Lincoln, Nebraska

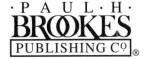
·P A U L·H·
BROOKES
PUBLISHING CO.®

Baltimore • London • Sydney

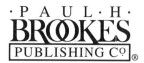

Paul H. Brookes Publishing Co.
Post Office Box 10624
Baltimore, Maryland 21285-0624
USA

www.brookespublishing.com

Typeset by Integrated Publishing Solutions, Grand Rapids, Michigan.
Manufactured in the United States of America by
Sheridan Books, Inc., Chelsea, Michigan.

The individuals described in this book are composites or real people whose situations are masked and are based on the authors' experiences. In most instances, names and identifying details have been changed to protect confidentiality. Real names and identifying details are used with permission.

Library of Congress Cataloging-in-Publication Data

Transition strategies for adolescents & young adults who use AAC / edited by David B.
McNaughton and David R. Beukelman.
    p.   cm.–(Augmentative and alternative communication series)
Includes index.
ISBN-13: 978-1-55766-997-1 (pbk.)
ISBN-10: 1-55766-997-X
1. People with disabilities—Means of communication.   2. Communication devices for people with disabilities.
3. Communication Disorders—rehabilitation.   I. McNaughton, David B. II. Beukelman, David R., 1943–.
III. Title.   IV. Series: AAC Series.
RC423.T59 2010
616.85′503–dc22   2009053994

British Library Cataloguing in Publication data are available from the British Library.

2014   2013   2012   2011   2010

10   9   8   7   6   5   4   3   2   1

Contents

Series Preface

The purpose of the *Augmentative and Alternative Communication Series* is to address advances in the field as they relate to issues experienced across the life span. Each volume is research based and practical, providing up-to-date and ground-breaking information on recent social, medical, and technical developments. Each chapter is designed to be a detailed account of a specific issue. To help ensure a diverse examination of augmentative and alternative communication (AAC) issues, an editorial advisory board assists in selecting topics, volume editors, and authors. Prominent scholars, representing a range of perspectives, serve on the editorial board so that the most poignant advances in the study of AAC are sure to be explored.

In the broadest sense, the concept of AAC is quite old. Gestural communication and other types of body language have been widely addressed in the literature about communication for hundreds of years. Only recently, though, has the field of AAC emerged as an academic discipline that incorporates graphic, auditory, and gestural modes of communicating. The series concentrates on achieving specific goals. Each volume details the empirical methods used to design AAC systems for both descriptive groups and for individuals. By tracking the advances in methods, current research, practice, and theory, we will also develop a broad and evolutionary definition of this new discipline.

Many reasons for establishing this series exist, but foremost has been the number and diversity of the people who are affected by AAC issues. AAC consumers and their families, speech-language pathologists, occupational therapists, physical therapists, early childhood educators, general and special educators, school psychologists, neurologists, and professionals in rehabilitative medicine and engineering all benefit from research and advancements in the field. Likewise, AAC needs are not delineated by specific age parameters; people of all ages who have developmental and acquired disabilities rely on AAC. Appropriate interventions for individuals across a wide range of disabilities and levels of severity must be considered.

Fundamentally, the field of AAC is problem driven. We, the members of the editorial advisory board, and all professionals in the field are dedicated to solving problems in order to improve the lives of people with disabilities. The inability to communicate effectively is devastating. As we chronicle the advances in the field of AAC, we hope to systematically dismantle the barriers that prevent effective communication for all individuals.

About the Editors

David B. McNaughton, Ph.D., Professor, Department of Educational and School Psychology and Special Education, and Department of Communication Sciences and Disorders, The Pennsylvania State University, 227 Cedar Building, University Park, PA 16802

Dr. McNaughton is a professor of education at The Pennsylvania State University. He teaches coursework in augmentative communication and assistive technology and collaboration skills for working with parents and educational team members. Dr. McNaughton's research interests include literacy instruction for individuals who use AAC and supports to employment for individuals with severe disabilities. He is a partner in the Rehabilitation Engineering and Research Center in Communication Enhancement (AAC-RERC), funded by the National Institute on Disability and Rehabilitation Research (NIDRR).

David R. Beukelman, Ph.D., Professor, Special Education and Communication Disorders, University of Nebraska, 118 Barkley Memorial Center, Lincoln, NE 68583

Dr. Beukelman is a speech-language pathologist who specializes in AAC and communication disorders associated with acquired medical conditions. He is the Barkley Professor of Communication Disorders at the University of Nebraska–Lincoln, a senior researcher in The Institute for Rehabilitation Science and Engineering at Madonna Rehabilitation Hospital in Lincoln, Nebraska, and a partner in the Rehabilitation Engineering and Research Center in Communication Enhancement (AAC-RERC).

Dr. Beukelman is an editor of the *Augmentative and Alternative Communication Series* published by Paul H. Brookes Publishing Co. and co-author of the textbooks *Augmentative and Alternative Communication: Supporting Children and Adults with Complex Communication Needs, Third Edition* (Paul H. Brookes Publishing Co., 2005) and *Management of Motor Speech Disorders in Children and Adults, Second Edition* (PRO-ED, 1999).

About the Contributors

Anthony Arnold, Prentke Romich Company, 2823 Knight Drive, Grand Forks, ND 58201

Mr. Arnold is an augmentative and alternative communicator who works in the AAC as a remote troubleshooter/beta tester.

Susan Balandin, Ph.D., Professor, Molde University College, Britvegen 2, Molde, Norway 6402

Dr. Balandin is a speech-language pathologist with both a clinical and research background in working with people with lifelong disability and complex communication needs. Her research focus is on inclusion and participation for people with lifelong disability in a range of community contexts including health care.

Laura J. Ball, Ph.D., Associate Professor, East Carolina University, 3310-U Allied Health Sciences, Mail Stop 668, Greenville, NC 27834

Dr. Ball is an associate professor in the Department of Communication Sciences and Disorders at East Carolina University. Dr. Ball completed her doctoral degree at the University of Nebraska with research interests in AAC and motor speech disorders. Dr. Ball has more than 25 years' clinical experience and is the author of numerous publications on topics related to AAC, dysarthria, and apraxia.

Elizabeth Benedek-Wood, M.Ed., Doctoral Candidate in Special Education, Department of Educational and School Psychology and Special Education, The Pennsylvania State University, 123 Cedar Building, University Park, PA 16802

Elizabeth Benedek-Wood is a doctoral candidate in special education at The Pennsylvania State University. Her current research interests include literacy instruction and language development for individuals with disabilities. Before entering her doctoral program, she worked as a special education teacher supporting the participation of students with disabilities in general education classrooms.

Erik W. Carter, Ph.D., Associate Professor, Department of Rehabilitation Psychology and Special Education, University of Wisconsin–Madison, Madison, WI 53706

Dr. Carter is an associate professor in the Department of Rehabilitation Psychology and Special Education at the University of Wisconsin–Madison. His research and teaching focuses on strategies for supporting meaningful school inclusion and promoting valued roles in school, work, and community settings for children and adults with intellectual and developmental disabilities.

Barbara Collier, Executive Director, Augmentative Communication Community Partnerships Canada, 131 Barber Greene Road, Toronto, Ontario, Canada M3C 3Y5

Barbara Collier is a speech-language pathologist and is currently executive director of Augmentative Communication Community Partnerships Canada, a nonprofit organization that promotes social awareness, justice, quality of life, and community partnerships for people with complex communication disabilities.

John Dattilo, Ph.D., Professor, Department of Recreation, Park and Tourism Management, The Pennsylvania State University, 801 Ford Building, University Park, PA 16802

Dr. Dattilo is a professor in the Department of Recreation, Park and Tourism Management at The Pennsylvania State University where he teaches courses on inclusive leisure for people with disabilities, therapeutic recreation, leisure education, and issues in higher education. Much of his research examines effects of interventions designed to enhance self-determination of people with disabilities relative to their leisure participation. Dr. Dattilo also solicits input from individuals with disabilities via interviews and observations to better understand their perceptions and to develop services based on their stated and observed interests and needs.

John Draper, Founder, *Together We Rock!*, 684 Glencairn Street, Oshawa, Ontario, Canada L1J 5A7

John Draper is founder of *Together We Rock!*, a business endeavor that promotes learning and leadership to build communities that are inclusive of and accessible to individuals with disabilities. He is a journalism graduate of Durham College and was honored by his alma mater with the Alumni of Distinction Award. He is the recipient of numerous awards, including the Possum-ISAAC Aspiration Award, for his efforts to make the vision of creating accessible and inclusive schools a reality.

Beth E. Foley, Ph.D., CCC-SLP, Professor and Head of the Department of Communicative Disorders and Deaf Education, Utah State University, Logan, UT 84322

For more than 2 decades, Dr. Foley's career has focused on using assistive technology to improve educational, social, and vocational outcomes for individuals with complex communication needs. Dr. Foley's primary research interests are language and literacy development in children with complex communication needs, and inclusion of students who use AAC in general education settings. Her numerous publications, conference presentations, and workshops on these topics communicate the critical need for integrating best practices in AT/AAC, language, and literacy intervention into educational programming for students with significant disabilities.

Denise Hazelrigg, M.S., B.S., Speech-Language Pathologist, Westside Community Schools, 1305 S. 90th Street, Omaha, NE 68124

Denise Hazelrigg is the assistive technology consultant for Westside Community Schools in Omaha, Nebraska. She serves the augmentative communication and literacy needs of a wide range of students.

Dave Hingsburger, M.Ed., Director of Clinical and Educational Supports, Vita Community Living Services, 4301 Weston Road, Toronto, Ontario, Canada, M9L 2Y3

Dave Hingsburger has worked with people with intellectual disabilities in the area of sexuality for more than 30 years. He is a prolific author and speaker. At present he is a director with Vita Community Living Services. In 2009, Dave was inducted into the Canadian Disability Hall of Fame in recognition of his groundbreaking work in the areas of sexuality and abuse prevention.

Christy A. Horn, Ph.D., ADA/504 Compliance Officer, University of Nebraska, 3835 Holdrege Street, Lincoln, NE 68583

Dr. Horn is the ADA/504 Compliance Officer for the University of Nebraska and holds a Ph.D. in cognitive psychology. She has been providing accommodation to individuals with disabilities in higher education for 25 years. Her work has centered on the creation of programs and environments that provide individuals with disabilities the opportunity to achieve their goals and realize their potential.

Pamela Kennedy, Writers Brigade Editor and Program Manager, Rehabilitation Engineering Researh Center on Communication Enhancement (AAC-RERC), 58 Amberley Way, Carrollton, GA 30116

Pamela Kennedy is an individual with complex communication needs who uses AAC. Pamela Kennedy is a journalist, advocate, and mentor who communicates via speech technology. She teaches journalism online to people with complex communication needs through the AAC-RERC Writers Brigade. Her interests include writing, research, assistive technology, and psychology.

Randy Joe May, B.S., Advocate
Randy May died in October 2005. He moved from Arkansas to attend University of Nebraska–Lincoln and graduated with a degree in political science. He worked for the Nebraska State Legislature as a researcher and established a physically challenged ministry at Christ Place Church. He was an advocate and a tremendous sports fan, and he was best known for his infectious smile and sense of humor.

Lateef McLeod, M.F.A., B.A., Consumer Consultant, DynaVox Mayer-Johnson, 2100 Wharton Street, Suite 400, Pittsburgh, PA 15203

Lateef McLeod has a budding career as a writer. He earned a B.A. degree in English from the University of California at Berkeley, then completed an M.F.A. degree in creative writing from Mills College in Oakland, California. He currently is a commissioner on the City of Oakland Mayor's Commission on People with Disabilities and is publishing his poetry book, *A Declaration of a Body of Love,* due out in 2010. He is also in the middle of writing his first novel.

Tracy Rackensperger, M.A., Outreach and Community Education Coordinator, University of Georgia, Institute on Human Development and Disability, 850 College Station Road, Athens, GA 30605

Tracy Rackensperger has worked in the field of AAC for more than a decade. She has conducted research and outreach with fellow scholars, families, and individuals who rely on AAC. A number of her published works can be found in the journal *Augmentative and Alternative Communication.* Ms. Rackensperger also has 28 years of personal experience with AAC.

Hazel Self, R.N., Community Services Coordinator, West Park Healthcare Centre, 100 Merton Street, Suite 105, Toronto, Ontario, Canada M4S 3G1

Hazel Self has had quadriplegia since 1978 and since then has been involved in using and developing different models of attendant services. She works at Gage Transition to Independent Living in Toronto, Canada. The Gage is a program providing experiential learning opportunities for people with physical disabilities who desire knowledge and skills for independent living. Hazel is presently Chair of the board of Augmentative Communication Community Partnerships Canada.

Sam Sennott, M.S., Doctoral Student, The Pennsylvania State University, 227 Cedar Building, University Park, PA 16802

Sam Sennott is a special educator and technology specialist who focuses his research and clinical practice on using innovative AAC systems. He has led inclusive school programs, camps, and assistive technology teams. He is the co-creator of Proloquo2Go applications for the iPhone and iPod Touch.

Elizabeth Serpentine, M.S., Speech-Language Pathologist, The Pennsylvania State University, 308 Ford Building, University Park, PA 16802

Elizabeth Serpentine is a doctoral candidate at The Pennsylvania State University and a speech-language pathologist for the Lower Merion School District in Ardmore, Pennsylvania. Her current research interests include the use of evidence-based practice for individuals with autism spectrum disorders (ASD), improving communicative competence for individuals with ASD, and transition/employment issues for life beyond the classroom for individuals with ASD.

Korey Stading, M.S., CCC-SLP, Speech-Language Pathologist, Munroe-Meyer Institute, University of Nebraska Medical Center, 985450 Nebraska Medical Center, Omaha, NE 68198

Korey Stading is a speech-language pathologist who specializes in AAC and children with severe communication disorders. She facilitates a preschool program at Munroe-Meyer Institute for young children who benefit from the use of differing levels of AAC support. She trains undergraduate and graduate students on the use of AAC strategies in this setting. She completes AAC evaluations for children and young adults at Munroe-Meyer Institute and also for various local school districts. She serves as a consultant to local school districts for AAC needs and provides training to teachers, speech therapists, and paraprofessionals to help implement AAC strategies and devices.

Annalu Waller, Ph.D., Rehabilitation Scientist and Senior Lecturer, School of Computing, University of Dundee, Perth Road, Dundee, Scotland DD1 4HN

Dr. Waller is a rehabilitation scientist and senior lecturer in the University of Dundee's School of Computing. Her research focuses on the design and evaluation of computer-based communication systems for people with little or no functional speech. She also has cerebral palsy, which affects her speech, mobility, and hand function.

Michael L. Wehmeyer, Ph.D., Professor, Director, Senior Scientist, The University of Kansas, 1200 Sunnyside Avenue, Room 3136, Lawrence, KS 66045

Dr. Wehmeyer is a professor of special education, the director of the Kansas University Center on Developmental Disabilities, and a senior scientist at the Beach Center on Disability—all at The University of Kansas. Dr. Wehmeyer has published extensively in the area of self-determination and is the author of several textbooks focused on self-determination.

Julie A. Wolter, Ph.D., CCC-SLP, Assistant Professor, Department of Communicative Disorders and Deaf Education, Utah State University, 1000 Old Main Hill, Logan, UT 84322

Dr. Wolter is an assistant professor in the Department of Communicative Disorders and Deaf Education at Utah State University. Dr. Wolter's teaching and research interests are in the areas of preschool and school-age language and literacy development, as well as evidence-based practice in the speech-language pathology clinical setting.

Sandra Wright, M.S., Instructor, University of Tulsa, 800 South Tucker Drive, Tulsa, OK 74112

Sandra Wright is an American Speech-Language-Hearing Association (ASHA) certified speech-language pathologist who has provided language intervention to people with complex communication needs resulting from developmental disabilities for 10 years. She is a doctoral candidate at The University of Kansas, under the mentorship of Dr. Jane Wegner, with a research emphasis in communicative competence and self determination of people who use AAC systems. Ms. Wright currently holds the position of Instructor at the University of Tulsa, where she is the graduate course instructor for the Communication Modalities course that allows graduate students hands-on opportunities to interact with a wide variety of AAC systems.

Foreword

As I read this excellent book on transitions in augmentative and alternative communication (AAC), I became aware of an insight I had many years ago: Communication disability is a unique dimension in disability because it compromises participation in the activities of life. Furthermore, the depth of its compromise is apt to be misunderstood, ignored, or discounted by people with other disabilities and professionals who serve people with disabilities.

Transition Strategies for Adolescents & Young Adults Who Use AAC has perceptive chapters about communicating with medical professionals and personal-care attendants. There are parts describing issues in school planning and employment. The difficulty of establishing personal independence is addressed as well as problems involved with friendships and intimacy. Nevertheless, I believe even a sincere reader of this book could underestimate two realities of life for people with complex communication needs. The first is the energy and focus required for an individual with significant speech and multiple disabilities to live in the community. The second is the impenetrability of the environmental and attitudinal barriers caused by the inability to communicate.

I am a communication aid system designer with a linguistics background who has served for 20 years as program chair of the Pittsburgh Employment Conference for Augmented Communicators (PEC@). During this time I have been inviting people who use AAC and their families, communication disability professionals, agency staff members, and other stakeholders in the AAC community to attend PEC@ and present their ideas, points of view, experiences, and formal research. Much of my experience with transitions in AAC comes from what individuals who use AAC have told me through my role at PEC@.

The first conference was well attended with interesting presentations on many levels. Decisions were made in planning and during the conference that were fateful. First was the decision to have all plenary sessions so that everybody would be part of all of the group discussions. At that time and even today, not much is known about overcoming barriers to employment for people with complex communication needs who use AAC. (See Chapter 6 about how much has been learned in the past 2 decades.) The second decision occurred during the first conference—all participants with complex communication needs had to be heard before oral speakers were called on. People who use AAC regularly say that PEC@ is their first conference experience where they feel they "really belonged" and did not feel like outsiders.

There have been 11 successful PEC@ conferences to date, and I continue to serve as program chair. I meet individuals who use AAC for whom employment is a strong life goal and others who are competent adults who have no interest in employment. Some years ago, I observed that the achievement of independence was itself a goal equal in dignity to employment for many people who use AAC. Controlling one's own life is experienced by people with complex communication needs as the psychological and symbolic equivalent of having a job, and justifiably so. For a person who use AAC, managing his or her own personal care and dwelling in the community are enormously complex and productive tasks. (Reading this book on AAC transitions will explain in detail why this is true.)

Allow me to introduce my thinking about the often unperceived power and scope of communication disability with an anecdote from 10 years ago. I was talking with a good friend of mine, RD, who was born without arms or legs and had risen to positions of significant authority in the world of government and social agencies. RD has been one of my guides in thinking about disability. He's a person whose mind and opinions I really respect. I was asking him to help me clarify my thinking around issues of employment for people who use AAC. I brought up the fact that many people with communication disabilities were terrifically driven toward employment, while a specific sector of this group had no interest in employment.

In most of the English-speaking world, having a job is a symbol of self-worth and key to independence, economic security, and a fulfilling adult life. I knew one man who, years ago, lived by himself in order to show that he was employable. This bold move cost him his life. He died of pneumonia one winter night in a freezing apartment. I reflected what a burden this man had taken upon himself, and how difficult it is for a person with cerebral palsy and unintelligible speech to organize life outside the support of a facility or a community living arrangement.

Discussing one sector's noninterest in jobs with my high-rolling friend, RD, whose disability (having no limbs) is considered challenging by any standards, I mentioned a particular employment-related conversation I had had with a woman who, owing to the severity of her cerebral palsy, communicated by eye blinks. Her arms and legs were tightly contracted against her torso with minimal use of either. Communication was physically stressful for her—I noticed the change in her breathing pattern and saw her upper torso extending up and out with each communicative effort.

Her conversational partner recites the alphabet in a certain way, and she signals by blinking both eyes to indicate the selected letter. The conversational partner starts out by saying, "Vowel . . . consonant." If "vowel" elicits a simultaneous blink of both eyes, the conversational partner then names the vowels: "a, e, i, o, u." The conversational partner then repeats the selected vowel. If "consonant" gets the two-eye blink, the next question is, "Before 'L'?" With a deep-blink answer, consonants are then recited: "b, c, d, f . . . *etc.*"

The eye-blink conversation I am speaking of took place in the foyer of an independent-living center. She worked hard teaching me her system with head nods, head shakes, and eye blinks. For nearly half an hour, this highly competent, determined woman and I had a conversation about the employment conference and whether or not she would attend, or perhaps, be interested in presenting (I had found her enormously impressive).

At the end of our exchange, she told me, "I am not interested in employment." I was surprised, particularly since I knew this woman's personal story. She was from another state and had been resident in a nursing home there. She had figured her way out of the nursing facility and had moved to Pittsburgh to live in a community living arrangement. She managed her own attendants and made the small and large decisions in her life—an amazing accomplishment! (See the wonderful opening passage from Ruth Sienkiewicz-Mercer in Chapter 2.)

"Upon reflection," I told RD, "it appeared that this woman already had a job." Achieving self-determination was her job and, by the way, probably saved the government thousands of dollars per year. RD said that he knew people with more profound disabilities than hers who, in fact, had paying jobs in the community. He then mentioned a gentleman I had recently seen in northern California traveling down a street, lying on a motorized hospital gurney. While he lay on the powered gurney, his small and slender body fully dressed, he drove backward through a crowded street of a major city by means of a mouth-stick system and several mirrors configured over his head.

It was improbable but serendipitous that both RD and I had had contact with this particular gentleman—mine, fleeting and his, professional. We reflected on the probabilities of our thinking of the same person when he said "more . . . disabled" and "paying job in the community." After a few moments of conversation, I asked whether the person in question could talk or not. "Certainly he can talk," RD answered somewhat defensively. I asked, "Could he hold down a job if he couldn't talk?"

After a few moments of silence, RD replied, "No, no, he couldn't." The conversation revealed something new for RD and clarified something for me—communication disability brings a major and often dominating dimension to any discussion of a disability situation and people in the disability field are not aware of its force. If RD hadn't fully recognized the often overwhelming effect of communication disabilities, I'm sure many people in the disability community hadn't either. Having disabilities can be very challenging, but having disabilities *and* being unable to communicate is another animal altogether.

Since that time, RD has been active in educating himself about AAC and solicitous in helping individuals with complex communications needs and all of their stakeholders in AAC. And I have continued to learn, from my interactions with people who use AAC and the many people who care about them, about how communication and self-determination are interwoven. I have also seen how AAC can help people with complex communication needs participate and interact in a broad range of settings and, perhaps most importantly, make decisions about what they want their lives to be. I am reminded of the words of Bob Williams, an individual who uses AAC and who served as a deputy assistant secretary for the Office of Disability, Aging, and Long-Term Care Policy under President Bill Clinton and who is an expert user of a variety of AAC techniques and strategies. He described the impact of AAC on his life:

> Having the power to speak one's heart and mind changes the disability equation dramatically. In fact, it is the only thing I know that can take a sledgehammer to the age-old walls of myths and stereotypes and begin to shatter the silence that looms so large in many people's lives. (2000, p. 249)

Transition Strategies for Adolescents & Young Adults Who Use AAC describes the particulars of going through major life changes while having multiple disabilities and complex communication needs. The authors approach their topics with a large amount of practical experience from the clinical, theoretical, and subjective points of view. The authors are all stakeholders in the AAC community—clinicians, scholars, and individuals who themselves use AAC. The book is well balanced but "tells it like it is" for general and professional audiences.

Bruce R. Baker, A.M.
Adjunct Associate Professor
University of Pittsburgh

REFERENCE

Williams, B. (2000). More than an exception to the rule. In M. Fried-Oken & H.A. Bersani (Eds.), *Speaking up and spelling it out: Personal essays on augmentative and alternative communication* (pp. 246–254). Baltimore: Paul H. Brookes Publishing Co.

Acknowledgments

We wish to thank Sarah Blackstone and Michael Williams (editors of *Augmentative Communication News* and *Alternatively Speaking,* respectively), Bruce Baker and the SHOUT board members (conference organizers for the Pittsburgh Employment Conference for Augmented Communicators), and Melanie Fried-Oken and Hank Bersani (editors of *Speaking Up and Spelling It Out: Personal Essays on Augmentative and Alternative Communication;* Paul H. Brookes Publishing Co., 2000) for their work in publishing the writings of individuals who use AAC. These first-person narratives from people who use AAC were invaluable sources of information for the authors of this book.

We are also grateful to the many students at our universities who have asked important questions and who have assisted with our research. There is much that is still to be learned about supporting effective transitions for individuals who use AAC, but their work has contributed to our understanding of what can help and what is needed.

We wish to acknowledge the external funding support that we have received and that has helped to build the AAC programs at our universities, including funding from the U.S. Department of Education, the National Institute on Disability and Rehabilitation Research, and the Barkley Trust.

We are grateful to the staff members at Paul H. Brookes Publishing Co. for their support of the *Augmentative and Alternative Communication Series* and for this volume specifically. Finally, we wish to thank our families—their generous love and encouragement provides the foundation for everything we do.

*This book is dedicated to the many individuals who use AAC
who have shared their transition experiences through
conversations, presentations, and publications.
Their stories have enriched and inspired
people who use AAC, their families, and professionals.*

I

Foundations for Successful Transitions

1

Supporting Successful Transitions to Adult Life for Individuals Who Use AAC

David B. McNaughton and Pamela Kennedy

> Being able to be independent and having the freedom to control my own destiny are the most important things to me. I am a very ambitious individual with lots of goals for my life. . . . I, and others who use augmentative communication, want good jobs, good places to live, and individuals who care about us and love us. It is important for the individuals who work with people who use augmentative communication to believe they can succeed at high levels. (Rackensperger, 2006)

Tracy Rackensperger, the author of the quote above, has a master's degree in communication and is pursuing a doctoral degree in the Social Foundations of Education program at the University of Georgia. She is also employed by the Institute on Disabilities at Temple University (Rackensperger, 2006).

Tracy has high expectations for participation in society, as do many young adults with complex communication needs. Following high school, Bobby O'Gurek took classes on software programming at a local community college. He now has a job as a web site developer, volunteers with his local fire department, and maintains friendships with his high school classmates (O'Gurek, 2007).

Working with an aide, Rebecca Beayni volunteers in an elementary classroom and helps as a guide at a local museum (Langille, 2007). She is also a member of a dance troupe that has performed internationally (Vereecke, 2004).

Beth Anne Luciani is completing her undergraduate degree in creative writing at the California University of Pennsylvania. She has successfully completed an internship with the university newspaper and maintains a strong grade point average as she works toward graduation (Luciani, 2009).

The individuals described in the preceding paragraphs have physical disabilities and complex communication needs. To overcome their speech challenges and participate in adult society, they communicate using multiple methods, including speech-generating devices (SGDs), gestures, speech and speech approximations, and facial expressions. These methods are collectively referred to as *augmentative and alternative communication* (AAC), and they can help support interaction with a wide variety of communication partners in a wide variety of settings.

TRANSITION GOALS

The experiences of the individuals just described show that people with communication challenges have new expectations regarding participation in society (Bryen & Moulton, 1998; McNaughton & Bryen, 2007). An emphasis on community living (Chapter 9), meaningful educational programs (Chapter 4), access to employment (Chapter 6), and increased community participation (Chapter 7) has led to new opportunities for many individuals who use AAC.

Fundamental to participation in society is the ability to communicate successfully—to interact with others for the purposes of expressing needs and wants, exchanging information, developing social closeness, and participating in social etiquette routines (Light, 1997). Many individuals with autism, cerebral palsy, and other disabilities experience difficulty with speech (Beukelman & Mirenda, 2005). For people with complex communication needs, reaching valued goals of adult life may pose special challenges (Hamm & Mirenda, 2006; Lund & Light, 2007a, 2007b; Mc-Naughton & Bryen, 2002, 2007).

In order to communicate successfully and participate in society, people with complex communication needs may use AAC. Because communication is a multimodal process, these individuals may make use of a wide variety of AAC techniques and strategies to fulfill a range of communication goals; for example, SGDs; picture, alphabet, and word boards; signs; gestures; facial expression; and speech and speech approximations (Beukelman & Mirenda, 2005). It is also important to remember that communication is an interactive process—successful communication requires that both the individual who uses AAC and his or her communication partner(s) make use of effective communication strategies (Light, 1997).

For the adolescent who uses AAC, there are unique communication challenges. For example, adolescence creates demands for both a large and rapidly growing vocabulary for academic participation and the ability to handle new expectations in social interactions with peers and others (Bryen, 2008; Murphy, Markova, Collins, & Moodie, 1996; Smith, 2005). Adolescence is also a time when many individuals begin to interact with a broader segment of society in pursuing opportunities for educational, vocational, and societal involvement (Wehman, 2006). At these times, those who use AAC need to learn strategies for communicating with familiar as well as unfamiliar partners in a wide range of environments.

For people with speech challenges, AAC can aid in negotiating living arrangements and communicating with personal assistants (Chapter 9); supporting interactions at school, at work, and in the community (Chapters 3–7); facilitating exchanges with coworkers, employers, and medical professionals (Chapters 6 and 10); and communicating with friends, family members, and significant others (Chapter 8). The use of AAC is not a goal in and of itself; rather, the use of AAC is the means by which successful communication is obtained and all of these other valued goals of adult life are pursued (Williams, Krezman, & McNaughton, 2008).

Like many transition-age youth, people with communication challenges identify new goals for their lives as they approach adulthood (Bryen & Moulton, 1998; Light et al., 2007). Although many of the issues they face are common to all transition-age youth, some challenges are unique. Many adolescents and young adults who have lived at home with family members are often interested in living more independently; however, people who use AAC need to consider issues of funding, accessibility, and attendant care as they plan their futures (Chapter 9). School provides an organized set of activities and a daily routine from an early age for all children; as adults, individuals with complex communication needs are responsible for finding the opportunities and support that will enable them to pursue educational, vocational, and recreation and leisure opportunities (Chapters 5–7). Although many youth enter the work force after completing their education and work to become financially independent, individuals who use AAC often find it difficult to obtain a reliable source of income and to access needed supports and medical services (Chapter 10). Finally, for many youth, adulthood is a time for new friendships and sometimes intimate relationships. However, many individuals with speech challenges experience difficulty gaining access to society and report feelings of loneliness (Bryen, Chung, & Segalman, 2009).

Successful transitions require paying attention to four major goals (Condeluci, 1995; Halpern, 1993; Wagner, Newman, Cameto, Garza, & Levine, 2005). As adults, all individuals have a need to

1.   Have a safe place to live

2.   Participate in meaningful activities

3. Maintain a reliable source of income and access to needed services

4. Develop friendships and intimate relationships

In the following sections, we describe the experiences of people who use AAC with respect to these goals and identify strategies to support positive transition outcomes in these areas.

Have a Safe Place to Live

> It was the best of highs. It was the worst of terrors. I was elated. I was depressed. I smiled with joy. I cried with sorrow. I knew everything. I knew nothing. What caused these swings of emotion? Moving out on my own. (Williams, 2001, p. 3)

In describing his first experience with independent living, Michael B. Williams—a man who uses AAC—captures the emotions of many people leaving home for the first time. For those with complex communication needs, however, there are additional challenges and considerations, including societal attitudes, the accessibility of the housing and the surrounding community, costs, and the availability of attendant care services (Williams, 2001).

There has been a dramatic change in the living environments of people with severe disabilities in the past 40 years (Lakin & Stancliffe, 2007). A majority of those with physical disabilities now live in community settings with a wide variety of support arrangements (Chapter 9). As it is for any individual, the perceived appropriateness of a living situation for someone with complex communication needs is a highly personal decision (Clarke, 2001; Lund & Light, 2006).

The shift to community-based group homes and independent living has clear advantages in terms of opportunities for social interaction. However, living in the community also means coming face to face with society's views on disability (Blackstone, Draper, & Draper, 2005). People with complex communication needs have described the challenges of dealing with societal discrimination in their efforts to obtain accessible housing (Williams, 2001), as well as the frustration of having only limited access to the resources they need to make independent living a reality (Davis, 2005).

For individuals with physical disabilities, the provision of attendant care services plays a critical role in their living experience. As Collier noted in Blackstone (2005, p. 3), "No matter where someone lives, their quality of life depends to a great extent on the degree to which they can direct the services of the person who provides attendant care." For many people who use AAC, this is a significant challenge. Based on a survey of adults with complex communication needs, Collier reported that individuals who use AAC may have to deal with as many as 15 different people to manage their personal care. However, few of these individuals reported being prepared to negotiate their own care, give feedback that was positive and constructive, and deal with conflicts and dangerous situations (Collier, as cited in Blackstone, 2005).

The inability to effectively direct the actions of others and to report inappropriate activity can have very damaging effects. After surveying 40 adults who used AAC, Bryen, Carey, and Frantz (2003) reported that 45% of the individuals had experienced crime or abuse. Of those individuals who had been victimized, 97% knew the perpetrators, 71% reported having been victimized multiple times, and 66% reported having experienced multiple types of victimization. The long-term effects of the crimes included significant physical and emotional harm as well as loss of property or money, yet only 28% of those who had been victimized had reported their experiences to the police.

Providing real choices in living arrangements for individuals with complex communication needs requires that options be available and accessible, both physically and financially. However, it is also important that the individual who uses AAC has the self-determination and communication skills necessary to manage his or her attendant care, including the ability to clearly and confidentially communicate concerns about inappropriate behavior by others.

Participate in Meaningful Activities

It is not terrible to have a disability. I've had a severe physical disability throughout my entire life, and it has never been terrible. Sometimes difficult and trying, but never, never, terrible. The worst part of the disability experience is the behavior that it produces in others around you. Sad, but true. . . . Society's reaction, rather than the disability itself, impedes effective interaction and inclusion. For some unknown reason, disability has become an acceptable excuse for the complete absence of civility between people. Disability has become a permissible reason to treat people as insignificant. Only society can change this by recognizing value in every—and I stress every—individual. (Dickerson, 1995, p. 30)

Nationwide studies of the life experiences of people with severe disabilities reflect Dickerson's sentiments and provide evidence that the transition to postschool activities can be difficult for individuals with severe disabilities (Blackorby & Wagner, 1996; Wagner, Newman, Cameto, Garza, & Levine, 2009). Many people with disabilities speak of their interest in being involved and making a contribution to society as adults, but they report significant barriers in gaining access to desired education, work, volunteering, and recreation experiences (Lund & Light, 2006; McNaughton & Bryen, 2007). Young adults with multiple disabilities, including those with complex communication needs, have the lowest level of participation of any disability group in school, work, or preparation for work activities (Wagner et al., 2005).

Individuals with speech disabilities face many challenges in assuming adult roles. Many individuals with disabilities leave school with limited academic and workplace skills (Wagner et al., 2005) and face negative societal attitudes while pursuing employment and education opportunities (Dickerson, 1995; McNaughton, Symons, Light, & Parsons, 2006). Despite these challenges, there is evidence that individuals who use AAC—even those with limited literacy skills—can successfully participate in meaningful social roles as employees, volunteers, students, and participants in recreation and leisure activities.

Employment   In an initial review of employment activity, Light, Stoltz, and McNaughton (1996) conducted a nationwide survey to identify individuals who used AAC and who were employed more than 10 hours per week in community-based activities. The authors identified 25 individuals who were employed in a variety of activities, including as clerical workers, laborers, public educators and consumer advocates, and educational/therapy aides.

Common barriers to employment included poor educational preparation, negative societal attitudes, and difficulties securing employment supports, such as transportation and attendant care services in the workplace (McNaughton, Light, & Arnold, 2002). Participants described a focused education—one that is centered on skills with high employment potential—and a strong work ethic as important to employment success. Although literacy skills were not required for employment, those individuals who had strong literacy skills described themselves as more satisfied with their opportunities for advancement and more satisfied with their jobs in general.

College   A growing number of individuals with disabilities are pursuing postsecondary education as a first step toward future employment opportunities (Wagner et al., 2009). Atanasoff, McNaughton, Wolfe, and Light (1998) described the communication experiences of seven individuals who used AAC and attended college. All participants described themselves as possessing strong literacy skills, and most reported that they had participated in competitive general education programs in high school. They had access to SGDs and used a variety of communication techniques to ask and answer questions; to lead and contribute to discussions; and, in one case, to complete a final oral examination using face-to-face communication. In an effort to address the challenges of communicating in a postsecondary setting, the participants reported using preprogrammed vocabulary and relying more on written communication or e-mail in place of face-to-face communication.

Volunteering   For many individuals, volunteering provides the satisfaction of contributing to society without having to deal with the negative social attitudes frequently encountered in employment situations. Ballin, Balandin, and Togher (2005) reported that the adults in their study who used AAC enjoyed volunteer activities and that these experiences reduced feelings of loneliness. Volunteering can be useful to individuals with a range of disabilities—Badger (2007) described how Rebecca Beayni, a young woman with severe cognitive and physical disabilities, pursues active societal participation through volunteer work in a variety of educational and social support settings.

Recreation and Leisure   Although work, education, and volunteer activities are an important part of a person's life, so too are recreation and leisure activities. These can provide opportunities for participation that may not be available through traditional educational or employment activities, including opportunities to interact with others, express talents, demonstrate capabilities, and experience enjoyment (Dattilo et al., 2008).

About three quarters of youth without disabilities participate in organized activities outside of school, including groups sponsored by the school or community. For these individuals, recreation provides an opportunity to build friendships, improve self-confidence, and simply experience enjoyment (Chapter 7).

The leisure and recreation experiences of many individuals with severe disabilities are markedly different. Less than one quarter of individuals with severe disabilities participate in organized community groups or volunteer activities. People with severe disabilities are also most likely to identify watching television as their major leisure activity (Wagner et al., 2009). Although some communities have appropriate supports that enable individuals with severe disabilities to participate in recreation and leisure activities, many communities face challenges associated with architectural and transportation barriers and—perhaps most limiting of all—negative societal attitudes (Chapter 7).

Despite these challenges, there is evidence of active social engagement among people who use AAC. Dattilo et al. (2008) described the recreation and leisure experiences of eight adults with complex communication needs. Through the appropriate use of supports, including maintaining positive personal attitudes, developing a broad network of friends, and making appropriate use of AAC technology, these individuals were able to participate in a wide variety of recreation and leisure activities, including attending movies and sports activities, dancing, and going to parties. Participants in the study had recommendations both for the individual who uses AAC as well as those who provide support. They suggested that the individual who uses AAC be willing to take risks and try new things. They also recommended that individuals who provide support consider ways that they can increase the self-confidence and independence of the person who uses AAC by preprogramming needed vocabulary and providing opportunities for that person to try new activities.

Maintain a Reliable Source of Income and Access to Needed Services

> I cried at the checkout counter because this is the freedom a paycheck will give me . . . picking out my own stuff will add value because nothing will feel like a hand-out, I won't have to wonder what medical assistance will and won't get for me. (Sam, as quoted in McNaughton et al., 2006, p. 185)

When he made a purchase with funds from his first paycheck, Sam, an individual who uses AAC, was overcome with emotion. Having even a part-time job provided a measure of financial independence he had never previously known, as well as an enhanced sense of self-worth. Unfortunately, this is not a typical experience for individuals with complex communication needs.

Because of negative societal attitudes and limited educational preparation, most people with communication challenges are unemployed (or underemployed) and have very limited incomes (Light et al., 1996). People with somewhat severe or very severe disabilities are three times more likely to live in poverty than people without disabilities (National Organization on Disability, 2000), which has adverse consequences for their living arrangements, medical services, and quality of life (McNaughton & Bryen, 2002). Government assistance typically provides little more than subsistence-level income. As a result, individuals with severe disabilities (and their support networks) must learn how to navigate a complex web of government agencies to obtain funding supports (Blackstone, 2005). Many adolescents and young adults are interested in enjoying greater financial self-sufficiency and living more independently. However, for many, leaving home has serious financial consequences. As Nancy Draper, a parent of a young adult with complex communication needs, wrote, "Being independent can often mean you have no quality of life. . . . When John moves out, he will live in poverty" (Blackstone et al., 2005, p. 9).

For adolescents and young adults with disabilities, learning to coordinate the medical and rehabilitation services they will receive as adults is a challenge. When they were children, parents and planning teams helped manage and coordinate their care and support services. In many countries there are government guarantees of pediatric rehabilitation services (Chapter 10). However, as adults, people with disabilities face new challenges as they become responsible for managing their own care. They must learn to define and describe their own care and rehabilitation goals, create networks of support, and identify and schedule needed services. They also need to interact with and coordinate information among multiple medical and rehabilitation professionals (e.g., general practitioners, dentists, vision specialists, speech-language pathologists, seating specialists). Of primary importance is the need to be able to advocate for themselves, as there are typically few guarantees of services, especially rehabilitation services, for adults with disabilities (Hamm & Mirenda, 2006). In the United States, even something as simple as nonemergency transportation to a medical appointment can take up to 6 months to schedule and can require making multiple phone calls and contacts (P. Kennedy, personal communication, December 7, 2009).

Develop Friendships and Intimate Relationships

I love college, even though the students don't associate with me much. It just comes with the territory of being handicapped. Students will occasionally come up and ask me about my [speech-generating device], but that will pretty much be the extent of it. I have no real friends from college, and that is something I have come to accept. Fortunately, though, I have about four good friends whom I have had for many years. They know the true me, and my disability comes second to them. (Luciani, 2009)

In the preceding passage, Beth Anne Luciani, an individual who uses AAC and who attends college, describes the challenges of dealing with negative societal attitudes and forming friendships with peers. Although family remains an important part of people's lives as they enter adulthood (Blackstone et al., 2005), peer friendships are essential to emotional well-being and are strongly associated with educational progress and other positive outcomes (Wentzel & Caldwell, 1997).

For most children, the process of developing friendships occurs seamlessly. More than 90% of adolescents without disabilities see friends outside of school at least once a week. These social supports are important not only for the positive impact of interaction with peers but also for the social support that peers provide in challenging times.

People with complex communication challenges report a wide variety of experiences with respect to friendship and intimacy. Some individuals report strong satisfaction with the quantity and quality of their friendships (Cooper, Balandin, & Trembath, 2009) and the development of rewarding intimate relationships (Williams, 2004). Others report that it can be difficult to make friends (Bryen et al., 2009; Light et al., 2007). As Beth Anne describes, society often shows little interest in individuals with differences. Close to one third of people with multiple disabilities reportedly never interact with friends outside of class (Cadwallader & Wagner, 2003). As individuals with severe disabilities get older, and especially during the high school years, it may become more difficult for them to build and maintain friendships. As the parent of a child with speech challenges commented, "When you are a cute disabled kid, the world stops and listens more. As you become an adult, they're not as patient" (Lund & Light, 2007b, p. 327).

Hunt, Doering, Maier, and Mintz (2009) described positive actions that can be taken by school personnel to increase the social interaction and friendship opportunities of students with disabilities while these students are still in school in an effort to prepare for adult life. They suggested designing and implementing social supports around three key areas. First, school personnel provide information to peers, which helps these students understand human diversity, the importance of friendships, and the means by which the student who uses AAC participates in conversations and activities. How they impart this information can range from hosting informal discussions to creating friendships groups, sometimes referred to as *circles of friends.* Second, school personnel identify and use interactive media to help ensure that there is support for positive social interactions. This may include recognizing communication modes used by all (e.g., facial expressions, gestures, vocalizations) as well as more sophisticated SGDs. Third, the teacher plays a role in arranging interactive activities and facilitating positive social interactions. This is a multistep process in which the teacher 1) develops rapport with the peers of the student with a disability; 2) sets up interactive activities; 3) shares information during these interactive activities; 4) models positive, respectful interactions with students who use AAC; 5) facilitates positive student-to-student interactions; and 6) fades the adult presence in order to avoid interfering with student-to-student social interactions.

As children become adults, they also develop an interest in more intimate relationships with significant others. There continue to be significant challenges to adult relationships for individuals with complex communication needs, including societal discrimination and policy barriers (Chapter 8). But at the same time, there are a growing number of success stories of individuals who use AAC who are in long-term intimate relationships (Creech & Williams, 2004; Williams, 2004).

SKILLS AND SUPPORTS FOR SUCCESSFUL TRANSITIONS

> It feels like you are led to the edge of a familiar place and then let go. Everything changes and the supports you once had are no longer available. (Nancy Draper, parent of a transition-age child with disabilities, in Blackstone et al., 2005, p. 9)

For families of adolescents and young adults, the end of school services can be a traumatic event. Even when families know that changes will occur, it can be difficult to plan for life after school when day-to-day activities pose many demands (Goldbart & Marshall, 2004). However individuals with disabilities and their family members often speak of the importance of starting early and taking a systematic approach to transition (Blackstone et al., 2005; Carlson, 1994).

Supporting successful transitions from school to the adult world for individuals who use AAC requires paying careful attention to desired adult outcomes in living arrangements; educational, vocational, and social activities; financial resources; and relationships. It is also necessary to give careful consideration to the skills and supports needed for an individual to pursue desired goals. This process should involve the collaborative efforts of a multidisciplinary team (the individual in question, family members, and professionals), thoughtful "sampling" of future environments to help shape educational goals, and attention to the development of the communication and self-determination skills that will be useful in any future environment.

Establish a Diverse and Committed Team

Just as with organizing an effective educational program, achieving desired transition outcomes requires the ongoing collaborative commitment of the person with complex communication needs, his or her family, teachers, the speech-language pathologist, the occupational therapist, the physiotherapist, and other specialists (Wehman, 2006). Preparing for the transition to adult life may also mean involving new professionals, such as vocational rehabilitation staff.

The composition of the team and the roles of participants will change over time. As their children approach adulthood, families may feel pressure to reduce their involvement. However, it is important to recognize the crucial long-term role of the family. As Nancy Draper noted,

> Professionals who view transition goals as a breaking away from the family are misguided. . . . Transition planning needs to start when a child is very young and should involve the family every step of the way. The reality is that adult services often have limited resources, so when anything goes wrong, the family is called upon to come to the rescue. Thus it is essential that family members know what is going on. The more prepared we are, the more able we can be to pitch in. (Blackstone et al., 2005, p. 8)

Teams dealing with the transition to life after high school need to consider four elements critical to effective team functioning: communication, goals, roles, and time. First, smooth team functioning requires the effective use of *communication* and problem-solving skills to promote active participation by all. When planning teams function well, both families and professionals feel as if their opinions are important and their contributions are valued (Thousand & Villa, 1992). Smooth team functioning cannot just be taken for granted (Beukelman & Mirenda, 2005); it requires planning and perhaps even training for all team members in communication and problem-solving skills (Robinson & Solomon-Rice, 2009). Salisbury, Evans, and Palombaro (1997) recommended the use of a five-step process for promoting collaborative problem solving, in which team members 1) identify the issue, 2) generate all possible solutions, 3) screen solutions for feasibility, 4) choose the solution to implement, and 5) evaluate the solution.

Second, the team will need to develop meaningful *goals* that address important adult outcomes (e.g., safe and accessible living arrangements, meaningful and enjoyable activities). Many people who use AAC report that while they were in school, they encountered low expectations for future employment and independent living from teachers and other professionals (McNaughton et al., 2002). John is an individual with complex communication needs who, after graduating from college, worked in the printing department of a major corporation, and then opened his own printing business. He commented, "After I turned 18, all they thought I could do was sit home or go into a [sheltered] workshop. Well, I guess I proved them wrong" (McNaughton et al., 2006, p. 187).

Third, careful planning is needed to ensure that team members are prepared to participate in appropriate *roles*. Especially important is that the individual who uses AAC is supported in assuming a greater leadership position in decision making and that families are helped to negotiate the transition from educational programs to adult services (Kim & Turnbull, 2004; McCarthy, Light, & McNaughton, 2007).

Fourth, it is important to devote sufficient *time* to the collaborative process—to start early, to ensure regular meetings, and to plan for the changes in team composition (and supports) after the individual leaves the educational system. Teachers, parents, and students frequently express the concern that transition planning starts too late (Hamm & Mirenda, 2006) and that inadequate time is given to planning and implementing transition activities (Lehmann, Bassett, & Sands, 1999). Hunt, Soto, Maier, and Doering (2003) reported that ensuring appropriate time for regular team meetings in which transition team members can reflect upon the impact of current approaches and problem-solve ongoing challenges is essential to the development of effective education programming for students with disabilities.

Sample the Next Environment

Living as an adult with complex communication needs means drawing upon a wide set of new skills and competencies that may include living independently and managing personal care attendants (Chapter 9), demonstrating appropriate workplace etiquette (Chapter 6), and participating in adult relationships (Chapter 8). Concerns have been expressed that most high school curricula do not adequately prepare individuals with complex communication needs for adult life—curricula are not appropriate for individuals' educational and vocational goals (McNaughton et al., 2006), there are low levels of peer interaction (Light et al., 2007), and there is little support for the development of needed AAC skills (Hamm & Mirenda, 2006).

It may be difficult for transition team members, many of whom are focused on the challenges of supporting participation in the current school environment, to have a clear sense of educational goals for participation in the adult world. Many transition specialists recommend sampling future environments (e.g., visiting anticipated residential or vocational settings) in order to get a better sense of needed skills and to help set education priorities to support a smooth transition. For example, Carter, Trainor, Ditchman, Swedeen, and Owens (in press) described how the summer job experiences of adolescents with severe disabilities helped teams determine appropriate educational goals. Similar sampling approaches have been implemented for living arrangements (Benedetti, 2002; Blackstone, 2005) and postsecondary educational environments (Luciani, 2009).

Older individuals with complex communication needs are another important source of information about the challenges of the adult world. As Bowe, Faye, and Minch noted, "Disabled individuals with several years of disability experience are frequently better aware of the needs of disabled people, and better informed about government benefits, than able-bodied professionals in the rehabilitation delivery system" (1980, p. 285).

The AAC Mentor Project (Light et al., 2007) investigated the impact of partnering experienced mentors who used AAC with younger individuals who were navigating important transitions. The project consisted of two phases. In the first phase, the older individuals received web-based instruction in the skills needed to be an effective mentor, including the use of effective sociorelational skills and problem-solving strategies. These adults later acted as mentors, via e-mail exchanges, to 32 adolescents and young adults who used AAC. The mentors provided social support and discussed transition-related problems such as planning living arrangements and looking for a job. In all, 100% of the adolescents and young adults indicated that they were "very satisfied" with their participation in the mentor program and with the quality of their mentors, and they planned to continue communicating with their mentor after the formal completion of the project.

Focus on the Development of Skills Needed in All Environments

Although the adult world presents many new demands for the individual with complex communication needs, two skills are fundamentally important: communication skills and self-determination skills. With these skills, individuals with complex communication needs will be able to develop other skills and access needed supports.

Unfortunately, however, there is strong evidence that many individuals with disabilities enter the adult world without appropriate communication systems and skills and with limited preparation to act in a self-determined manner. For example, Hamm and Mirenda (2006) examined the postschool outcomes of eight individuals with developmental disabilities and complex communication needs. They reported a positive correlation between scores for quality of communication and scores for quality of life. However, they also noted that a majority of the individuals who used AAC experienced difficulty in communicating, and that they—and their caregivers—were very dissatisfied with the AAC services and supports available for young adults (ages 19–24).

It is critical that educational programs make it a priority to ensure that transition-age youth receive appropriate communication services. Essential outcomes include both the individual leaving school with a solid understanding of his or her AAC system, and family members and caregivers understanding how best to support that individual's communication development and participation. Instruction must go beyond simply the technical operation and upkeep of a device.

Interventions must address the need for linguistic, operational, social, and strategic skills (Light, 1997). Communication interventions must recognize the multimodal nature of communication and ensure that individuals have access to a wide variety of modes of communication to convey a wide variety of content. As John Draper, a young adult who uses AAC, noted, it is "important to realize that technology is not a miracle, and it won't solve all your communication needs" (Blackstone et al., 2005, p. 9).

The ability to effectively communicate is intertwined with the ability to act in a self-determined manner (Chapter 2). Opportunities to develop self-determination skills should begin at an early age and should be formally recognized as part of an individual's transition program (Palmer, Wehmeyer, Gipson, & Agran, 2004). Lund and Light (2006) used The Arc's Self-Determination Scale (Wehmeyer & Kelchner, 1995) to measure self-determination in seven young men ages 19–23 who had used AAC for more than 15 years. Participants reported a wide range of self-determination scores; however, those with the highest self-determination scores were the most likely to report a higher quality of life.

CONCLUSION

> I think that right from the time that a young person is about 12 . . . we need to start thinking about where they're going to be. . . . You need to start having those discussions earlier rather than later because the actual transition is stressful enough, but if it's done with some certainty and some natural expectations it's a much easier step to take. (The mother of "Josh," a young man who uses AAC, as quoted in Lund & Light, 2007b, p. 329)

Individuals who use AAC expect to be full participants in society (Blackstone, 2005; Bryen & Moulton, 1998). In today's world, however, it still remains enormously challenging for individuals with complex communication needs to obtain appropriate housing, engage in ongoing meaningful activities, receive a reliable income and needed services, and gain access to opportunities for social interaction.

Although individual examples of positive transition outcomes exist, transition team members need to work to make desired goals a reality for all individuals with complex communication needs. Planning for the transition from school to the adult world can help to promote positive outcomes for individuals with complex communication needs. Although much about the future is unknown and unpredictable, at every age steps can be taken to prepare for life in the adult world and to develop needed competencies in communication and self-determination.

There is no single definition of what constitutes a "good" outcome; it must be defined on an individual basis by the key stakeholders involved (Lund & Light, 2006). Yet for all individuals, a good outcome should involve safe housing, meaningful activities, financial support, access to services, and positive social relationships.

Successful transitions require the efforts of a collaborative team over an extended period of time, appropriate sampling of future environments to help shape educational goals, and a focus on skills needed in all environments. The transition process can seem extensive and complicated; however, Scott, a young man who uses AAC, lives in his own apartment with supports, and who has started his own business, provides a useful summary:

> I learned that beside faith, you need a clear view of your goal, a lot of stamina, and a huge amount of self-advocacy. I have learned that you can't listen to other people's fears because that is their garbage, not mine. I have learned to not let them hold me back from my successes. I have learned to listen to my own instincts and make my own decisions and have found an incredible support team that can envision my dream. (Palm, 2007, p. 74)

Scott's summary of the key components of a successful transition provides a fitting end to this introduction and lays the foundation for the rest of this book.

REFERENCES

Atanasoff, L.M., McNaughton, D., Wolfe, P.S., & Light, J. (1998). Communication demands of university settings for students using augmentative and alternative communication. *Journal of Postsecondary Education and Disability, 13*(3), 32–47.

Badger, C. (2007). *Cerebral palsy can't slow social justice advocate.* Retrieved October 14, 2009, from http://www.catholicregister.org/content/view/829/849/

Ballin, L., Balandin, S., & Togher, L. (2005). Community connection: The role of employment in reducing the experience of loneliness. In S. Osgood, R.V. Conti, & Z. Sloane (Eds.), *Proceedings of the Tenth Pittsburgh Employment Conference* (pp. 32–37). Pittsburgh: Shout Press.

Benedetti, D. (2002). Conference outlines how to create transition programs for students with challenges. *Outreach Communications, 3*(1). Retrieved November 25, 2009, from http://www.outreach.psu.edu/news/magazine/vol_3.1/transitions.html

Beukelman, D.R., & Mirenda, P. (2005). *Augmentative and alternative communication: Supporting children and adults with complex communication needs* (3rd ed.). Baltimore: Paul H. Brookes Publishing Co.

Blackorby, J., & Wagner, M. (1996). Longitudinal post-school outcomes of youth with disabilities: Findings from the National Longitudinal Transition Study. *Exceptional Children, 62,* 399–414.

Blackstone, S.W. (2005). The coming of age transition. *Augmentative Communication News, 17*(1), 1–4.

Blackstone, S.W., Draper, J., & Draper, N. (2005). Do not work on me! *Augmentative Communication News, 17*(1), 8–11.

Bowe, F., Faye, F., & Minch, J. (1980). Consumer involvement in rehabilitation. In E.L. Pan, S.S. Newman, T.F. Backer, & C.L. Vash (Eds.), *Annual review of rehabilitation* (pp. 279–303). New York: Springer Publishing Co.

Bryen, D.N. (2008). Vocabulary to support socially-valued adult roles. *Augmentative and Alternative Communication, 24,* 294–301.

Bryen, D.N., Carey, A., & Frantz, B. (2003). Ending the silence: Adults who use augmentative communication and their experiences as victims of crimes. *Augmentative and Alternative Communication, 19,* 125–134.

Bryen, D.N., Chung, Y., & Segalman, R. (2009). *Depression, social isolation, and ACOLUG.* Retrieved December 3, 2009, from http://aac-rerc.psu.edu/documents/Bryen_PEC_09.pdf

Bryen, D.N., & Moulton, B. (1998). Why "employment, independence, marriage, and sexuality"? Because we want it all. In R.V. Conti (Ed.), *The Sixth Annual Pittsburgh Employment Conference for Augmented Communicators* (pp. 1–11). Pittsburgh: Shout Press.

Cadwallader, T.W., & Wagner, M. (2003). Interactions with friends. In M. Wagner, T. Cadwallader, & C. Marder (Eds.), *Life outside the classroom for youth with disabilities: A report from the National Longitudinal Transition Study-2* (pp. 3.1–3.7). Menlo Park, CA: SRI International.

Carlson, F. (1994). How can you expect to get a job if you don't start in preschool. In R.V. Conti & C. Jenkins-Odorisio (Eds.), *Proceedings of the Second Annual Pittsburgh Employment Conference for Augmented Communicators* (pp. 32–38). Pittsburgh: Shout Press.

Carter, E.W., Trainor, A.A., Ditchman, N., Swedeen, B., & Owens, L. (in press). Evaluation of a multi-component intervention package to increase summer work experiences for transition-age youth with severe disabilities. *Research and Practice for Persons with Severe Disabilities.*

Clarke, G. (2001). Alternative housing for augmentative communicators. *Alternatively Speaking, 5*(3), 7.

Condeluci, A. (1995). *Interdependence: The route to community.* Boca Raton, FL: CRC Press.

Cooper, L., Balandin, S., & Trembath, D. (2009). The loneliness experiences of young adults with cerebral palsy who use alternative and augmentative communication. *Augmentative and Alternative Communication, 25,* 154–164.

Creech, R., & Williams, M. (2004). Friends and relations. *Alternatively Speaking, 7*(2), 5.

Dattilo, J., Estrella, G., Estrella, L.J., Light, J., McNaughton, D., & Seabury, M. (2008). "I have chosen to live life abundantly": Perceptions of leisure by adults who use augmentative and alternative communication. *Augmentative and Alternative Communication, 24,* 16–28.

Davis, R.L. (2005). *Reflections of nine participants regarding their experiences of being African American and using augmentative and alternative communication across their lifespan at home, school, vocation, and community.* Unpublished doctoral dissertation, The Pennsylvania State University, University Park.

Dickerson, L.A. (1995). Techniques for the integration of people who use alternative communication devices in the workplace. In R.V. Conti & C. Jenkins-Odorisio (Eds.), *Proceedings of the Third Annual Pittsburgh Employment Conference for Augmented Communicators* (pp. 27–34). Pittsburgh: Shout Press.

Goldbart, J., & Marshall, J. (2004). "Pushes and pulls" on the parents of children who use AAC. *Augmentative and Alternative Communication, 20,* 194–208.

Halpern, A.S. (1993). Quality of life as a conceptual framework for evaluating transition outcomes. *Exceptional Children, 59,* 486–498.

Hamm, B., & Mirenda, P. (2006). Post-school quality of life for individuals with developmental disabilities who use AAC. *Augmentative and Alternative Communication, 22,* 134–147.

Hunt, P., Doering, K., Maier, J., & Mintz, E. (2009). Strategies to support the development of positive social relationships and friendships for students who use AAC. In G. Soto & C. Zangari (Eds.), *Practically speaking: Language, literacy, and academic development for students with AAC needs* (pp. 247–264). Baltimore: Paul H. Brookes Publishing Co.

Hunt, P., Soto, G., Maier, J., & Doering, K. (2003). Collaborative teaming to support students at risk and students with severe disabilities in general education classrooms. *Exceptional Children, 69,* 315–333.

Kim, K.H., & Turnbull, A. (2004). Transition to adulthood for students with severe intellectual disabilities: Shifting toward person-family interdependent planning. *Research and Practice for Persons with Severe Disabilities, 29,* 53–57.

Lakin, K.C., & Stancliffe, R.J. (2007). Residential supports for persons with intellectual and developmental disabilities. *Mental Retardation and Developmental Disabilities Research Reviews, 13,* 151–159.

Langille, D. (2007). *Toronto social justice award.* Toronto: Center for Social Justice.

Lehmann, J.P., Bassett, D.S., & Sands, D.J. (1999). Students' participation in transition-related actions: A qualitative study. *Remedial and Special Education, 20,* 160–169.

Light, J. (1997). "Communication is the essence of human life": Reflections on communicative competence. *Augmentative and Alternative Communication, 13,* 61–70.

Light, J., McNaughton, D., Krezman, C., Williams, M., Gulens, M., Galskoy, A., et al. (2007). The AAC Mentor Project: Web-based instruction in sociorelational skills and collaborative problem solving for adults who use augmentative and alternative communication. *Augmentative and Alternative Communication, 23,* 56–75.

Light, J., Stoltz, B., & McNaughton, D. (1996). Community-based employment: Experiences of adults who use AAC. *Augmentative and Alternative Communication, 12,* 215–229.

Luciani, B. (2009). *AAC and college life: Just do it!* Retrieved November 12, 2009, from http://aac-rerc.psu.edu/index.php/webcasts/show/id/5

Lund, S.K., & Light, J. (2006). Long-term outcomes for individuals who use augmentative and alternative communication: Part I—What is a "good" outcome? *Augmentative and Alternative Communication, 22,* 284–299.

Lund, S.K., & Light, J. (2007a). Long-term outcomes for individuals who use augmentative and alternative communication: Part II—Communicative interaction. *Augmentative and Alternative Communication, 23,* 1–15.

Lund, S.K., & Light, J. (2007b). Long-term outcomes for individuals who use augmentative and alternative communication: Part III—Contributing factors. *Augmentative and Alternative Communication, 23,* 323–335.

McCarthy, J., Light, J., & McNaughton, D. (2007). The effects of Internet-based instruction on the social problem solving of young adults who use augmentative and alternative communication. *Augmentative and Alternative Communication, 23,* 100–112.

McNaughton, D., & Bryen, D.N. (2002). Enhancing participation in employment through AAC technologies. *Assistive Technology, 14,* 58–70.

McNaughton, D., & Bryen, D.N. (2007). AAC technologies to enhance participation and access to meaningful societal roles for adolescents and adults with developmental disabilities who require AAC. *Augmentative and Alternative Communication, 23,* 217–229.

McNaughton, D., Light, J., & Arnold, K.B. (2002). "Getting your wheel in the door": Successful full-time employment experiences of individuals with cerebral palsy who use augmentative and alternative communication. *Augmentative and Alternative Communication, 18,* 59–76.

McNaughton, D., Symons, G., Light, J., & Parsons, A. (2006). "My dream was to pay taxes": The self-employment experiences of individuals who use augmentative and alternative communication. *Journal of Vocational Rehabilitation, 25,* 181–196.

Murphy, J., Markova, I., Collins, S., & Moodie, E. (1996). AAC systems: Obstacles to effective use. *International Journal of Language & Communication Disorders, 31,* 31–44.

National Organization on Disability. (2000). *Key findings: 2000 N.O.D./Harris Survey of Americans with Disabilities.* Retrieved December 18, 2009, from http://www.nod.org/index.cfm?fuseaction=Feature.showFeature&FeatureID=862#inco

O'Gurek, R. (2007, November). *2007 Edwin and Esther Prentke AAC distinguished lecturer* [Presentation at the annual convention of the American Speech-Language-Hearing Association, Boston, MA]. Retrieved November 12, 2009, from http://www.aacinstitute.org/Resources/PrentkeLecture/2007/RobertO%27Gurek.html

Palm, S. (2007). The therapeutic value of one augmented communicator helping another augmented communicator is without parallel. In R.V. Conti, P. Meneskie, & C. Micher (Eds.), *Proceedings of the Eleventh Pittsburgh Employment Conference for Augmented Communicators* (pp. 70–74). Pittsburgh: Shout Press.

Palmer, S.B., Wehmeyer, M.L., Gipson, K., & Agran, M. (2004). Promoting access to the general curriculum by teaching self-determination skills. *Exceptional Children, 70,* 427–440.

Rackensperger, T. (2006, November). *2006 Edwin and Esther Prentke AAC distinguished lecturer* [Presentation at the annual convention of the American-Speech-Language-Hearing Association, Miami, FL]. Retrieved December 20, 2009, from http://www.aacinstitute.org/Resources/PrentkeLecture/2006/TracyRackensperger .html

Robinson, N.B., & Solomon-Rice, P.L. (2009). Supporting collaborative teams and families in AAC. In G. Soto & C. Zangari (Eds.), *Practically speaking: Language, literacy, and academic development for students with AAC needs* (pp. 289–312). Baltimore: Paul H. Brookes Publishing Co.

Salisbury, C., Evans, I., & Palombaro, M. (1997). Collaborative problem solving to promote the inclusion of young children with significant disabilities in primary grades. *Exceptional Children, 63,* 195–209.

Smith, M.M. (2005). The dual challenges of aided communication and adolescence. *Augmentative and Alternative Communication, 21,* 67–79.

Thousand, J.S., & Villa, R.A. (1992). Collaborative teams: A powerful tool in school restructuring. In R.A. Villa, J.S. Thousand, W. Stainback, & S. Stainback (Eds.), *Restructuring for caring and effective education: An administrative guide to creating heterogeneous schools* (pp. 73–108). Baltimore: Paul H. Brookes Publishing Co.

Vereecke, R. (2004). *Dance—Boston College.* Retrieved November 11, 2009, from http://www.rebecca beayni.com/portfolio_Dance.html

Wagner, M., Newman, L., Cameto, R., Garza, N., & Levine, P. (2005). *After high school: A first look at the postschool experiences of youth with disabilities.* Retrieved November 29, 2009, from http://www.nlts2.org/ reports/2005_06/nlts2_report_2005_06_complete.pdf

Wagner, M., Newman, L., Cameto, R., Garza, N., & Levine, P. (2009). *The post-high school outcomes of youth with disabilities up to 4 years after high school.* Retrieved November 4, 2009, from http://www.nlts2.org/ reports/2009_04/nlts2_report_2009_04_complete.pdf

Wehman, P. (2006). *Life beyond the classroom: Transition strategies for young people with disabilities* (4th ed.). Baltimore: Paul H. Brookes Publishing Co.

Wehmeyer, M., & Kelchner, K. (1995). *The Arc's Self-Determination Scale.* Arlington, TX: Arc National Headquarters.

Wentzel, K.R., & Caldwell, K. (1997). Friendships, peer acceptance, and group membership: Relations to academic achievement in middle school. *Child Development, 68,* 1198–1209.

Williams, M.B. (2001). Give me shelter. *Alternatively Speaking, 5*(3), 1–3.

Williams, M.B. (2004). Message from the editor. *Alternatively Speaking, 7*(2), 2.

Williams, M.B., Krezman, C., & McNaughton, D. (2008). "Reach for the stars": Five principles for the next 25 years of AAC. *Augmentative and Alternative Communication, 24,* 194–206.

2

Self-Determination and Young Adults Who Use AAC

David B. McNaughton, Tracy Rackensperger, Michael L. Wehmeyer, and Sandra Wright[1]

> I had never had a place of my own. As a result, I had never worried about buying groceries and planning meals, paying the rent and the phone bills, balancing a checkbook, making appointments, figuring out how to keep the appointments I made—all of the things adults just do. But starting out in society at the age of twenty-eight, after living at a state institution for the mentally retarded for 16 years, I found these everyday tasks confusing, and wonderful, and frightening. (Sienkiewicz-Mercer & Kaplan, 1989, p. 202)

Ruth Sienkiewicz-Mercer was born with cerebral palsy in 1950. In 1978, a Massachusetts court enabled her to leave a state institution and move into her own community apartment. She left behind a life in which virtually every aspect of her care and daily activities had been controlled by institutional staff to join a world in which she was suddenly responsible for making many "confusing, and wonderful, and frightening" decisions. Her liberation was due, in equal measure, to her increased capacity to communicate using augmentative and alternative communication (AAC) and to her *self-determination*—her desire to take a larger role in both large and small life decisions.

Today, many adolescents and young adults who use AAC live in community settings and attend schools in those same communities. Few will experience the same sharp transition from institutional care to personal responsibility encountered by Ruth; however, careful planning is needed to ensure that people who use AAC are meaningfully involved in guiding their daily lives and routines, as well as their future employment and community participation. All people at all ages have a need and a right to live self-determined lives.

In this chapter we focus on three main issues that lead AAC users such as Ruth to be able to direct their lives: 1) conceptualizations of self-determination, with a particular focus on the application of theories of self-determination to people with severe disabilities; 2) skills that are used to act in a self-determined manner, and formal and informal activities to support the development of those skills; and 3) future research directions to support the development of self-determination within people who use AAC.

SELF-DETERMINATION

> [Self-determined people] know how to choose—they know what they want and how to get it. From an awareness of personal needs, self-determined individuals choose goals, then doggedly pursue them. This involves asserting an individual's presence, making his or her needs known, evaluating progress toward meeting goals, adjusting performance, and creating unique approaches to solve problems. (Martin & Marshall, 1995, p. 147)

---

[1]All authors contributed equally to the content of this chapter and, as such, are listed alphabetically.

The self-determination construct emerged from the philosophical doctrine of *determinism,* which suggests that all actions are caused by events or natural laws that precede or are antecedent to the occurrence of the action. Obviously, causes of human behavior are varied, from genes to environment; the meaning of self-determination (or self-determinism) is that one's actions are caused by oneself as opposed to something or someone else (e.g., other-determination). People who are self-determined make or cause things to happen in their own lives. They act based on their own will, preferences, choices, and interests instead of being coerced or forced to act by others or by circumstances (Wehmeyer, 2005).

People who are self-determined, as embodied in the quote from Martin and Marshall (1995), act in ways that enable them to solve problems in their lives, set and attain goals, make decisions, advocate on their own behalf, and generally improve the quality of their own lives. They act volitionally and are causal agents in their lives. The ideas of *volitional action* and *causal agent* are central to understanding what is meant by being self-determined.

By acting volitionally, we mean that people who are self-determined act based upon their preferences and interests and not upon coercion or someone else's preferences and interests. However, there is more to being self-determined than simply doing what one wants rather than what someone else wants one to do. *Volition* is the exercise of the capability of a person to make a conscious choice or decision with intention. Self-determined behavior, therefore, is not just acting to gratify instant needs or acting recklessly for short-term pleasure; it is acting consciously and with intention based upon one's preferences and interests to choose, make decisions, advocate, and, generally, self-govern and self-regulate one's behavior in pursuit of one's goals.

People who are self-determined are causal agents in their lives. The adjective *causal* means to express or indicate cause, or showing the interaction of cause and effect. The noun *agent* refers to one who acts or has the authority to act. Self-determined people act with authority to make or cause something to happen in their lives. However, causal agency implies more than just causing action; it implies that the individual who makes or causes things to happen in his or her life does so with an eye toward *causing* an effect to accomplish a specific end or to cause or create change; in other words, the individual acts volitionally and intentionally.

People too often equate self-determination with being physically independent, acting without help, and controlling one's own life. People with intellectual disabilities often have limitations to their capacity to solve difficult problems or make complex decisions and, in many meaningful ways, to control their lives. People with physical disabilities may be unable to perform some activities of daily living and will need to direct others to provide needed care. The important point to understand, particularly as it pertains to people with more severe disabilities, is that being self-determined is *not* about doing things independently but instead is about making things happen in one's life by acting volitionally and being a causal agent. Such actions lead, in turn, to an enhanced quality of life (Wehmeyer, Gragoudas, & Shogren, 2006). Rousso provided an excellent illustration of just this point:

I know a sculptor who is quadriplegic. She sculpts by giving precise instructions to her assistants, who serve as her hands. While it is tempting to think that her assistants are the true artists, she is, in fact, the sculptor in charge. When she has given the same directions to two assistants who have had no contact with each other, they both produce identical pieces of sculpture. Through the experience of disability, this woman has learned to articulate her vision and her needs in direct, specific ways—so much so, that she gets precisely the help she needs in forms that are replicable. (1997, p. 134)

BENEFITS OF SELF-DETERMINATION

The importance of enhanced self-determination is frequently highlighted by adults who use AAC (Creech, 1992; Kitch, 2005) and cited in the professional literature. Lund and Light (2006) reported that in their follow-up study of seven adults who use AAC, those people who reported the highest levels of self-determination also reported the highest quality of life. Shogren, Faggella-Luby, Bae, and Wehmeyer (2004) reported that when students with disabilities are provided with opportunities to make choices, reductions in problem behavior and increases in adaptive behavior are observed. Finally, Wehmeyer and Schwartz (1997) and Wehmeyer and Palmer (2003) found that young adults with disabilities who left school as more self-determined were more likely than young adults who were less self-determined to live independently, be employed, and earn higher wages, and Sowers and Powers (1995) showed that instruction on multiple components related to self-determination increased the participation and independence of students with severe disabilities in performing community activities.

BARRIERS TO SELF-DETERMINATION

Unfortunately, however, many people who use AAC are routinely denied the opportunity to communicate their preferences and decisions and to play a role in shaping their living environments. People who use AAC frequently describe being ignored and being denied opportunities to participate in many situations, including educational decision making (Seals, 2005), activities of daily living (McNaughton et al., 2008), and decisions about community living (Creech, 1992).

For people who use AAC, acting in a self-determined manner is often complicated by the communication challenges encountered while sharing personal opinions (Light & Gulens, 2000). Whereas adults who use AAC and who have effective communication skills face many challenges in making decisions and managing their lives (Williams, 2000), people with more significant cognitive challenges (and more limited communication skills) are even more likely to be routinely denied the opportunity to acquire and exercise decision-making skills, express preferences and make choices, and set and work toward goals (Wehmeyer, 2005).

SUPPORTS TO PROMOTE SELF-DETERMINATION

A person's capacity to act in a self-determined manner is clearly context dependent and interacts with a number of other variables. For example, the extent to which people make decisions about their lives is related to the opportunities for decision making that are available and to the availability of communication systems to support such participation. For people with complex communication needs, full and meaningful participation in decision-making and goal-setting activities will be closely tied to three often interrelated factors: 1) the communication skills of the person and the communication partner; 2) the belief of the person and the partner that the person who uses AAC has a right to act as a primary causal agent in his or her life; and 3) the shared ability of the person and the communication partner to recognize and develop decision-making, problem-solving, goal-setting, and choice-making opportunities.

Although people with complex communication needs are often denied opportunities to influence their environment, it is still relatively easy to think of examples of self-determined behavior for people with severe disabilities such as Ruth Sienkiewicz-Mercer (Sienkiewicz-Mercer & Kaplan, 1989) who can spell or who otherwise have access to large vocabularies. Self-determination, however, is a legitimate expectation for all people regardless of the severity of the disability. As in communicative interaction, the successful expression of self-determination may rest in part on the skills of the partner in supporting communication and providing appropriate decision-making opportunities. For example, an individual with severe physical and cognitive disabilities who needs assistance with eating can still be described as acting as the primary causal agent if he or she selects the food to be eaten (e.g., eye gaze to a preferred item) and/or provides feedback on an appropriate pace for feeding (e.g., smile when pace is appropriate, vocalize when pace is too slow). As in many communication situations, the ability of an individual to act in a self-determined manner may also be closely tied to the recognition of both the person who uses AAC and the partner that all individuals have a right to act as personal causal agents in their own lives.

Supports also may be needed to help an individual act in ways that maintain or improve his or her quality of life. Wehmeyer (1998) described the story of a person with severe cognitive challenges who had formed a friendship with a community volunteer. In the hope that the community friend would come and visit, the person with cognitive disabilities spent entire days standing by the window, watching for his arrival. Although the individual in this situation was acting as a primary causal agent, this cannot be considered self-determination because it has little chance of improving that person's quality of life—there is no reason to think that standing by a window for hours will help the person achieve the desired goal of social interaction. The individual in this situation should be provided with the supports, including instruction and practice with goal-setting and problem-solving strategies, to attain the desired goal of social interaction in a variety of ways. Self-determination does not just mean that an individual acts independently—he or she needs to do so in ways that have a reasonable chance of success (Light & Gulens, 2000).

SKILLS TO SUPPORT SELF-DETERMINED BEHAVIOR

The term *self-determination* is used to describe a wide range of actions and behaviors that enable an individual to act as the primary causal agent in his or her life and to maintain or improve his or her quality of life. It should not be conceptualized as a set of specific or isolated skills—although the behaviors are important, it is the integrated use and function of these component elements to act as the primary causal agent that is critical (Wehmeyer, 1996).

In order to exercise self-determination, people need to have skills in the following domains: 1) self-knowledge (including self-awareness, self-evaluation, and self-regulation), 2) decision making (including choice making and problem solving), 3) communication (including self-advocacy and meta-representation), and 4) goal setting and attainment (see Table 2.1). These four domains are best thought of as interrelated areas and not stages of development. For example, although self-knowledge will help in goal setting, the process of setting goals and attaining them will help an individual develop a better sense of who he or she is and will provide important opportunities to develop and practice new skills in decision making and communication.

Table 2.1.   Self-determination domains and skills

Domain	Skill
Self-knowledge	Understanding of personal strengths and needs and how to use these unique attributes to enhance one's quality of life
Self-awareness	Understanding of one's strengths and limitations
Self-evaluation	Ability to identify needed areas for change
Self-regulation	Ability to change behavior based on evaluation of progress toward a goal
Decision making	Ability to use information to identify a course of action
Choice making	Ability to select from alternatives
Problem solving	Ability to use an organized approach to identify a solution to a problem
Communication	Ability to interact with others to express needs and wants, transfer information, establish and maintain social closeness, and/or demonstrate social etiquette
Self-advocacy	Ability to ensure that one's opinions are known in important situations
Meta-representation	Ability to conceptualize problems and to create abstract representations to assist in thinking about problem states and possible solutions
Goal setting and attainment	Ability to set goals, identify appropriate strategies for attaining goals, and monitor progress (and adjust behavior) to reach goals

In this section, we describe both informal and formal opportunities to support the acquisition of skills in each of these domains. Again, these should not be thought of as isolated behaviors but rather as skills that are used and developed in an integrated manner throughout the day and across the life span. At the same time, for adolescents and young adults who are often denied the opportunity to acquire and exercise these skills, it is important to target specific opportunities to support the development of these behaviors.

Self-Knowledge

To act in a self-determined manner, adolescents and young adults who use AAC must enjoy a strong sense of personal identity. They must know who they are with regard to strengths and needs and be able to evaluate how changes in behavior have an impact on desired progress toward goals. This is often difficult for people who have grown up with labels and diminished expectations that continue to be communicated to adults with complex communication needs. Peg Johnson is a college graduate and is employed at the Minnesota Public Library. However, she described how many people underestimate her abilities:

> People frequently assume that a person's mental capability is directly related to their physical limitations or their physical appearance. There are a few people who are able to communicate with me on an adult basis. Some people attempt to communicate with me but retreat after not understanding my speech. There are others who are unable to deal with the situation at all and simply pat me on the head or say, "It's nice you could get out today." (Johnson, 2000, p. 53)

The need for assistance with activities of daily living can make it difficult for people with complex communication needs to develop an understanding of who they are and what they can do. As Michael B. Williams (2005) has noted, caregivers who do not provide opportunities for choices and who do not create appropriate and respectful assistance relationships can unwittingly communicate inappropriate expectations to those who need help:

> Sometimes a real need for help in doing the tasks of daily living leads to the false impression that people who rely on AAC are child-like, asexual, and dependent. Children don't work. Children don't have adult relationships. Children aren't relied on to make their own decisions. Thus a paternalistic pat on the head or a juvenile nickname is not harmless. It steals away our opportunities for adult roles.

In addition, communication challenges and negative reactions from communication partners can lead to reduced expectations for communication on the part of both the young adult with complex communication needs and his or her communication partner. These reduced communication opportunities can have a profound effect on an adolescent's self-image. Jan Staehely, a person with cerebral palsy who lives with dysarthric speech, wrote, "I had become so used to not being able to say something in depth to a person that I started to believe that I was a person who didn't have much to tell people" (2000, p. 9).

Self-knowledge is typically acquired slowly, through an adolescent's growing awareness of his or her skills and needs and through communicative interactions with other people. The development of self-knowledge is best supported by opportunities to participate in a range of activities and environments; the provision of structured learning experiences to help adolescents acquire new, socially valued skills; and the facilitation of interaction with a wide range of partners, especially peers.

It may be challenging to identify skills and activities that young adults with physical disabilities can perform independently, even with assistive technology, but making a tangible contribution to the home and school environment is important to the development of self-knowledge (Hurd, 2007). It may be a useful task to analyze activities at home and school to identify those areas in which individuals with disabilities can play a role. Perhaps they cannot independently sort the recycling at home, but they can guide a partner to place the item in the appropriate bin. They may not be able to present an entire lecture at school, but they can prerecord and deliver their segment in front of the class (Williams, 1998).

One should not underestimate the impact of the chance to demonstrate valued skills and receive feedback from others. Scott Palm, an individual who uses AAC, described his first experience with public speaking using an AAC device as part of a workplace transition program:

> My job developer came up with the idea of me giving a speech to the city council about my job. I was scared to death. . . . Then the night of the speech came. My scared feeling was replaced with a blend of emotions. I was excited but nervous. I was excited because I knew I could do it. I was nervous about how it would turn out. I invited my speech-language pathologist to be there, and she was in the audience. After some technical issues with the mike, I did the speech. Something started to happen. I began to have the feeling that I was in charge of the entire room. Everybody was listening to me. It was really intoxicating. I never had a full room of people listening to me before. The speech was a huge success. (2007, p. 70)

An understanding of one's strengths and needs is strongly shaped by the demands of a particular environment. Effective high school transition programs should support the development of self-knowledge by providing structured opportunities for participation in targeted adult environments (e.g., independent living, job placements) so that individuals can develop a better sense of their skills and needs. Rick Creech, a person with cerebral palsy who operates his AAC device using a head pointer, described how his stay at a managed care facility as a young man, although stressful, contributed to his sense of self-efficacy:

> I am not the same person that I would have been if I had not stayed at the CP Hospital. Even if I had learned nothing else, I learned that I could rely on my own abilities, and that made me able to try anything. Leaving me at the CP Hospital was perhaps the hardest thing my parents have done and perhaps the best. (1992, p. 43)

Adolescents who use AAC can develop a stronger sense of self by participating in a range of activities and receiving clear feedback on their performance at these times. The challenge is to create activities and goals that are challenging but achievable—people may have a false sense of achievement if they receive significant praise for minimal achievements. As Michael B. Williams, an adult who uses AAC, has commented, "It's easy to be an overachiever in the land of lowered expectations" (1997, p. 9). False feedback can lead to difficulties as people proceed into higher education and the workplace. One individual who uses AAC commented that it was only during his first job that he received honest feedback about the quality of his performance—he was "mad as hell" to be told for the first time, at age 23, to do something over because his first attempt was inadequate. On reflection, the individual noted that the feedback was justified, and he stated that he believed that school could have better prepared him for the workplace by providing him with honest feedback at an earlier age (McNaughton, Symons, Light, & Parsons, 2006).

Self-knowledge, especially self-image, is strongly influenced by interactions with peers. The teenage years are often especially challenging for people with complex communication needs. Many people who use AAC report difficulties in establishing and maintaining friendships with peers without disabilities, and they experience difficulty developing a positive self-image (Smith, 2005). As Rick Creech has written,

> In order not to take this reaction of people personally, the augmented speaker needs to be able to separate oneself from one's disability and accept a negative reaction to the disability as only being to the disability, and not as reaction to the person. (1992, p. 35)

Interactions with other people who use AAC, including older people, may be useful at these times. The Mentor Project (Light et al., 2007) partnered adolescents and young adults who use AAC (protégés) with *mentors*—older people who use AAC and who had successfully addressed

> ## BOX 2.1.   Mentor Project case study
>
> A mentor can provide important guidance and support, especially when he or she has confronted and addressed challenges encountered by the protégé. Many people who use augmentative and alternative communication (AAC), however, have only limited contact with older people who also use AAC and who could act as mentors. In order to investigate the impact of mentoring on addressing important adolescent and young adult transition issues, the Mentor Project (Light et al., 2007) partnered 30 adults who used AAC (mentors) with 32 adolescents and young adults who also used AAC (protégés). (Some mentors worked with more than one protégé.)
>
> As a first step in the process, the mentors were provided with web-based instruction in interpersonal communication skills, problem-solving and goal-setting skills, and strategies for accessing disability-related resources and services. Once training was completed, mentors were eligible to be selected by protégés, who picked their mentors based on brief biographical descriptions.
>
> Throughout the year-long mentoring program, which took place entirely via e-mail, the protégés had the opportunity to interact socially with their mentors, solve problems, and work toward individual goals. Topics that were frequently discussed across dyads included education, relationships, AAC, and family. The protégés set a total of 80 goals across a wide variety of domains, including education, vocation, independent living, personal relationships, and assistive technology. Data indicated that they made progress toward or attained 84% of these goals. The overwhelming majority of the mentors (97%) and the protégés (96%) reported high levels of satisfaction with the mentoring program.

many of the same challenges that confronted the protégés (see Box 2.1). The Mentor Project enabled the protégés to talk about and work though the challenges they experienced in their own lives. Both mentors and protégés viewed the experience positively, and 100% said they would recommend the project to others.

Decision Making

> Imagine sitting in a nice fancy restaurant. The waiter comes to take your order. You order a juicy steak, medium rare. After 30 minutes the waiter returns with a full fluffy salad. You confront the waiter stating that you ordered a steak not a salad. The waiter responds back that a survey was given to 1,000 brothers-in-law of people with disabilities and the results were that people with disabilities need to eat salad, so . . . Adults with disabilities have experienced this situation all of their lives from make and model of wheelchairs to one's augmentative communication devices. (Watson, 1999, p. 36)

Making decisions, communicating choices, and solving problems are important ways that people who use AAC can exercise control over their lives. Often these decisions are preempted by caregivers or educational staff, sometimes out of the belief that they are helping, sometimes out of the belief that the young adult with complex communication needs does not have the cognitive capacity or communication skills to make choices. However, even people with severe cognitive disabilities have demonstrated the ability to exercise control of their environment when provided by caregivers with structured choice-making opportunities (McNaughton & Light, 1989). Even these individuals have a right to make decisions about their daily lives.

Increasing the participation of adolescents who use AAC in decision-making and problem-solving activities will require interventions with both the young adults who use AAC (to learn effective problem-solving strategies) as well as their communication partners (to learn to provide appropriate opportunities and support). As part of the Mentor Study, adolescents who used AAC (protégés) identified problems they encountered in their daily lives (Light et al., 2007). Some were common to all adolescents: education, planning future employment, family, and social relationships. Other problems were unique to people with complex communication needs: communication and AAC, other equipment and technologies, personal care attendants, and specialized transportation issues. Protégés worked in partnership with their mentors, who had received training in the five-step problem-solving strategy DOIT! (based on the problem-solving strategy developed by Wehmeyer & Lawrence, 1995). Protégés viewed these interactions very positively and reported making significant progress toward attaining or addressing a majority of their goals (see Figure 2.1).

In a follow-up study, McCarthy, Light, and McNaughton (2007) investigated the use of an Internet-based training program to teach young adults who used AAC (ages 18–20) to learn to use the DOIT! strategy to analyze problems and generate solutions for problems in their own lives. All five participants learned to successfully use the strategy after an average of 8 hours of online instruction, and participants maintained their skills 3 months after instruction ended. All participants reported that they had enjoyed the instructional program and would recommend similar instruction to adolescents who use AAC.

Instruction in problem-solving strategies and the provision of additional opportunities can be a key first step in introducing adolescents to more important decision-making activities. However, caregivers and educational staff must also become comfortable with the idea that "not every decision a person makes turns out to be an optimal decision, nor is every choice the perfect selection or every goal the right goal" (Wehmeyer, 1998, p. 11). People may occasionally experience negative outcomes from their decisions, but, within reason, these are important learning opportunities. The challenge is for educational staff and family members to allow for risk while being prepared to provide additional supports if it is clear that a behavior has little chance of providing benefit. It is important to realize that if people are denied the opportunity to make meaningful decisions as adolescents, they will be poorly prepared to make important decisions as adults. It is difficult for a parent or caregiver to watch loved ones expose themselves to risk, but risk is critical to the pursuit of valued life goals. As Rick Creech has written,

> Going on to college, leaving their [my parents'] home, building an independent life for myself was something I had to do, and I paid the price with hard work, physical discomfort, fear, and even pain. However, I also experienced the rewards of that life: friendships, opportunities, responsibilities, knowledge, and useful work. (1992, p. 25)

Describe the specific problem or goal and explain why this is a problem or a goal.

Outline lots of different ways to solve the problem or meet the goal.

Identify the consequences of each plan and choose the best plan.

Take action toward solving the problem or meeting the goal.

! Celebrate success! when the problem is solved or the goal is achieved.

Figure 2.1.   DOIT!: A collaborative problem-solving strategy. (Light et al., 2007, from Wehmeyer, M., & Lawrence, M. [1995]. Whose future is it anyway? Promoting student involvement in transition planning. *Career Development for Exceptional Individuals, 18,* 69–83; adapted by permission.)

Communication

If I could not express myself clearly and accurately, I could not tell my physician and others how I feel or describe the health problems I may be having. Similarly, I could not let others know what I know or what I am capable of learning. Nor could I go to work or vote. Furthermore, if I could not express myself, I would become like the tree in the forest—the one for which it does not matter if it makes a sound when it comes crashing down, because there is no one around to hear it. Unfortunately, there are still a great many silent fallen trees all around us if we stop and look. (Williams, 2000, p. 250)

Communication skills are fundamental to self-determination. Although choices and decisions can be communicated via a variety of modes (e.g., eye gaze, pointing, AAC devices), communicating complex decisions requires elaborate cognitive and collaboration skills (Light & Gulens, 2000). People who use AAC describe the importance of the effective use of AAC systems both to communicate their decisions but also to make clear to others that they are capable of speaking their minds. Communication approaches viewed by communication partners as difficult to understand or unconventional may be ignored, and people who use AAC will need to develop a variety of modes and strategies to communicate successfully with others.

Light (1989) suggested that for people who use AAC, communicative competence rests on knowledge, judgment, and skills in four interrelated domains—linguistic, operational, social, and strategic (see Table 2.2). Randy Kitch (2005), who as a young adult communicated by sitting on the floor and spelling out words with his toe on a letterboard, provides a vivid example of the coordinated use of these skills. Randy was linguistically and operationally competent with this system; however, interacting with people in the community who were unfamiliar with his system often meant needing to bring other skills into play. Randy described his use of social and strategic skills with a record store clerk who had previously ignored his communication attempts:

I decided to type him a note explaining how I communicated with my letter board and went back to the store the next day to give it to him. I went up to him, sat on the floor and footed him the note. It said, "I communicate by spelling words out on a letter board with my big toe and I would appreciate it if you would communicate with me." It also said "I would like to purchase some head cleaner for my cassette player." He got the cleaner, I gave him the money, and after he handed me the cleaner, I spelled out, "THANK YOU" on the letter board and he said, "You're welcome." (p. 49)

Communication includes not only the ability to interact with others but the ability to talk to oneself about problems. *Meta-representation* describes the ability to conceptualize problems to create abstract representations to assist in thinking about problem states and possible solutions. Meta-representation can pose significant cognitive demands, especially in situations in which people are expected to keep a large number of variables (i.e., problems, possible solutions) in their head. As part of the problem-solving strategy taught in the Internet-based training program described in

Table 2.2.   Communicative competence

Domain	Examples of knowledge, judgment, and skills
Linguistic	Develop skills in the native language(s) spoken in the individual's family and social community
	Develop skills in the "linguistic codes" of AAC systems
Operational	Produce unaided symbols (convention gestures, pantomime, signs) as required
	Operate aided AAC systems accurately and efficiently as required
Social	Develop appropriate sociolinguistic skills
	Develop appropriate sociorelational skills
Strategic	Use appropriate strategies to bypass limitations in the linguistic domain
	Use appropriate strategies to bypass limitations in the operational domain
	Use appropriate strategies to bypass limitations in the social domain

Source: Light and Gulens (2000).

McCarthy et al. (2007), adolescents who used AAC learned to write down alternative solutions rather than just trying to keep them "in their head." Writing the solutions down may have reduced the cognitive load associated with this task and may have facilitated the consideration of the strengths and weaknesses associated with various options.

Finally, *self-advocacy* describes the ability to speak up for oneself and to ensure that one's opinions are known in important situations. The ability to speak one's mind is, as noted by Hurd (2007), a character trait that is important for helping children who use AAC become self-sufficient adults. But it is also not necessarily looked upon as a good thing by professionals and service providers. As noted by Williams, "Professionals often expect clients to be compliant. An adult who knows what he or she wants may be perceived as noncompliant" (2004, p. 3).

Sometimes a young adult's desire to self-advocate can be confounded by a lack of appropriate vocabulary:

> A part of growing up and being an adult is saying what you want and expecting others to respect your decisions about yourself. It is very frustrating for the non-verbal person and the personal assistant when the AAC device doesn't have enough adult words to discuss some of the more personal aspects of personal care. (Lever, 2003, p. 4)

Lack of vocabulary and self-advocacy affects not only personal care but also issues of personal safety and the ability to report abuse:

> Sometimes even when we want to speak out, we don't have the right words to do so. Most communication aids don't come with vocabulary necessary to end the silence about crime and abuse. Many of us don't have easy access to the right vocabulary in our communication devices. Not having adequate vocabulary raises the risk of people who rely on AAC being victimized because we are identified as unable to tell anyone when crime or abuse occurs. It allows those who would commit crimes against us to continue undeterred. We need adequate vocabulary to talk about crime and abuse, and we need to know how to use that vocabulary. (Lever, 2003, p. 4)

Transition programs must work to prepare students who use AAC to advocate for themselves in a variety of postschool environments, including in situations involving activities of daily living, employment, and transportation. These experiences will lead to additional opportunities for individuals to learn and make use of self-advocacy skills. Randy Horton, a young adult who uses a Pathfinder (Prentke Romich Company) to communicate, described his use of prestored messages to advocate for his personal safety while riding on public transportation:

> I tell the driver politely, at first, what needs to be done. If the driver does not heed my directions, I say, "Company rules say that it is your responsibility." Then if there is still no compliance, I say, "You need to call your supervisor," followed by, "All right I will call them myself." And, "Please send a supervisor," if the driver refused to tie my chair down. (2005, p. 85)

For people who are unable to independently spell out or otherwise generate new vocabulary, it is critical that caregivers anticipate and plan for the unthinkable (e.g., abuse situations, criminal activity), ensuring that people who use AAC have the vocabulary and the skills to report inappropriate behavior by others (Williams, Krezman, & McNaughton, 2008).

Goal Setting and Attainment

Bob Segalman and Neil Jacobson are two adults with complex communication needs. Bob is employed as a statistical analyst for the State Department of Rehabilitation in California, and Neil is a vice president in charge of computer operations at a bank. Only a small number of people with complex communication needs are employed (Light, Stoltz, & McNaughton, 1996), and experts have only a limited understanding of how to achieve success for this population. After speaking with both Bob and Neil, Michael B. Williams was interested to note the following similarities:

> In talking to these two people I see they are a lot alike. Both of them have "the will to win" or "that killer instinct." They are not afraid to take risks or accept new challenges. They grab hold of new opportunities when they come along, not accepting that old adage that says "good things come to those who wait." Both men make things happen knowing that if you wait for things to happen, you could be waiting a long time. (1994, p. 6)

Setting goals, and working aggressively to reach those goals, is a key feature of self-determined behavior. However, many people who use AAC report that they were rarely asked to set goals or make plans for their adult life while they were in school (Blackstone, 1993). Structured interventions to support goal setting and attainment for transition-age youth with complex communication needs were a key feature of the Augmentative Communication Employment Training and Supports program (Bryen, Cohen, & Carey, 2004). Eight young adults who used AAC received training in goal setting and attainment with respect to employment activities during a 1-week intensive training session at Temple University and year-long follow-up activities. Participants worked with program staff to identify goals and activities related to obtaining a job and then provided updates on their progress during the year using an online reporting form. All participants reported improvements in their job-hunting skills and in their ability to translate personal interests into employment goals. At the end of the year, five of the eight participants reported an increase in their monthly income as well as achievement of a variety of individualized job-related goals (e.g., one person obtained a high school equivalency certificate).

FUTURE RESEARCH

Supporting adolescents and young adults who use AAC in the development of self-determination skills requires two critical elements (Light & Gulens, 2000): 1) These young adults must have regular opportunities to act as primary causal agents in ways that maintain or improve their quality of life, and they must receive appropriate feedback at these times; and 2) they must have the knowledge, judgment, and skills to communicate effectively during these opportunities. Most of the existing intervention programs addressing self-determination are designed for students with mild to moderate disabilities (Karvonen, Test, Wood, Browder, & Algozzine, 2004). Future research should examine the factors involved in the provision of needed opportunities and the instructional activities necessary to ensure the acquisition of needed skills.

Developing Opportunities to Act as Primary Causal Agents

Whereas self-determination is typically ranked highly by people who use AAC and is strongly associated with a good quality of life, it is typically viewed as a low priority by education personnel (Wehmeyer, 2005). This may be due in part to the misconception that self-determination means independent control, which teachers view as an unrealizable and inappropriate goal. However, as Wehmeyer noted,

> The role of teachers is not to teach students to control their lives. It is to enable students with severe disabilities to become more self-determined, even if it is just a little bit more. . . . The goal is not to promote control, but to enable students to act volitionally and to become causal agents in their lives, to make things happen in their lives. (2005, pp. 119–120)

There is sometimes a misconception that self-determination refers only to large, high-stakes decisions such as choosing living arrangements or a career, but opportunities for behaving in a self-determined manner—for acting as a primary causal agent—occur throughout the day. Educators can help students to become more self-determined by teaching them to express preferences (McNaughton & Light, 1989), by implementing instruction that promotes involvement in problem solving and decision making (McCarthy et al., 2007; Wehmeyer, 1998), and by promoting self-advocacy and student-directed learning (Agran, Blanchard, & Wehmeyer, 2000).

The recognition that opportunities for the development of self-determination skills occur regularly throughout the day should help educators see that self-determination, like communication, is not an additional skill to be learned in isolation but rather an integral part of every activity. The critical challenge is to recognize and develop appropriate opportunities and to provide a responsive context to assist in the development of new skills. Turnbull and colleagues (1996) described responsive contexts as including the following key features: 1) opportunities for enjoyable and reciprocal relationships, 2) nonjudgmental and informative feedback, 3) a reasonable degree of successive challenges, 4) negotiation of reasonable and constructive limits, 5) open and honest communication, 6) facilitating but not controlling support, and 7) celebratory affirmations of progress. Future research should investigate instructional strategies to ensure that adolescents and young adults receive multiple opportunities to act in a self-determined manner throughout the day and to ensure that educators and family members provide responsive contexts, including appropriate feedback, at these times.

Developing Communication Skills

Self-determination and communication are closely intertwined—communication skills are of critical importance if an individual is to act as a primary causal agent. In order to be maximally effective, AAC interventions must be two pronged (Beukelman & Mirenda, 2005). They must consider not only the skill development of the people with complex communication needs but also the skills of the significant others in their lives and those of members of society generally. Intervention with people who require AAC ensures that they have the knowledge, judgment, and skills required to communicate effectively. Intervention with their typical communication partners, and with society generally, ensures that the people who use AAC have the opportunity to communicate and to act as primary causal agents in their lives.

When considering the communication skills needed to support self-determination, special attention should be given to teaching students how to advocate for themselves and how to communicate their perspective. Adolescents and young adults need to learn how to negotiate, to compromise, and to deal with systems and bureaucracies. Consideration of the four major reasons for communicating—expression of needs and wants, information transfer, social closeness, and social etiquette (Light, 1989)—reminds one that many targeted self-determination skills involve the integrated use of a variety of communication competencies. For example, when advocating with a teacher for extended test time, a student must not only express needs and wants but must do so in a way that is viewed as appropriate by the teacher (social etiquette). When informing a friend of his or her perspective (information transfer), an individual must communicate in a way that maintains the friendship (social closeness).

These skills are best learned in the context of real-world opportunities, and opportunities to act in a self-determined manner and for self-advocacy should be embedded throughout the school day by allowing students to set up a class schedule, work out their supports with a resource room teacher or other support provider, or participate in individualized education program and transition meetings (Wehmeyer et al., 2006). Future research should examine 1) interventions that support the acquisition of communication skills needed for participation in structured and unstructured self-determination opportunities and 2) ways to develop the provision of meaningful communication opportunities throughout the day and across multiple environments.

CONCLUSION

Tracy Rackensperger, a young woman who grew up in Florida and who uses a Pathfinder to communicate, attended an inclusive high school program and obtained both an undergraduate and master's degree. Like many young people, Tracy was aware that she would have adult responsibilities one day, but she was still surprised by the amount of planning required for successful independent living.

> I knew the day would come when I would have to manage supports because I have always had dreams of moving into my own place, having a career, and living independently in the community. Knowing this, it would have made sense for me to plan ahead and work out how exactly I would accomplish everything I planned to do. Yet, due to my laid back nature and my notion that everything eventually comes out okay in the end, I conducted very little pre-planning. Thus, until I was 27 years old, my parents were the sole providers of the physical support I required each day. (Rackensperger, 2007, p. 1)

When she obtained a full-time job in another state, Tracy was forced to quickly learn how to take charge. Her initial efforts at living in an apartment and arranging supports provided her with insights into the challenges of managing personal care.

> Well, the apartment living situation was a disaster. Due to very poor planning, I waited way too long to advertise for a roommate and to garner additional support. Additionally, my family suffered a severe medical crisis. The only solution at that time was to move back in with my family.
>
> In the meantime, I found that building and relying on natural supports was challenging for me. I grew up in a very conservative family, where the ideas of self-reliance and independence were instilled. Sure, it was okay to ask friends to help with small tasks (e.g., pouring you a drink everyday at lunch), but you didn't ask them for major assistance (e.g., driving the van). I still value these concepts. However, friends kept offering to do things for me and gradually I have learned to use natural supports more regularly. I have friends who I know I can call upon for assistance in the same way they can ask me for assistance. (p. 1)

Tracy noted that, as many do, she has learned through a process of trial and error how to make it work. She acknowledged that although everything is not perfect,

> It's working adequately. I now know that managing the supports I need to live is a challenging and long-term process. I know I have to plan ahead and have contingencies. I need to be prepared for the "what ifs." While I'm still learning how to integrate the natural and paid supports in my life, I am empowered and supported by others who are living independently with various types of supports. By listening and talking with others about their experiences with managing support, I am inspired to try new approaches in fitting together the assistance I need to live my life. (p. 1)

Tracy's story provides important supports for the key principles associated with the development of self-determination skills: that attention must be paid to supporting the development of a wide range of self-determination skills from an early age; that these skills are best acquired in responsive and supportive contexts; and that overcoming problems, if appropriate supports are available, can provide important learning experiences.

The benefits of supporting self-determined behavior—both in Tracy's situation and for all individuals who use AAC—are clear. High levels of self-determination are associated with high measures of quality of life (Lund & Light, 2006; Wehmeyer & Palmer, 2003), and every individual has the right and should have the opportunity to make important decisions about his or her life. Providing effective support for the development of self-determination skills, however, will require that educators and caregivers carefully consider how they view themselves and their expectations for people with disabilities. Although many educators view people with severe disabilities as inappropriate candidates for self-determination, there is almost always some aspect of even the most complex activity, from decision making to goal setting, in which people with significant cognitive disabilities can participate with adequate support and accommodations (Wehmeyer, 1998).

Emphasizing the promotion of self-determination and encouraging people to act as primary causal agents in their own lives may also require that adolescents and young adults who use AAC change how they view themselves and their futures. Michael B. Williams (1998) has written that many people who use AAC have come to accept society's reduced view of their skills and interests. Moreover, he has noted that regular meaningful opportunities to exercise self-determination will be needed to help people develop a sense of self and an interest and belief in their ability to act in a self-determined manner.

The importance of the goal is clear, however. Although every life involves unique choices and decisions, what is common—and what is critical—is that every person has an opportunity to act in a self-determined manner and to influence his or her life. As noted by Light and Gulens,

> Communicative competence and self-determination are at the core of our existence as human beings. Together they allow us to define who we are, what dreams we have, how these dreams are realized (or not), and what connections and relationships we build with others. (2000, p. 138)

REFERENCES

Agran, M., Blanchard, C., & Wehmeyer, M.L. (2000). Promoting transition goals and self-determination through student self-directed learning: The self-determined learning model of instruction. *Education & Training in Mental Retardation & Developmental Disabilities, 35,* 351–364.

Beukelman, D.R., & Mirenda, P. (2005). *Augmentative and alternative communication: Supporting children and adults with complex communication needs* (3rd ed.). Baltimore: Paul H. Brookes Publishing Co.

Blackstone, S. (1993). For consumers: What do you want to be when you grow up? *Augmentative Communication News, 6*(4), 1–2.

Bryen, D.N., Cohen, K.J., & Carey, A. (2004). Augmentative Communication Employment Training and Supports (ACETS): Some employment-related outcomes. *Journal of Rehabilitation, 70,* 10–19.

Creech, R. (1992). *Reflections from a unicorn.* Greenville, NC: RC Publishing.

Horton, R. (2005, August). Communicating in public places. In R.V. Conti, P. Meneskie, & C. Micher (Eds.), *Proceedings of the Thirteenth Pittsburgh Employment Conference for Augmented Communicators* (pp. 85–86). Pittsburgh: Shout Press.

Hurd, R. (2007, August). Getting children who use AAC ready for the "real world", and getting the "real world" ready for them! In R.V. Conti, P. Meneskie, & C. Micher (Eds.), *Proceedings of the Thirteenth Pittsburgh Employment Conference for Augmented Communicators* (pp. 60–62). Pittsburgh: Shout Press.

Johnson, P.L. (2000). If I do say so myself! In M. Fried-Oken & H.A. Bersani, Jr. (Eds.), *Speaking up and spelling it out: Personal essays on augmentative and alternative communication* (pp. 48–55). Baltimore: Paul H. Brookes Publishing Co.

Karvonen, M., Test, D.W., Wood, W.M., Browder, D., & Algozzine, B. (2004). Putting self-determination into practice. *Exceptional Children, 71,* 23–42.

Kitch, R. (2005, August). Identifying the barriers of community interaction and knocking them down. In R.V. Conti, P. Meneskie, & C. Micher (Eds.), *Proceedings of the Thirteenth Pittsburgh Employment Conference for Augmented Communicators* (pp. 48–51). Pittsburgh: Shout Press.

Lever, S. (2003). Speaking out: Access to vocabulary. *Alternatively Speaking, 6*(3), 4–5.

Light, J. (1989). Toward a definition of communicative competence for individuals using augmentative and alternative communication systems. *Augmentative and Alternative Communication, 5,* 137–144.

Light, J.C. (2003). Shattering the silence: Development of communicative competence by individuals who use AAC. In D.R. Beukelman & J. Reichle (Series Eds.) & J.C. Light, D.R. Beukelman, & J. Reichle (Vol. Eds.), *Augmentative and alternative communication series. Communicative competence for individuals who use AAC: From research to effective practice* (pp. 3–40). Baltimore: Paul H. Brookes Publishing Co.

Light, J.C., & Gulens, M. (2000). Rebuilding communicative competence and self-determination. In D.R. Beukelman, K.M. Yorkston, & J. Reichle (Vol. Eds.), *Augmentative and alternative communication series. Augmentative and alternative communication for adults with acquired neurologic disorders* (pp. 137–179). Baltimore: Paul H. Brookes Publishing Co.

Light, J., McNaughton, D., Krezman, C., Williams, M., Gulens, M., Galskoy, A., et al. (2007). The AAC Mentor Project: Web-based instruction in sociorelational skills and collaborative problem solving for adults who use augmentative and alternative communication. *Augmentative and Alternative Communication, 23,* 56–75.

Light, J., Stoltz, B., & McNaughton, D. (1996). Community-based employment: Experiences of adults who use AAC. *Augmentative and Alternative Communication, 12,* 215–229.

Lund, S.K., & Light, J. (2006). Long-term outcomes for individuals who use augmentative and alternative communication: Part I—What is a "good" outcome? *Augmentative and Alternative Communication, 22,* 284–299.

Martin, J.E., & Marshall, L.H. (1995). ChoiceMaker: A comprehensive self-determination transition program. *Intervention in School and Clinic, 30,* 147–156.

McCarthy, J., Light, J., & McNaughton, D. (2007). The effects of Internet-based instruction on the social problem solving of young adults who use augmentative and alternative communication. *Augmentative and Alternative Communication, 23,* 100–112.

McNaughton, D., & Light, J. (1989). Teaching facilitators to support the communication skills of an adult with severe cognitive disabilities: A case study. *Augmentative and Alternative Communication, 5,* 35–41.

McNaughton, D., Rackensperger, T., Benedeck-Wood, E., Krezman, C., Williams, M., & Light, J. (2008). "A child needs to be given a chance to succeed": Parents of individuals who use AAC describe the benefits and challenges of learning AAC technologies. *Augmentative and Alternative Communication, 24,* 43–55.

McNaughton, D., Symons, G., Light, J., & Parsons, A. (2006). "My dream was to pay taxes": The self-employment experiences of individuals who use augmentative and alternative communication. *Journal of Vocational Rehabilitation, 25,* 181–196.

Palm, S. (2007). The therapeutic value of one augmented communicator helping another augmented communicator is without parallel. In R.V. Conti, P. Meneskie, & C. Micher (Eds.), *Proceedings of the Fifteenth Pittsburgh Employment Conference for Augmented Communicators* (pp. 70–74). Pittsburgh: Shout Press.

Rackensperger, T. (2007). Support and AAC. *Alternatively Speaking, 9*(2), 1.

Rousso, H. (1997). Seeing the world anew: Science and disability. In N. Kreinberg & E. Wahl (Eds.), *Thoughts and deeds: Equity in mathematics and science education* (pp. 131–134). Washington, DC: American Association for the Advancement of Science.

Seals, D. (2005). Rewind, pause and fast forward (past, present, and future). In R.V. Conti, P. Meneskie, & C. Micher (Eds.), *Proceedings of the Tenth Pittsburgh Employment Conference for Augmented Communicators* (pp. 5–12). Pittsburgh: Shout Press.

Shogren, K.A., Faggella-Luby, M.N., Bae, S.J., & Wehmeyer, M.L. (2004). The effect of choice-making as an intervention for problem behavior: A meta-analysis. *Journal of Positive Behavior Interventions, 6,* 228–237.

Sienkiewicz-Mercer, R., & Kaplan, S.B. (1989). *I raise my eyes to say yes.* Boston: Houghton Mifflin.

Smith, M.M. (2005). The dual challenges of aided communication and adolescence. *Augmentative and Alternative Communication, 21,* 67–79.

Sowers, J., & Powers, L. (1995). Enhancing the participation and independence of students with severe physical and multiple disabilities in performing community activities. *Mental Retardation, 33,* 209–220.

Staehely, J. (2000). Prologue: The communication dance. In M. Fried-Oken & H.A. Bersani, Jr. (Eds.), *Speaking up and spelling it out: Personal essays on augmentative and alternative communication* (pp. 1–12). Baltimore: Paul H. Brookes Publishing Co.

Turnbull, A.P., Blue-Banning, M.J., Anderson, E.L., Turnbull, H.R., Seaton, K.A., & Dinas, P.A. (1996). Enhancing self-determination through Group Action Planning: A holistic emphasis. In D.J. Sands & M.L. Wehmeyer (Eds.), *Self-determination across the life span: Independence and choice for people with disabilities* (pp. 237–256). Baltimore: Paul H. Brookes Publishing Co.

Watson, R. (1999). The economics of dating. In R.V. Conti, P. Meneskie, & C. Micher (Eds.), *Proceedings of the Third Pittsburgh Employment Conference for Augmented Communicators* (pp. 36). Pittsburgh: Shout Press.

Wehmeyer, M.L. (1996). Self-determination as an educational outcome: Why is it important to children, youth, and adults with disabilities? In D.J. Sands & M.L. Wehmeyer (Eds.), *Self-determination across the life span: Independence and choice for people with disabilities* (pp. 17–36). Baltimore: Paul H. Brookes Publishing Co.

Wehmeyer, M.L. (1998). Self-determination and individuals with significant disabilities: Examining meanings and misinterpretations. *Journal of The Association for Persons with Severe Handicaps, 23,* 5–16.

Wehmeyer, M.L. (2005). Self-determination and individuals with severe disabilities: Re-examining meanings and misinterpretations. *Research and Practice for Persons with Severe Disabilities, 30,* 113–120.

Wehmeyer, M.L., Gragoudas, S., & Shogren, K. (2006). Self-determination, student involvement and leadership development. In P. Wehman (Ed.), *Life beyond the classroom: Transition strategies for young people with disabilities* (4th ed., pp. 41–69). Baltimore: Paul H. Brookes Publishing Co.

Wehmeyer, M., & Lawrence, M. (1995). Whose future is it anyway? Promoting student involvement in transition planning. *Career Development for Exceptional Individuals, 18,* 69–83.

Wehmeyer, M.L., & Palmer, S.B. (2003). Adult outcomes for students with cognitive disabilities three years after high school: The impact of self-determination. *Education and Training in Developmental Disabilities, 38,* 131–144.

Wehmeyer, M., & Schwartz, M. (1997). Self-determination and positive adult outcomes: A follow-up study of youth with mental retardation or learning disabilities. *Exceptional Children, 63,* 245–255.

Williams, B. (2000). More than an exception to the rule. In M. Fried-Oken & H.A. Bersani, Jr. (Eds.), *Speaking up and spelling it out: Personal essays on augmentative and alternative communication* (pp. 245–254). Baltimore: Paul H. Brookes Publishing Co.

Williams, M.B. (1994). Going to work. *Alternatively Speaking, 1*(3), 5–7.

Williams, M.B. (1997, December). Transitions to success. *Team Rehab Report, 8,* 8–9.

Williams, M.B. (1998). Heading for work. *Alternatively Speaking, 4*(1), 8.

Williams, M.B. (2004). Love and marriage. *Alternatively Speaking, 7*(2), 1–3.

Williams, M.B. (2005). Who is that masked man? *Alternatively Speaking, 8*(2), 1–3

Williams, M.B., Krezman, C., & McNaughton, D. (2008). "Reach for the stars": Five principles for the next 25 years of AAC. *Augmentative and Alternative Communication, 24,* 194–206.

II

Education and Transition Programs

3

Literacy Instruction for Transition-Age Youth Who Use AAC

What Is and What Could Be

Beth E. Foley and Julie A. Wolter

> Adolescents entering the adult world in the 21st century will read and write more than at any other time in human history. They will need advanced levels of literacy to perform their jobs, run their households, act as citizens, and conduct their personal lives. They will need literacy to cope with the flood of information they will find everywhere they turn. They will need literacy to feed their imagination so they can create the world of the future. (Moore, Bean, Birdyshaw, & Rycik, 1999, p. 3)

The need to prepare transition-age youth who use augmentative and alternative communication (AAC) for adult life after leaving school is a vital component of secondary special education. As part of the Individuals with Disabilities Education Act Amendments (IDEA) of 1997 (PL 105-17), the individualized education program process specifically requires planning for this transition from school to adulthood for all students with special education needs. The most critical transition planning process, however, is for students with AAC needs and their families to create a vision for the future and, in collaboration with school personnel, to take action toward realizing their vision for employment, postsecondary education, independent living, and community participation (Wehman, 1992). A closer examination of the skills required to be a full participant in these postschool environments reveals the importance of conventional literacy skills, and thus the need for ambitious goals and appropriate literacy instruction cannot be overstated.

Conventional literacy, defined here as the ability to read and write fluently for a variety of purposes, is a major key to communicating effectively, accessing knowledge, gaining independence, and exercising life choices (Houston & Torgesen, 2004). In middle and high school settings, literacy is the primary medium through which students acquire information and by which their academic performance is assessed. Given the importance of conventional literacy skills to adolescents who use AAC, it is unfortunate that most of these students are unable to read, write, or spell at grade level and that up to 90% of them will enter adulthood without acquiring functional literacy skills (Berninger & Gans, 1986a, 1986b; Erickson, Koppenhaver, & Yoder, 1994; Foley, 1993; Foley & Pollatsek, 1999; Foley & Staples, 2003; Mirenda & Erickson, 2000).

Explanations for such literacy deficits include both intrinsic and extrinsic factors. Intrinsic factors include the type of disability; degree of physical impairment; and cognitive, linguistic, or perceptual abilities (e.g., Berninger & Gans, 1986b; Foley & Pollatsek, 1999; Smith, 1989, 2005; Vandervelden & Siegel, 2001). Extrinsic factors contributing to poor literacy outcomes include access to, and features of, AAC systems; the amount and quality of language and literacy experiences; parent, teacher, and learner expectations; and, perhaps more important, the lack of an evidence base to guide literacy instruction (Koppenhaver, Evans, & Yoder, 1991; Light & Kelford Smith, 1993).

There is a need for research that addresses the problem of low literacy among adolescents and young adults who use AAC (e.g., Berninger & Gans, 1989a, 1989b; Foley, 1993; Foley & Pollatsek, 1999; Koppenhaver & Yoder, 1992, 1993). The AAC field has made important progress in documenting the impact of organized instructional activities on the literacy skills of individuals with complex communication needs (Coleman-Martin, Heller, Cihak, & Irvine, 2005; Erickson, Koppenhaver, Yoder, & Nance, 1997; Light, McNaughton, Weyer, & Karg, 2008; Truxler & O'Keefe, 2007). Although there are a few descriptions of case studies and small-scale research projects (Foley & Staples, 2003; McNaughton & Tawney, 1993), the evidence base on effective literacy intervention for older students who use AAC remains exceedingly slim, and literacy outcomes for these individuals have improved very little over the past 2 decades (Koppenhaver, 2000).

Teachers and practitioners charged with improving the literacy skills of transition-age youth who use AAC can ill afford to wait any longer for a comprehensive evidence base to accumulate. They need immediate information to help them identify and effectively address the individual literacy-learning needs of their students. The purpose of this chapter is to respond to that need by 1) describing research-based literacy intervention strategies demonstrated to be effective with both individuals who require AAC and other at-risk populations and 2) suggesting adaptations to make these strategies more accessible to students who use AAC.

LITERACY AND TRANSITION

For students who use AAC, better literacy outcomes translate into greater educational, vocational, and social opportunities throughout life. Literate transition-age youth are much more likely to graduate from high school and participate in postsecondary and vocational education programs (Newman, 2005). As a result, compared with their nonliterate peers, these youth tend to have better employment outcomes; are more likely to find paid employment as adults; and, when employed, are more likely to report satisfaction with their jobs (Light, Stoltz, & McNaughton, 1996). Literate individuals are better able than their nonliterate peers to access distance communication and information technologies such as e-mail, cell phones, instant messaging, word processing, and the Internet (Bryen, Carey, & Potts, 2006; Bryen, Potts, & Carey, 2007; McNaughton, Symons, Light, & Parsons, 2006)—technologies that are critical to gaining employment, developing and maintaining social networks (Carey, Potts, Bryen, & Shankar, 2004; Dattilo et al., 2007; McNaughton, Light, & Arnold, 2002; Rackensperger, Krezman, McNaughton, Williams, & D'Silva, 2005), and overcoming some of the challenges associated with face-to-face communication (Atanasoff, McNaughton, Wolfe, & Light, 1998). Transition-age students who do not learn to read and write have fewer educational, vocational, and social opportunities as adults, and poor literacy skills threaten their economic security, citizenship, and general well-being (McCardle & Chhabra, 2004).

How Are Literacy Initiatives Affecting
Transition-Age Youth Who Use AAC?

Several K–12 educational initiatives at national and state levels influence the content of literacy instruction for all students, the methods used to teach specified skills, and the contexts in which literacy instruction is delivered. IDEA 1997 mandates that *all* students, including those with significant disabilities, 1) be educated in the least restrictive educational environment, 2) have access to the general education curriculum, and 3) receive the instruction they need to successfully achieve core curriculum standards. The No Child Left Behind Act (NCLB) of 2001 (PL 107-110) further requires that such instruction be founded on scientifically based research to improve student performance. In addition, the National Reading Panel (NRP; 2000), a group charged by Congress and the Secretary of Education to review the effectiveness of reading and writing approaches, identified several essential and interrelated components of literacy instruction that shape state K–12 curriculum, including the following:

1. *Phonemic awareness*—the ability to hear, identify, and manipulate individual speech sounds (phonemes) in spoken words

2. *Phonics*—the ability to understand and use relationships between letters of written language and the sounds of spoken language

3. *Fluency*—the ability to read a text accurately; quickly; and with appropriate stress, pauses, and intonation

4. *Vocabulary*—the ability to use words to communicate effectively in speaking and listening (oral vocabulary) and to recognize or use words in print (reading vocabulary)

5. *Text comprehension*—the ability to gain understanding and information from print

6. *Writing*—the ability to compose meaningful written texts for a variety of purposes

The NRP report provides detailed descriptions of instructional activities that effectively develop each of these key literacy components in both typical and at-risk learners. These evidence-based practices are described briefly later in this chapter within an integrated model of literacy development and instruction.

What Are the Barriers to Implementing Evidence-Based Literacy Instruction?

Despite these national and state initiatives, most transition-age youth who use AAC are not yet receiving research-based literacy instruction as mandated by NCLB and as described in the NRP synthesis report. For instance, the majority of literacy instruction provided to transition-age students who use AAC addresses only one of the NRP components—vocabulary, through sight word instruction (Browder, Wakeman, Spooner, Ahlgrim-Delzell, & Algozzine, 2006). Other key components of literacy instruction have rarely been addressed empirically in this population, and incorrect assumptions about required cognitive abilities have prevented children from receiving appropriate literacy instruction (Browder et al., 2006; Foley & Pollatsek, 1999; Foley & Staples, 2003). Moreover, transition-age youth with AAC needs are not always provided the assistive technology (AT) they need to function in the least restrictive environment.

Zascavage and Keefe (2004) examined factors preventing the implementation of literacy initiatives and thus impeding the literacy achievement of students who use AAC. These researchers interviewed stakeholders such as parents, teachers, university faculty, and school administrators involved in the literacy education of students who use AAC and identified a number of barriers to implementing literacy initiatives. These barriers are identified and discussed here.

Prerequisites and Expectations   Conceptualizations of literacy development acknowledge that literacy learning begins at birth and develops along a continuum from emergent to conventional literacy. Some educators, however, still operate from a reading readiness perspective, believing that certain levels of linguistic and cognitive ability must be reached before students can benefit from literacy instruction. By these standards, many students with significant cognitive disabilities would never be considered ready for formal literacy instruction—this despite evidence that they can and do develop literacy skills when provided with systematic and intensive literacy instruction (Browder et al., 2006; Browder & Xin, 1998; Foley & Staples, 2003; Light et al., 2008). In addition, by the time students who use AAC reach transition age, key decision makers such as parents, school personnel, or even the students themselves may no longer believe that conventional literacy is attainable. Consequently, they may have low expectations for literacy achievement or may consider conventional literacy a low priority.

Consider the case of Josh, a 15-year-old boy with cerebral palsy and moderate cognitive impairment. Since age 5, Josh has been using a DynaVox (DynaVox Mayer-Johnson) to communicate and participate in academic instruction. Now in eighth grade, Josh is educated in both resource and general education settings. Josh reads and writes at a mid–second-grade level, and his parents have struggled to get him the intensive instruction needed to improve his literacy skills and increase his access to the general education curriculum. School personnel have suggested that, at his age, Josh should focus on developing functional life skills, not literacy, because, as one special education teacher said, "his literacy skills have probably reached a plateau." His father Jim commented, "Josh is often misread, in that his physical appearance and demeanor portray a poor intellect. On the contrary, he's a very bright, caring individual. It's as if it's already predetermined what he'll be able to accomplish" (personal communication, May 10, 2008).

Assistive Technology Policies   Despite the IDEA (1997, 2004 [PL 108-446]) mandate that all students have access to the curriculum, the cost of purchasing the high-tech devices required to fully accommodate the oral and written language needs of students who use AAC is often perceived as prohibitive. Many school systems either still claim to be unable or are reluctant to provide adequate funding for high-tech AAC devices, thereby limiting critical language- and literacy-learning opportunities for transition-age youth who need such supports and are entitled by law to receive them. Without high-tech AT devices, transition-age youth cannot access distance communication and information technologies critical to employment options, residential support, and participation in 21st-century life (Kamil, 2003; Pierce & Porter, 1996; Steelman, Pierce, & Koppenhaver, 1993).

> The school administrators always cry poor. I know their resources are strained but so are mine. I am tired of always having to pay for the AT my son needs. I feel like in some ways NCLB has hurt Josh because more resources are going toward low-achieving kids without disabilities and there is even less money left for kids like him than there was before. (Jim, father of Josh, personal communication, May 10, 2008)

Assistive Technology Knowledge   Educators and other service providers are not always computer literate, current on available AAC/AT supports for literacy instruction, or even aware of a particular learner's need for such devices and services (Foley & Staples, 2006; Resta, Bryant, Lock, & Allan, 1998). In addition, rapid changes in technology necessitate ongoing continuing education, which few school districts routinely provide.

> Josh has Wi-Fi on his AAC device. He surfs the Internet every day after school. On his own, he e-mails his brother and sister, finds web sites on topics of interest, reads multimedia books, looks for games and toys on eBay, and learns new vocabulary with an online dictionary. At school Josh has no way to really participate in the core curriculum despite year after year of addressing this issue during his [individualized education program] meetings. No one really knows how his AAC device or his Wi-Fi setup works and he doesn't even have access to a computer. (Jim, father of Josh, personal communication, May 10, 2008)

Segregation Policies   Despite legislative mandates requiring that students with disabilities be educated in the least restrictive environment, many school districts continue to segregate students who use AAC in separate schools or self-contained units without first considering more inclusive options. In 2005, more than 65% of students with multiple disabilities spent more than 60% of their day outside of the general education classroom (National Center for Education Statistics, 2009). Placement in segregated environments limits students' opportunities for peer interaction and restricts their access to the general education curriculum, including research-based literacy instruction (Kliewer, 1999; Kliewer & Biklen, 2001; Ryndak, Morrison, & Sommerstein,

1999; Sturm, 1998). Jim, Josh's father, said, "We feel like Josh is a victim of one of the last forms of segregation in the United States" (personal communication, May 10, 2008).

Limitation on Instructional Time
Whereas their peers in general education settings typically spend more than 3 hours a day engaged in literacy-related activities, students who use AAC typically receive 30 minutes (or less) of such instruction a day (Koppenhaver & Yoder, 1993; Mike, 1995). Reduced time for literacy instruction is sometimes seen as the inevitable consequence of students' needs for services from occupational therapy, physical therapy, and speech-language pathology providers. Poorly managed transitions among therapies, toileting, and other activities reduce instructional time even further (Ford, Davern, & Schnorr, 2001; Kliewer, 1999; Koppenhaver & Yoder, 1993; Mike, 1995).

> Josh's [individualized education program] specifies 30 minutes a day of literacy instruction but half of that time is lost in coming and going. Traveling to different locations all over the school, being pulled out for special services and toileting, all these things disrupt his day. (Jim, father of Josh, personal communication, May 10, 2008)

Lack of Transdisciplinary Programming
When large portions of time are allotted to different therapies and related services, educational programs for students who use AAC tend to become fragmented and inconsistent. Research has indicated that emphasizing therapy over academics is not conducive to students' development of cognitive and literacy skills (Koppenhaver & Yoder, 1993; Mike, 1995). Traditional school organizational structures are not designed to accommodate the continuum of literacy and other services required to adequately address the needs of adolescents who use AAC.

> The greater number of people involved [in Josh's education] leads to the "law of diminishing returns." This has progressively been the case in Josh's educational experience. His last [individualized education program] involved fourteen school personnel, and with us made seventeen. Accountability wanes, communication gets fragmented, and this raises the level of complexity and thus places more demands on the parents and child. (Jim, father of Josh, personal communication, May 10, 2008)

Life Skills/Functional Skills Instruction
It is common practice to educate transition-age youth who use AAC in special education classrooms using a life skills/functional skills curriculum. Literacy instruction within this curriculum focuses almost exclusively on the acquisition of sight words, thereby limiting students' opportunities to develop other essential literacy skills such as phonemic awareness, phonics, and text comprehension (Browder et al., 2006) and to engage in authentic, relevant, and age-appropriate literacy experiences (Koppenhaver & Yoder, 1993; Mike, 1995).

> The school administration early on imposed low expectations on Josh and encouraged an emphasis on life skills. Unfortunately, as unsuspecting parents we initially bought into it somewhat. This reduced an already small window of opportunity for literacy learning at a time when we should have been maximizing our effort. (Jim, father of Josh, personal communication, May 10, 2008)

Limited Research Evidence
An additional barrier to implementing evidence-based literacy instruction is the existence of limited research-based information to guide educators in developing instructional activities appropriately modified for transition-age youth who use AAC. In the absence of an evidence base, best practices in literacy instruction for students without disabilities or those at risk for literacy-learning difficulties may be used as a guide (Browder et al., 2006; Foley & Staples, 2003; Koppenhaver, 2000; Light & McNaughton, 2009). Although it is not yet clear whether this knowledge translates directly to adolescents who use AAC, Koppenhaver (2000) and others (e.g., Foley & Staples, 2003) have suggested that instructional strategies effective with typically developing learners and other at-risk populations are likely to benefit students who use AAC as well.

Quality of Teacher Preparation   Most general education teachers at the middle and high school levels are unaccustomed to teaching students with severe disabilities. Although these teachers may be highly qualified to integrate literacy into their content area instruction, they often lack the knowledge and skills or the confidence needed to effectively adapt instruction for students who use AAC. Information on how to accommodate the learning needs of these students within general education settings is not yet a core component of preservice training for secondary education teachers. Another issue is time—many middle and high school educators teach more than 120 students a day over multiple class sections, thus limiting their ability to effectively accommodate the learning needs of their students with more severe disabilities. Karen, a middle school English teacher, described her experiences working with Annie, a 12-year-old student with muscular dystrophy:

> I am passionate about literacy and have three different literacy endorsements. When Annie was placed in my classroom I knew nothing except that her parents had decided to take her out of special education. I knew of Annie because I'd seen her zipping up and down the hall, but that's all I knew. Nobody gave me a manual with her. I would have liked to have known more about her device (an ECO [Prentke Romich Company]). I didn't even know how to turn it on. No one took me aside and showed me even the basics of how to use it. I would have to ask Annie what to do. To be honest, in the beginning I didn't expect much from her, but in spite of that, she's done amazingly well, she's just really determined. . . . Now I expect her to do what everyone else is doing. She just needs her AAC device and a computer to write with and extra time. (personal communication, February 4, 2008)

Special educators are trained to teach students with disabilities, and they are more likely than general educators to have experience using AAC/AT in the classroom. However, most special educators have limited preservice training in literacy, and the training they do have focuses primarily on sight word instruction (Browder et al., 2006; Katims, 2000a, 2000b). In addition, special educators may have inadequate knowledge of subject matter addressed in general education content area classes, making it difficult for them to collaborate effectively with general education teachers. It is not surprising that many special educators feel ill prepared to respond to NCLB and NRP mandates to provide their students who use AAC with high-quality literacy instruction that is aligned with the general education content area standards. Jason, a middle school special educator responsible for resource instruction, described his preservice literacy training:

> When I was in school more than 10 years ago, we didn't even have a class in reading. We were pretty much taught that we were going to be working with these kids that were going to be severely handicapped and that we wouldn't really try to teach [them] reading and writing, and now it's like that's all we are expected to do. (personal communication, January 18, 2008)

Angie, a special education teacher in a high school life skills classroom, reported similar challenges:

> The most frustrating thing is when you have a student who is nonverbal and you have to figure out a way to know if they are understanding what's on the page...being able to know whether they know the sounds, the letter names. If they have a device that's one thing, but if a student doesn't have a device and they're using the [Picture Exchange Communication System] or something and they're nonverbal....A lot of it is we're just pointing to letters. . . . I don't know, that's when I think "what do I do?" So with one of my students who is nonverbal, basically what I do is get pictures of different signs and have her match them to the words. That's kind of where I go and then it's like, now what do I do? So . . . it's a real challenge. I mean I always hit that roadblock of what do I do. (Personal communication, January 9, 2008)

Motivation   Student engagement is a positive predictor of desirable outcomes: graduation rates, grades, satisfaction with school (Guthrie & Davis, 2003). Unfortunately, after years of struggling with literacy, older students who use AAC may experience feelings of frustration or discouragement that reduce their motivation to continue with literacy instruction. Because of the lack of age-appropriate texts for adolescents with low reading levels, teachers often use instructional materials designed for much younger children. This may understandably increase students' resistance to literacy instruction during the middle and high school years. Another issue affecting motivation is the widening gap between the literacy levels of students who use AAC and those of their peers without disabilities. Tonya, the parent of a 12-year-old girl who suffered a traumatic brain injury at age 1, described her daughter's increasing resistance to literacy activities in the general education classroom:

> Kaya has severe problems with writing and spelling, so even though she is smart and has a lot to say with her DynaVox, writing takes a long time and is physically exhausting. When she sees how much her peers have written in the same amount of time, she gets discouraged. Sometimes she refuses to write at all. (personal communication, September 29, 2007)

Summary

The challenge for content area teachers, reading specialists, speech-language pathologists, special educators, parents, and others is to provide transition-age youth with developmentally appropriate, accessible, and intensive literacy instruction in the least restrictive environment and in a coordinated and efficacious manner. In the following section we provide a developmental framework for literacy development and instruction as well as suggestions for adapting the NRP instructional components in age- and developmentally appropriate ways for use with transition-age students who use AAC.

AN INTEGRATED MODEL OF LITERACY DEVELOPMENT AND INSTRUCTION

As discussed earlier, phonemic awareness, phonics, fluency, vocabulary, text comprehension, and writing are key components of literacy. Yet these key components are not taught, nor are they acquired, sequentially. Rather, effective instruction addresses *all* components to some extent throughout *all* phases of development. It is only the degree to which each component is emphasized at various developmental phases that changes. The development of these components is highly interrelated and reciprocal; for example, the development of phonics facilitates and enhances development of fluency, text comprehension, and spelling (Cooper, Roth, Speece, & Schatschneider, 2002). Therefore, when planning instruction, it is useful to know how these components interact at various phases of reading, writing, and spelling development.

Bear and Barone (1998) described an *integrated model of literacy*, one of the only models to highlight the *synchronous* development of reading, writing, and spelling. The model lays out distinct phases along a continuum of literacy development, from emergent to intermediate/advanced. Bear and Barone proposed that reading, writing, and spelling develop in an orderly and interrelated fashion, with constellations of literacy behaviors appearing at each developmental phase. At each of these phases, educators can observe literacy behaviors in one area, such as reading, and reasonably predict the behaviors that should be occurring in other areas, such as writing and spelling. Armed with this flexible developmental framework, educators can more effectively match instructional strategies and activities to a student's development. Educators can also note when one aspect of literacy development is out of balance with another, as is often the case with students who use AAC, and respond with targeted remediation. In addition, by looking at students' reading, writing, and spelling in developmental terms, educators can combine their understanding of literacy development with effective teaching practices to facilitate progress from one developmental stage to another.

The integrated literacy model can be applied to students of widely varying literacy abilities, ages, or grade levels and is thus useful for considering the literacy-learning needs of transition-age students who use AAC. The model helps educators identify students' current literacy skills and determine what skills are expected to develop next or in an interrelated manner and would therefore be appropriate to target for intervention. As students move from one developmental phase to another, boundaries between these phases become blurred. That is, students carry over behaviors associated with a previous phase as they develop more complex understandings.

Emergent Phase of Literacy Development

Most children go through a long and gradual process of acquiring literacy that begins within their first year of life at home and continues into their preschool, kindergarten, and early elementary years (Teale & Sulzby, 1986). During this emergent phase of literacy development, children develop their language skills and begin to make connections between spoken and written language. Emergent literacy instruction highlights the interrelationships among speaking, listening, reading, and writing, typically through scaffolded interactions with adults and peers in natural contexts (see Table 3.1).

Emergent Reading

Characteristics   Students in this phase of development engage in pretend reading and have limited understanding of concepts of print (e.g., directionality, word boundaries, conventions of print). Given appropriate learning opportunities in print-rich environments, students begin to acquire knowledge of letters, particularly the letters in their names (Bear, Invernizzi, Templeton, & Johnston, 2000, 2008), and may demonstrate an initial awareness of the phonological structure of words (e.g., sensitivity to rhyme and alliteration). Students in this phase often recognize some very familiar words by sight (e.g., names of family members, McDonald's logo) based on their visual features and the contexts in which these words typically occur.

Recommended Best Practices   One of the primary goals of best practice emergent literacy instruction is to develop students' oral language abilities. Students develop vocabulary and language comprehension through participation in thematic shared-reading experiences. As teachers read stories to children on a daily basis, they use a variety of strategies to develop vocabulary, including preteaching difficult vocabulary, pairing new words with words students already know, modeling the use of new words in context, and providing multiple exposures to new words across instructional activities (Bryant, Goodwin, Bryant, & Higgins, 2003; NRP, 2000). Teachers also employ before-, during-, and after-reading strategies to improve students' story comprehension. Before reading, for example, they activate students' background knowledge and help them to relate personal experiences to stories being read. During reading, they model effective use of comprehension strategies such as using picture cues to make predictions, asking and answering factual and inferential questions, and using simple graphic organizers and other visual supports to aid in comprehension. After reading, they provide multiple means for students to retell and reenact stories.

Other best practice goals at this level include developing students' understanding of concepts of print and increasing their phonological awareness and alphabet knowledge. Teachers facilitate this through the use of predictable books featuring rhythm, rhyme, and repetition. They think aloud about print conventions, point to words and have students point to words as they read, encourage students to engage in pretend reading of memorized texts, talk about letters and the sounds they make, point out rhyming words, and have students clap out the number of words in sentences and the number of syllables and sounds in words.

Instructional Adaptations for Transition-Age Youth   Research has indicated that students with AAC needs who are beginning communicators tend to 1) lack operational competence with AAC systems, 2) produce a limited range and frequency of communicative intents, and

3) produce primarily single-word utterances (e.g., Kent-Walsh & Binger, 2009; Kent-Walsh & Mc-Naughton, 2005). These issues can be addressed, at least in part, by including students in shared reading and other emergent literacy activities. For example, before reading the teacher can relate new vocabulary to AAC symbols, or during reading he or she can provide students with opportunities to add AAC symbols to story maps or graphic organizers. Postreading activities might include having students retell a story with pictures, rate a story (thumbs up or thumbs down), or put symbol–sentence strips in order to demonstrate knowledge of story sequence (Foley & Staples, 2007). Additional AAC/AT strategies and supports for emergent readers, such as providing accessible, age-appropriate reading materials, are summarized in Table 3.1.

Emergent Writing

Characteristics   Emergent writing development progresses from earlier forms, such as drawing, scribbling, and letter-like forms, to letter strings and invented spelling, to more conventional copying and writing (Sulzby, 1990). When children first start to copy words they see, they may write letters backward, leave letters out, or run one word into another. Children's emergent writings are context- or situation-dependent and may be difficult to interpret by those unfamiliar with the children's experiences.

Recommended Best Practices   Effective emergent writing instruction highlights the many forms and functions of print. Teachers model the writing process for emergent writers when they create language experience stories and think aloud while doing so. They encourage experimentation with different kinds of writing (e.g., names, labels, lists, book responses) via drawing, scribbling, copying, and invented spelling. Emergent writing is supported by print-rich writing environments that include a wide variety of writing materials (e.g., different kinds of paper, sign-in sheets, journals, junk mail, stationery, sticky notes), tools (e.g., pencils, markers, stamps, magnetic letters), and supplies (e.g., staplers, scissors, envelopes, tacks, tape, labels).

Instructional Adaptations for Transition-Age Youth   Transition-age youth with AAC may be considered emergent writers for a long period of time, even into adulthood, depending upon their particular disabilities (e.g., severe cognitive impairment, limited physical ability), reduced access to writing tools and instruction, and/or low expectations for literacy development (Foley, Koppenhaver, & Williams, 2009). Frequent age- and developmentally appropriate experiences with varied forms and functions of print help develop the understanding that writing, including messages constructed using AAC symbols, has communicative value and is useful in everyday life. Challenges for emergent writers with AAC needs include their need for accessible writing tools (see Foley et al., 2009, for an extensive list) and the fact that they cannot read aloud the non-conventional texts that they produce. Consequently, a variety of directed writing tasks are useful in increasing the interpretability of the texts they produce. These tasks include writing names, labeling pictures, and spelling dictated words (Foley et al., 2009).

Emergent Spelling

Characteristics   Spelling at the beginning of this phase is primarily pretend spelling. It is referred to as *prephonemic* because children do not represent words using sound–symbol strategies and cannot reread their own written text (Bear et al., 2000). Students draw, scribble, make letter-like forms, and, later, write the alphabet, copy words, and engage in invented spelling.

Recommended Best Practices   Bear et al. (2000) suggested that emergent spellers have opportunities to develop concept sorts (e.g., sort words by semantic category, rhyme, size); play with speech sounds to develop phonological awareness; explore the alphabet to develop letter recognition and naming; sort pictures by initial sound; and point to words in memorized rhymes, dictations, and simple pattern books. Use of invented spelling is also encouraged.

Table 3.1. Characteristics, recommended best practices, and AAC adaptations for the emerging literacy phase

Characteristics	Recommended best practices	Adaptations
Reading		
Recognize some environmental print Limited concepts of print (e.g., directionality) Pretend reading	Print-rich environment	Use visual schedules, social stories, orthographic labels on objects and areas, and literacy tools (e.g., computer with expanded keyboard; Foley & Staples, 2003; Koppenhaver & Erickson, 2003).
	Teacher read-alouds/guided reading	Provide easy access to core and topic-specific vocabulary to promote participation (Erickson & Clendon, 2009).
	Story retells	Use story maps and props to increase participation during shared reading (Foley & Staples, 2003; Soto & Hartmann, 2006; Soto, Yu, & Henneberry, 2007; Soto, Yu, & Kelso, 2008).
		Provide generic phrases on AAC displays to facilitate story retelling (e.g., FIRST, THEN, NEXT, AT THE END) and reader response (e.g., I LIKED THAT, THAT WAS FUNNY, READ IT AGAIN).
	Predictable texts	Have student produce age-appropriate predictable texts and patterned books for repeated reading (Foley & Staples, 2003).
		Write lines from predictable texts on sentence strips, then cut sentence strips into individual words and have student reorder the words (Foley & Staples, 2003).
	Language experience stories	Use visual schedules within and across daily activities to support language comprehension (Bopp, Brown, & Mirenda, 2004).
		Create talking photo albums to document shared/home experiences.
	Self-selected reading	Provide a wide variety of age-appropriate, high-interest, accessible books (e.g., adapted books, multimedia texts, photo albums, video painting; Koppenhaver & Erickson, 2003).

44

Writing		
Drawing with pretend writing	Journals	Use an AAC device or computer for "scribbling" and invented spelling (Foley et al., 2009).
	Book responses	Assemble a book response journal on paper or electronically. Add a picture of a book cover for each response; student indicates thumbs up or down or marks a rating scale next to the picture.
Spelling		
Prephonemic stage: scribbling, random letters or numbers	Phonological awareness	Have student match orally presented phonemes or initial/final sounds to picture or AAC symbol (Fallon, Light, McNaughton, Drager, & Hammer, 2004; Light & Mc-Naughton, 2007).
		Program AAC device with "sound" page and preprogrammed phrases (e.g., THE WORD STARTS WITH ____, ENDS WITH ____, RHYMES WITH ____, DOESN'T RHYME WITH ____).
	Explore letters	Program AAC device with alphabet page or dictionary pages (i.e., pictures of words that start with specific letters).
		Encourage invented spelling using known words and word processor or AAC device with speech feedback.
	Concept sorts	Have student locate categories of words (e.g., food, clothing, words that start or end with a target sound), highlighting AAC device retrieval strategies.

45

Instructional Adaptations for Transition-Age Youth   Transition-age emergent writers benefit from print-rich environments; opportunities to explore letters and sounds with auditory feedback; and engagement in a variety of naturally occurring, functional writing opportunities. A variety of AT/AAC supports for emergent spellers with AAC needs are described in Table 3.1.

Case Example: Emergent Phase   Foley and Staples (2003) described an emergent literacy intervention with Allen, a young adult with Down syndrome, autism, and severe/profound cognitive impairment. During his transition years, Allen used a Picture Exchange Communication System and spent most of his day in a functional life skills classroom where he received no literacy instruction. At the point when Allen was preparing to transition out of the public school system, he had some concept of print (e.g., how to turn pages, reading a book from front to back) and enjoyed looking at family photo albums, picture books, and food circulars from the grocery store. He scribbled from left to right when asked to write his name. Developmentally, Allen was functioning at the emergent phase of literacy development.

During a transition planning meeting at Allen's school, his parents expressed a desire to see him enter a supported employment program rather than a local sheltered workshop, where he would be segregated from the community. They considered possible supported employment options and thought Allen might enjoy stocking shelves at the neighborhood grocery store. Thus, his literacy intervention goals were designed to be relevant to working in a vocational context such as a grocery store and to build upon his emergent literacy abilities. Allen's literacy instruction focused on increasing his awareness of environmental print in ways that led to the development of necessary job skills. For example, he learned to match identical product logos (e.g., two cans of Pepsi) so that he could help refill soda vending machines at local convenience stores. He learned to match a printed logo to a specific product as a way of requesting the correct type of soda needed to complete this job. Allen used pictures of products cut from grocery store circulars to make shopping lists and consulted these lists when locating and purchasing items from the market with his parents. He used a name stamp to fill out a time card at work and to sign his paycheck. Allen also received direct instruction using high-utility sight words; given his age, low literacy level, and functional needs, word recognition was prioritized over phonemic awareness instruction.

Allen's emergent literacy instruction helped him to develop the understanding that print is useful for communicating and functioning in everyday life. It broadened his employment options and participation in community life while also providing him with a strong foundation for further literacy development.

Beginning Phase of Literacy Development

During the emergent literacy phase, instruction focuses on developing spoken language and listening skills, concepts of print, and some awareness of the alphabetic principle. Instruction during the beginning phase of literacy development (typically during first and second grade) builds on these foundational skills and marks a period during which students learn to read, write, and spell in more conventional ways (Bear & Barone, 1998).

Beginning Reading

Characteristics   Students in this phase acquire the ability to decode simple texts accurately (Juel, 1991) and increase their phonemic awareness. They learn to isolate phonemes in words, blend phonemes together into words (/s/-/u/-/n/ = *sun*), and segment words into their constituent phonemes (/b/-/a/-/t/ = *bat*). They also develop knowledge of letter–sound correspondence (phonics) and use this knowledge to decode words they have never seen before in print. Students also build a store of high-frequency (e.g., *the, of*) and/or irregularly spelled (e.g., *eight*) words that they can recognize by sight.

Recommended Best Practices   Beginning readers learn to read high-frequency words and patterns that allow them to decode many other words using analytic decoding strategies. The NRP (2000) review of K–12 literacy instruction suggested that phonemic awareness, phonics, and decoding skills be taught together. Research at the K–12 level suggests that the best strategies for teaching phonemic awareness focus on only a few specific skills, including

- *Phoneme blending:* listening to a sequence of separately spoken sounds and combining them to form a recognizable word (e.g., "What word is /s/-/u/-/n/?")

- *Phoneme segmentation:* breaking a word into its sounds by tapping out or counting the sounds or by positioning a marker for each sound (e.g., "How many sounds are there in *ship*?" [three: /sh/, /i/, /p/]).

Phonemic awareness instruction is most effective when letters (phonics), not just sounds, are used for instruction, and research has indicated that systematic phonics instruction improves the reading and spelling abilities of both younger and older students (Blevins, 2001; Curtis, 2004; Curtis & Longo, 1999). Those students with weak phonological skills benefit most from this type of instruction (Juel & Minden-Cupp, 2000; Moats, 2001). Effective strategies include systematic and explicit instruction in letter–sound correspondence, with a focus on teaching learners how to convert individual *graphemes* (letters and letter combinations) into *phonemes* (sounds) and then blend them together to form a word. Alternatively, the instructional focus is on converting larger letter combinations such as word families (e.g., *-at, -up, -in*) and common spelling patterns (e.g., *-ing, -able, -tion*) into sounds. High-frequency words (e.g., *of, the*) and irregularly spelled sight words (e.g., *eight*) are also included in instruction.

Commonly used instructional activities for developing phonemic awareness, phonics, and decoding skills include saying the sounds associated with letters and letter combinations; orally blending and segmenting words; sorting words by initial, final, and medial sounds and consonant–vowel–consonant patterns; sounding out unfamiliar words; and developing automatic sight word recognition by fluently reading high-frequency, irregularly spelled words aloud. Word Wall and word bank activities are also widely used (Cunningham & Cunningham, 1992), as are decodable books that provide students with opportunities to practice reading learned words in context.

Instructional Adaptations for Transition-Age Youth   Beginning readers who use AAC, including those with moderate to severe cognitive disabilities, often develop word-level reading skills much more slowly than their typically developing peers (Browder et al., 2006). Research supports the use of direct, explicit, and systematic instruction for teaching decoding, phonemic awareness, and phonics to transition-age youth who struggle with these skills (Curtis, 2004; Kamil, 2003; Nokes & Dole, 2004). However, alternatives to these traditional tasks are needed to accommodate those students who cannot produce verbal responses. An alternative to a rhyme production task is to provide a display of pictures and ask the student to point to a word that rhymes with a target word. A phoneme blending activity can be modified by providing four AAC symbols (e.g., FISH, FAN, MAN, and FAT) and having the student indicate which of the pictures corresponds to the blended word (e.g., /f/-/a/-/t/ = *fat;* Blischak, Shah, Lombardino, & Chiarella, 2004). Students can demonstrate phoneme segmentation skills using AAC devices with speech output programmed to produce individual sounds (e.g., "What is the first sound in *mat*?" "What is the last sound?" "Tell me all the sounds in *lamp*"; Fallon et al., 2004; Light & McNaughton, 2007). These and other AAC adaptations for beginning readers are summarized in Table 3.2.

Table 3.2. Characteristics, recommended best practices, and AAC adaptations for the beginning literacy phase

Characteristics	Recommended best practices	Adaptations
Reading		
Focus on decoding	Teacher read-alouds	Use a variety of adapted pre-, during-, and post-reading strategies to increase comprehension (Erickson, 2003; Foley & Staples, 2003; Light & McNaughton, 2007).
	Story retells using story grammar elements	Provide visual supports such as story maps and templates to support production of meaningful narratives (Bedrosian, Lasker, Speidel, & Politsch, 2003; Soto & Hartman, 2006; Soto et al., 2007, 2008).
	Guided reading–thinking activity	Have student listen for specific information (e.g., main character, setting, problem) and indicate to instructor when he or she hears it.
	Charting ideas	Create computer-generated graphic organizer templates (e.g., Kidspiration [Inspiration Software] or Inspiration software; Bedrosian et al., 2003; Foley & Staples, 2003).
	Dictation	Create dictated stories or texts by writing down what student says using AAC device, then expanding (e.g., student says MOVIE, write the word and then the expanded sentence "I went to a movie"; Foley & Staples, 2003).
	Patterned stories	Have student fill in patterned story template using AAC device, Boardmaker [Dyna-Vox Mayer-Johnson] symbols, Clicker 5 [Crick Software] (Foley & Staples, 2003).
	Single-word reading (regularly spelled words and irregularly spelled sight words)	Provide student with opportunities to match AAC symbols to single written words (Eikeseth & Jahr, 2001; Fallon et al., 2004; Fossett & Mirenda, 2006; Light & McNaughton, 2007).
	Decoding in context	During shared reading, have student point to an AAC symbol representing the target word in a sentence (Fallon et al., 2004; Foley & Staples, 2003; Light & McNaughton, 2007).
	Self-selected/independent reading	Provide age-appropriate text types, including browsing (e.g., catalogs, photo journals, wordless picture books, magazines), beginning reading (e.g., language experience texts, decodable books), and information gathering (e.g., nonfiction books with simple text, simplified content area texts, web-based resources; Fallon et al., 2004; Foley & Staples, 2003, 2007; Light & McNaughton, 2007).

Writing	
Writing letter by letter	
Develop knowledge of world and text genres	Increase background knowledge using real-world experiences and virtual Internet experiences (Foley & Staples, 2003).
	Provide computer-generated templates (e.g., outlines, paragraph organization) of various text types to support planning and composing.
Write patterned stories/texts	Create patterned sentences using student's AAC device or word processor for the student to label pictures or fill in the blank (e.g., MY FAVORITE FOOD IS ___, I HAVE A PET ___; Foley & Staples, 2003).
Daily teacher modeling of prewriting, writing, rewriting, editing, and post-writing	Have student generate list of writing topics using pictures or AAC device (Foley, 2007).
Spelling	
Semiphonetic, letter-name stages: initial and final consonants (*b, bd/bed*), later vowels included (*pat/pet*)	Use AAC device or speech-supported computer software (e.g., WordMaker, Leap Into Phonics, Simon Sounds It Out) during word sort activities and real-word, nonword spelling dictation (Foley & Staples, 2003; Hanser & Erickson, 2007).
Contrastive word sorts: initial consonants, blends, and diagraphs; then short vowel patterns	
Word banks	Create word banks on AAC device containing key words representing VC, CV, CVC, CVCC, and CCVC patterns and high-frequency sight words to assist student with spelling (Hanser & Erickson, 2007; Kinney, Vedora, & Stromer, 2003; Light & McNaughton, 2007).
Encourage invented spelling	Have student spell dictated words or picture labels using AAC device, magnetic letters, or word processor (Foley & Staples, 2003; Millar & Light, 2001; Millar, Light, & Schlosser, 2004); systematically teach letter–sound correspondence (Light & McNaughton, 2009).

Beginning Writing

Characteristics   In this phase, students label their drawings and learn to produce phrases and full sentences. They write word by word and typically write only a few words or lines. Unless encouraged to use *invented spelling* (i.e., spelling words as they sound), beginning writers often write using only the few words they know they can spell correctly.

Recommended Best Practices   Beginning writers are often introduced to the writing process (planning, drafting, revising, and editing) through writer's workshop activities. Students are taught via modeling and explicit instruction to write using a variety of forms, including patterned stories and simple texts. In addition, beginning writers are encouraged to focus on the content, not the form, of their writing and therefore are encouraged to use invented spelling when they do not know how to spell a word.

Instructional Adaptations for Transition-Age Youth   In order to participate fully in the writing process, beginning writers who use AAC typically require supports (Sturm & Clendon, 2004; Sturm & Koppenhaver, 2000). Some AT supports (e.g., alternative keyboards) provide physical access, whereas others allow for communication during writing. Low-tech AAC supports, such as simple communication boards, enable students to choose topics to write about, create patterned stories, or make comments about other students' writing (e.g., THAT'S FUNNY, I LIKE THAT, I DON'T UNDERSTAND). Beginning writers with limited spelling ability may benefit from graphic support for translating their ideas into text. Software programs such as Writing with Symbols (Widgit) and PixWriter (Slater Software) allow students to compose using a combination of picture symbols and text.

Beginning Spelling

Characteristics   During this phase, *semiphonetic* or *letter–name* spelling strategies are used (Bear et al., 2000). Students in the semiphonetic spelling stage begin using initial and final sounds, as well as some blends and digraphs in their spelling (e.g., *b* or *bd/ bed, cn* or *chnl chain*). Later, short vowel patterns are also included (e.g., *bad/bed, can* or *chan/chain*). Beginning spellers often omit preconsonantal nasals (*bop* or *bup/bump*).

Recommended Best Practices   Beginning spelling instruction is highly coordinated with instruction in phonemic awareness, phonics, and decoding. Students engage in word sorts that call attention to features of words encountered during reading activities. These sorts focus first on initial and final sounds, then on vowels in single-syllable words. Students develop sight word vocabulary through word banks and Word Wall activities. Making Words is another instructional approach that integrates reading and spelling; it has been used successfully with children both with and without disabilities (Cunningham & Cunningham, 1992; Cunningham, Hall, & Sigmon, 1999; Hanser & Erickson, 2007; Stahl, Duffy-Hester, & Stahl, 1998).

Students in this phase are expected to spell the words and features they have studied in conventional ways, but when they engage in independent writing, they are encouraged to use invented spelling for words they do not know how to spell. Students can usually spell unfamiliar words phonetically, representing all salient sounds in a one-to-one linear fashion (e.g., *majikol/magical;* Bear et al., 2000).

Instructional Adaptations for Transition-Age Youth   Beginning spellers can use AAC devices or word processing to engage in word-making activities. Additional opportunities for individualized instruction, repeated practice, and auditory feedback can be provided to beginning spellers via computer software designed for that purpose (e.g., Leap Into Phonics, Leap into Learning, Simon Sounds It Out, WordMaker, and Balanced Literacy [Don Johnston Incorporated]). Word processing programs with text-to-speech can also provide feedback on students' spelling, and some programs, such as Co:Writer (Don Johnston Incorporated), have a flexible spelling option that recognizes and corrects phonetic spelling.

Case Example: Beginning Phase   Foley and Staples (2003) described an integrated communication and literacy intervention developed for Frank, a 23-year-old man with autism and severe intellectual disability who had literacy skills characteristic of the beginning phase of development. Frank recognized some environmental sight words, knew all of the letters of the alphabet, and could identify the sounds associated with more than half of the letters. He had an awareness of basic concepts of print, which he demonstrated by holding a book correctly and looking through it a page at a time from front to back.

Frank's intervention included participation in shared-reading activities, during which he was taught through modeling and repeated practice to use his AAC device to respond to simple *wh-* questions (e.g., Q: Who is this story about? A: MR. HATCH; Q: Where did he go? A: WORK; Q: What did the mailman bring? A: CANDY). Over time, Frank's growing awareness of story structure became evident in his ability to correctly sequence three to four pictured events from familiar stories with minimal facilitator prompting (e.g., "Then what happened?").

Frank displayed an interest in magazines and texts related to his favorite movie (*Star Wars*). He pointed to different characters when asked and copied their names into his journal during writing activities. High-frequency sight words and pictures of *Star Wars* characters were combined in simple books with repeated sentence patterns (e.g., "This is Yoda. This is Darth Vader. This is Luke Skywalker"). Frank used a DynaMyte (DynaVox Mayer-Johnson) to read these texts aloud by matching words on the communication display to the text. Later, he was able to read the sentences silently and match them to appropriate pages of a version of the book containing the pictures but no text.

When offered choices of writing activities, Frank often elected to write captions for photos of his community experiences. He also produced patterned books and dictated sentences using a combination of known high-frequency sight words and invented spellings (I LIKE PETZ for I LIKE PIZZA). Other writing activities included the use of graphic organizers to relate information learned through shared-reading activities.

Integrated phonological awareness, phonics, and decoding instruction focused on teaching Frank to use an AAC device with speech output to read and spell by analogy. Using high-frequency words he already recognized as the rimes (e.g., *-at, -in, -up*), Frank was shown how to add different initial sounds to spell new words (e.g., *fat, cat, hat*). New word families were added as Frank mastered the reading and spelling of previous words. By the end of the second year, Frank could read and spell approximately 100 of these decodable words. In addition, he added about 50 high-frequency words to his personal word bank. Gains in phonemic awareness were evident in his inclusion of both beginning and ending sounds and some vowel sounds in his invented spellings (e.g., *vacm/vacuum, spoj/sponge, brum/broom*).

Transitional Phase of Literacy Development

Whereas the focus of beginning literacy instruction is on teaching students how to read and write, literacy instruction in the transitional phase emphasizes the use of reading and writing as vehicles for learning and expressing what students know. This shift typically occurs between third and fourth grade in students without disabilities. Students in the transitional phase begin to exhibit more mature, and more fluent, reading, writing, and spelling behaviors (see Table 3.3).

Transitional Reading

Characteristics   During the transitional phase, which typically occurs between Grades 1 and 4, decoding skills are applied with greater automaticity, using a combination of phonemic,

Table 3.3. Characteristics, recommended best practices, and AAC adaptations for the transitional literacy phase

Characteristics	Recommended best practices	Adaptations
Reading		
Expanded sight vocabulary More fluent decoding Focus on meaning	Repeated readings Reader's Theater	Have student select reading partner for repeated reading. Encourage student to use "inner voice" during choral reading and partner reading activities. Program student's AAC device with lines of dialogue to contribute.
	Literature groups, book clubs	Preprogram AAC device with appropriate starters (MY FAVORITE PART WAS, I LEARNED ABOUT).
	Independent/wide reading	Use electronic texts and multimedia texts with built-in learning supports (e.g., Start-to-Finish books [Don Johnston Incorporated], Pair-It books [Steck-Vaughn]).
Writing		
Writing one or two paragraphs Approaching fluency Focus on meaning	Authentic and engaging tasks in different genres	Provide computer-generated templates of various text types to support planning and composing.
	Supportive writing environment	Have student use AAC device to generate a list of motivating topics and consult the list during writing assignments. Provide extra time to complete writing assignments. Encourage writing support via peer scaffolding (Bedrosian et al., 2003).
	Explicit strategy instruction	Provide computer-generated templates of various text types to support planning and composing (e.g., Inspiration, Draft:Builder). Teach use of spell check option with speech support. Teach student to access content dictionaries in word prediction program.
Spelling		
Within-word stage: including familiar patterns in words (*bed/bad, chane, chain*)	Word sorts: long vowel patterns	Provide student with speech feedback during spelling instruction (e.g., student types MAT, listens, adds an *e* to hear *mate*) to help solidify knowledge of long vowel patterns.
	Coordinate spelling with word study	Provide structured spelling instruction and opportunities for independent practice; use computer software with speech feedback (e.g., WordMaker, Leap into Phonics, Simon Sounds It Out).

orthographic, and contextual analyses. Students in this phase, who are approaching fluency, typically prefer to read silently (Barrs, Ellis, Hester, & Thomas, 1989; Routman, 1988). They can read and comprehend longer books and explore new genres (e.g., poetry, expository text) in both their reading and writing.

Recommended Best Practices   Students in the transitional phase of reading development must change their focus from *learning to read* to *reading to learn.* Although appropriate for students at all levels of development, direct instruction in the use of text comprehension strategies is particularly important when students increase the volume and complexity of what they read (Alverman & Eakle, 2003; Kim, Vaughn, Wanzek, & Wei, 2004; Underwood & Pearson, 2004). Research supports the use of several effective comprehension strategies: answering questions, asking factual and inferential questions, writing summaries, monitoring comprehension, using graphic and semantic organizers, using text structures, and *learning cooperatively* (in which students work together while learning strategies). The NRP (2000) has noted that effective reading comprehension instruction includes not only the teaching of multiple comprehension strategies but also training on when to use them.

Another focus of transitional best practice literacy instruction includes increasing reading fluency. Research has demonstrated that reading fluency and text comprehension are highly correlated (Fuchs, Fuchs, Hosp, & Jenkins, 2001; Meyer & Felton, 1999), presumably because fluent readers devote little conscious effort to decoding and instead focus their cognitive resources on deriving meaning from text. However, fluency varies based on a number of factors, including the level of difficulty of the text; the reader's familiarity with the words, content, and genre; and the amount of practice the reader has with the text. Research supports a systematic approach to improving fluency in students with and without disabilities, with practice being the most essential component of fluency instruction. The more frequently and regularly students practice reading, the more fluent they become. NRP (2000) suggestions for increasing reading fluency include

- Providing fluent models of reading

- Engaging students in repeated readings of texts written at students' independent reading level (i.e., the level of text students can read with 96%–100% accuracy)

- Engaging students in *choral reading* (in which students read the same text aloud at the same time)

- Engaging students in partner reading, pairing fluent readers with less fluent readers

- Providing books on tape or multimedia texts for students with low literacy skills to follow along as text is read aloud

Instructional Adaptations for Transition-Age Youth   Depending upon the topics, genres, or text types they encounter during their independent reading, transitional readers who use AAC may have limited background or prior knowledge to support their reading comprehension. AT supports such as movies, videos, and multimedia texts from the Internet can help such students learn about topics before they read about them and can also help students to organize or summarize what they have read (Foley & Staples, 2007).

Students who use AAC in middle and high school settings are expected to learn and use new vocabulary they encounter in content area studies. Many transition-age students have reduced vocabularies and must be assisted in connecting new words to words they understand and/or words they can produce using their AAC devices. Some strategies for this include asking students who have high-tech AAC devices to find synonyms, antonyms, or other words in the system that relate to the new vocabulary word; adding AAC symbols to semantic maps to reinforce meaning; providing access to online dictionaries with text-to-speech feedback; and giving students multiple opportunities and multiple means (e.g., AAC device, content area writing assignments) for using new words. Students who use AAC can also learn vocabulary by going beyond text to experience other media such as graphic representations, hypertext, or online dictionaries.

Fluency is another literacy component that warrants special attention in transitional readers who use AAC. Despite mastery of word-level decoding, transitional readers who use AAC may have persistent difficulty generating and retrieving phonological representations when they read (Bishop & Robson, 1989a, 1989b; Dahlgren Sandberg, 2001, 2006; Dahlgren Sandberg, & Hjelmquist, 1996a, 1996b, 2002; Foley & Pollatsek, 1999; Vandervelden & Siegel, 2001). Such difficulty may reduce reading fluency and negatively affect processing and recall of extended text. Because students who use AAC are unable to read aloud, assessing and monitoring their fluency is problematic. In the beginning reading phase, students are sometimes asked to read text word by word using voice output AAC devices. At higher levels of reading development, however, this practice inhibits fluent reading. It also prevents students from developing the internal sense of *prosody* (intonation, stress, and expression) that characterizes fluent reading and that is a desired outcome of fluency instruction (Erickson & Koppenhaver, 2007). An alternative and more effective strategy is to have students read silently, encouraging them to actively employ their inner voices as their partner or group reads aloud. Instructional follow-up activities, such as having students answer true/false questions about a text, will help assess how successfully these students are reading and understanding. Additional strategies for helping students who use AAC develop an internal sense of prosody were described by Erickson and Koppenhaver, who suggested, for example, that a teacher can record herself reading a short passage one sentence at a time with a pause between each sentence that allows the student to echo "in his head" what was read. They suggested that using live, recorded, or digitized human voices during fluency practice may be preferable to using the synthesized speech of computers or most AAC devices because the latter do not provide appropriate models of fluency and expression.

Transitional Writing

Characteristics   During this phase, students can write more fluently and explore genres other than the more familiar narrative story form, such as *expository* (nonfiction) writing and poetry. Students' writing tends to be several paragraphs long and more complex and better organized than in earlier phases (Graves, 1994).

Recommended Best Practices   Several instructional strategies are effective at improving writing skills in transitional writers. These include providing direct, explicit, and systematic instruction in the specific aspects of the writing process (planning, drafting, revising, and editing) and in skills relevant to editing and revision (De La Paz & Graham, 2002; Fountas & Pinnell, 2001). Direct instruction in word processing and spelling skills can also increase writing quality during this phase (Schlagel, 2007).

Instructional Adaptations for Transition-Age Youth   Transitional writers who use AAC typically have deficits across multiple domains that influence the generation of written text and underlie well-developed composing processes. These domains include 1) cognitive/linguistic (e.g., conceptual ability, linguistic, metalinguistic, metacognitive, content knowledge, processing speed, working memory), 2) production (e.g., graphomotor skills, mode and speed of output), 3) social/rhetorical (e.g., knowledge of text schema and genre, environment), and 4) beliefs and attitudes (e.g., self-efficacy, goals, affect; Foley, 2007; Koppenhaver & Yoder, 1993; Singer & Bashir, 2004). These writers may fatigue quickly and have difficulty sustaining attention to a physically demanding task. Phonological processing impairments may make the use of inner speech less efficient as a self-regulatory mechanism. In addition to direct instruction in the NRP writing strategies described previously, explicit instruction in executive function and self-regulation strategies is likely to benefit transitional writers who use AAC by providing them with greater control over the selection and use of compensatory strategies (e.g., rate enhancement features, graphic organizers; Foley, 2007).

Because writing is so challenging, transition-age students who use AAC need a supportive instructional environment in order to flourish as writers. Suggested NRP (2000) strategies for creating such an environment include

- Planning daily writing activities across content areas

- Providing opportunities for authentic writing, allowing for the recursive nature of writing practice over a period of days or weeks

- Making teacher and peer response an integral part of writing instruction

- Conveying the ways in which writing will be useful to students in their lives outside of school

- Connecting writing to reading and other academic subjects

- Displaying students' writing in prominent places

Introducing transitional writers who use AAC to new digital multimedia technologies is another way to increase engagement in the writing process. Such technologies enable students to share what they know with peers in a variety of formats, such as PowerPoint presentations, web page downloads, DVDs, or podcasts. Students who use AAC can learn to determine the best mode of presentation for the content and the audience and the best technology tools for producing and presenting their work. Proficiency in the use of information technologies can potentially increase students' educational and vocational options. Melanie, the mother of a middle school student with muscular dystrophy, explained the critical role of technology, motivation, and social engagement in her daughter's writing development:

> Learning reading and writing in the regular classroom has been so important in Annie's development, both socially as well as educationally. We have found that for her the most realistic place to learn these skills is not in a resource room one-on-one with an adult, but from actually interacting with age-appropriate peers in a learning environment. It has been very important for her writing and language skills to share her work with other students, sometimes working one-on-one with them, sharing thoughts and ideas. She has been able to edit her peers' writing and have her work edited by others. She has listened as others have shared their "published" work and has been excited to share her finished work with her classmates as well. She has been motivated to increase both her writing and reading skills to keep up with the other students in her class. It is definitely a challenge for her as well as her teacher and peers to keep her in the classroom setting for this learning time, as her communication device and computer typing speed hold her to a slower pace, but it is worth the extra effort as we see the progress that she makes from year to year. (personal communication, July 13, 2008)

Transitional Spelling

Characteristics   Spelling reflects the *within-word* stage, when students' representations of long vowel patterns within words are beginning to stabilize. Students begin to develop mental–graphemic representations, or visual images, for these patterns to distinguish among them and facilitate their correct use (e.g., *play* versus *plai*), and they can spell many words conventionally (Templeton, 1995).

Recommended Best Practices   Instruction with transitional spellers begins with an exploration of long vowel patterns to increase their understanding that there are many possible spellings of long vowels (e.g., the long *a* vowel in *ate, play, wait, weigh, puree, chalet*). As students explore long vowels, they notice *homonyms* (e.g., *to, too, two*), which sound the same but are spelled differently, and *homophones* (e.g., *spring*), which sound and are spelled the same but have multiple meanings. Students engage in word sorts and record in word study notebooks examples of words containing targeted long vowel patterns they encounter in their reading.

Instructional Adaptations for Transition-Age Youth   Transitional spellers who use AAC may have well-developed phonemic awareness skills yet still have persistent difficulty applying these skills to spelling tasks (Dahlgren Sandberg, 2001; Dahlgren Sandberg & Hjelmquist, 1996a, 1996b; Foley & Pollatsek, 1999; Hart, 2006; Vandervelden & Siegel, 1999, 2001). They must learn to recognize quickly patterns of letters, associate them with sounds, and recombine the sounds. Students benefit from explicit instruction and repeated practice using spelling software that provides auditory feedback. A published phonics curriculum is useful for planning a systematic sequence of instruction for transitional spellers (e.g., Bear et al., 2000; Cunningham, Moore, Cunningham, & Moore, 2004).

Transitional spellers who use AAC may lack spelling fluency but have spelling abilities that are sufficient for word prediction. Teachers and learners can also create topic dictionaries or electronic word banks containing content area words that may be necessary for writing but difficult for students to spell.

Case Example: Transitional Phase   Seth is a young adult with cerebral palsy who uses a high-tech AAC device for communication and computer access. He attends general education classes, and his plans for the future include going to college. Seth was attending high school when he was referred to the first author for a literacy assessment. His primary concern at that time was his increasing difficulty with the volume and complexity of content area reading and writing assignments—Seth reported that he experienced language comprehension problems when reading but not when listening to grade-level text.

Seth's literacy assessment revealed age-appropriate listening comprehension but markedly reduced comprehension and recall of grade-level text. His poor comprehension appeared to stem, at least in part, from his difficulty applying decoding skills fluently. Although his single-word reading skills were accurate, they were not yet automatic, especially when he encountered multisyllable words and unfamiliar content area vocabulary. Consequently, Seth read and processed extended text slowly and thus had difficulty with comprehension and recall. The assessment also revealed deficits in spelling, difficulty planning and organizing information in content area writing assignments, and slow writing speed.

Based on these findings, Seth appeared to be in the transitional phase of literacy development. Considering his educational goals (which included postsecondary education) and his identified skill levels, Seth's literacy instruction focused on improving his reading and spelling fluency as well as on developing the more advanced language and literacy skills he needed to be successful in high school and college. While he was receiving explicit instruction in reading, writing, and spelling, Seth accessed grade-level text using compensatory strategies to support text comprehension and recall. He learned to use AT supports, including Read:OutLoud (Don Johnston Incorporated) and the CAST eReader (CAST). Both programs enabled him to select multisyllable words or even pages of text to be read aloud. He used the eReader to take notes and drag and drop important information into a study guide and used the software program Draft:Builder (Don Johnston Incorporated) to help him negotiate the process of planning and writing research papers. Use of word prediction and content-specific dictionaries helped his spelling. These literacy skills and tools helped prepare Seth for postsecondary education. Seth now attends a local university that provides extensive AT and other support services (e.g., learning labs with accessible computer stations, notetakers, literacy tutors, electronic text books) to students with disabilities.

Intermediate/Advanced Phase of Literacy Development

Students typically develop into intermediate/advanced readers in fourth through sixth grades, although some may not reach this phase until the secondary grades or beyond. During the intermediate/advanced phase, students significantly increase the volume and complexity of their reading and writing. Intermediate and advanced readers and writers differ mostly in experience and depth of knowledge of reading and writing styles and practices (see Table 3.4).

Intermediate/Advanced Reading

Characteristics   Students in this phase learn to use a variety of strategies for analyzing text and reading critically. Decoding familiar vocabulary is automatic and effortless; students only consciously apply decoding strategies when they encounter unfamiliar or technical words. Students increase the volume of what they read and write and widen their repertoire of reading and writing styles. There is no endpoint to this phase because students' language comprehension and general knowledge become increasingly sophisticated through exposure to written text (Bear & Barone, 1998) and thus continue to develop through life. Students continue to grow as they are challenged to read and write texts of increasing linguistic and cognitive complexity.

Recommended Best Practices   Teaching explicit strategies for decoding multisyllabic words remains important because such words encompass most of the new vocabulary students encounter in their content area reading. Specifically, teaching strategies for applying phonemic awareness and phonics knowledge to the task of decoding multisyllabic words help learners to decode other unknown words, build a more extensive sight vocabulary, and learn how to spell longer words (Bear et al., 2000; Moats, 2001; Torgesen, 2004). Many text- or web-based resources are available to guide advanced decoding, phonemic awareness, and phonics instruction (e.g., Bear et al., 2000).

Shared reading and direct instruction in comprehension strategies continue to be effective. Students also benefit from explicit instruction in strategic reading skills (Bear et al., 2000), such as scanning text for specific information; using textual graphs, tables, and outlines; and learning and using study- and test-taking skills and routines.

Instructional Adaptations for Transition-Age Youth   The reading comprehension ability of intermediate/advanced readers who use AAC is often depressed relative to their language comprehension (Foley & Pollatsek, 1999). Comprehension difficulties often relate to 1) difficulty decoding multisyllabic words, 2) slower than typical reading rates, 3) poor visual tracking while reading extended text, and 4) difficulty processing and recalling information in extended text (Foley & Pollatsek, 1999; Iacono, Balandin, & Cupples, 2001). Intervention strategies that help improve text comprehension in intermediate/advanced readers who use AAC include

- Having a summary of the text provided before the text is read

- Having difficult words spoken aloud when selected, or having access to text-to-speech output

- Having meanings for words available (e.g., selecting a word and hearing a definition)

- Having text presented cumulatively, one word at a time, to facilitate keeping place in the text

- Using larger print when necessary

- Having the entire text read aloud after reading

Educators can provide students with reading software that enables them to hear selected words spoken aloud and that provides definitions (e.g., Thinking Reader [Tom Snyder Productions]). Other software programs, such as Read:OutLoud and CAST eReader, enable students who use AAC to read back any kind of text via text-to-speech synthesis. Students can open a web site, highlight a portion of the text to be read (a single word, a sentence, a paragraph or longer), and

Table 3.4. Characteristics, recommended best practices, and AAC adaptations for the intermediate/advanced literacy phase

Characteristics	Recommended best practices	Adaptations
Reading		
Reading with fluency and expression	Read-alouds to introduce new genres, content area topics	Provide access to topic-specific vocabulary and preprogrammed phrases that facilitate participation.
Familiarity with different styles and genres of text		Preview/preteach difficult vocabulary; link to vocabulary in AAC device.
	Charting ideas with clusters, maps, and webs	Provide computer-generated templates of graphic organizers.
	Guided reading (predict–read–confirm)	After reading, have student match questions with answers presented on sentence strips in random order (Erickson, 2003).
	Strategic reading (study skills and routines, test-taking strategies)	Provide text electronically; teach student to highlight critical information and/or drag and drop to outlines or graphic organizers.
	Information literacy	Teach student to use locate and use web-based information resources (e.g., libraries, dictionaries, content-specific web sites; Foley & Staples, 2003).
	Reading reflections	Preprogram AAC device with language needed to express opinions (e.g., I AGREE/DISAGREE WITH THE AUTHOR, I DIDN'T UNDERSTAND THE SECTION DEALING WITH ___).
		Have student select best summary of text from three or more written summaries (Erickson, 2003).
		Have student highlight confusing sections in text (e.g., abstract and figurative language, unfamiliar vocabulary) so he or she can request clarification from instructor (Foley & Staples, 2003).

Writing

Experience with different styles and genres Sense of audience and voice		Provide multiple examples of good writing, opportunities to write, corrective feedback, and specific skills instruction (e.g., combining sentences, organization, punctuation).
	Prepare for state-mandated assessments	Arrange for untimed tests.
	Revising and editing	Provide editing/revising checklists.
	Note-taking strategies	Provide text electronically; teach student to highlight critical information and/or drag and drop to outlines or graphic organizers (e.g., CAST eReader, SOLO [Don Johnston Incorporated]).

Spelling

Syllable juncture and derivational-constancy stage: morphological analysis, including inflectional (e.g., -ed, -ing) and derivational morphemes (e.g., un-, pre-, -tion, -ness)	Strategy instruction	Provide guided practice in the use of spelling strategies (e.g., use context, sound it out, use word prediction, check word bank).
	Examine morphology	Provide AAC display that enables student to experiment with adding prefixes and suffixes to root and base words (Foley & Staples, 2003). Use content area vocabulary for word study.

hear it read back to them clearly and distinctly. They can also open two or more other windows to reference additional documents at the same time or take advantage of drag-and-drop notetaking. These software programs enable users to create assignment templates, outlines for reading assignments, and other effective reading comprehension scaffolds.

Intermediate/Advanced Writing

Characteristics   In this phase, students develop competence in writing mechanics and can write fluently with expression and voice in different writing styles and genres. Students can now use more sophisticated language to express opinions, summarize events, and evaluate information in cohesive texts. Writing fluency rates increase significantly and are flexible to purpose (Bear & Barone, 1998).

Recommended Best Practices   Students in this phase are engaged in more complex writing (e.g., book reports, essays, and synthesis reports) and in preparing for high-stakes testing (Nelson & Calfee, 1998). They continue to benefit from explicit instruction in the writing process, as well as the use of executive function and self-regulation strategies (e.g., asking "How does this sentence sound?" "How should this essay be organized?" "How much time do I need to complete this assignment?"; Singer & Bashir, 2004). Instruction in the use of prewriting strategies (e.g., brainstorming, creating outlines, mapping ideas), peer conferencing, and revising/editing checklists is emphasized.

Instructional Adaptations for Transition-Age Youth   As discussed previously, many intermediate/advanced writers who use AAC lack the cognitive or linguistic foundations that underlie more advanced writing. Careful measures of their writing abilities (e.g., syntactic complexity, productivity, fluency, cohesion) provide direction for planning interventions (Foley et al., 2009). Intermediate/advanced writers who use AAC will continue to require direct instruction in the writing process as they learn to produce longer, more cohesive texts in different genres. Teaching these students to use executive function and self-regulatory strategies is critical (Foley, 2007; Singer & Bashir, 2004), as is teaching the development of self-advocacy (e.g., requesting take-home tests, requesting additional time to complete assignments). High-tech AAC devices are essential for writers in the intermediate/advanced phase (as well as in earlier phases); they offer word processing and word prediction functions, as well as access to generative communication and prestored, generic messages during writing activities (e.g., I'M HAVING TROUBLE GETTING STARTED, CAN YOU HELP ME? HOW DO YOU LIKE THE ENDING OF MY STORY? or I DON'T KNOW WHAT TO WRITE ABOUT NEXT).

Software programs such as Inspiration (Inspiration Software), Draft:Builder, and the CAST eReader provide a variety of scaffolds for planning and organizing ideas across texts and genres. Students in every genre and curriculum area and at any stage of writing development are guided through planning, notetaking, organizing, citing resources, and preparing a rough draft. Teachers can use these software programs to easily create assignment templates and graphic organizers, such as semantic webs, time lines, story maps, or cuing charts, which students can use to construct more cohesive texts. Use of the advanced features and utilities of word processors (e.g., graphics, spell checker, grammar checker, and thesaurus) may also lead to improvements in student writing.

Intermediate/Advanced Spelling

Characteristics   Early in this stage, students are in the *syllable-juncture* stage of spelling development (Bear et al., 2000), when they learn to examine external features of multisyllabic words, including prefixes and suffixes, and rules governing syllable boundaries (e.g., consonant doubling, open versus closed syllables). Later, students enter the *derivational-constancy* stage of spelling, when they explore the internal structure of words, their morphology, and in particular their roots and derivations (Bear et al., 2000).

Recommended Best Practices   As students enter the derivational-constancy phase, vocabulary study is integrated within instruction to underscore spelling–meaning connections. Word study focuses on multisyllabic words and connects closely with vocabulary and reading instruction (Bear et al., 2000). Students learn about word origins (e.g., Greek and Latin roots) and explore the impact of a range of prefixes and suffixes on word meaning. Systematic, sequential phonics instruction (Bear et al., 2000; Cunningham, 2002) remains important during this phase.

Instructional Adaptations for Transition-Age Youth   Many students who use AAC lag behind their peers in acquiring morphological markers and syntactic forms (Binger & Light, 2008; Blockberger & Johnston, 2003; Sutton, Soto, & Blockberger, 2002), and this may contribute to their persistent difficulty reading and spelling multisyllable words (Foley & Pollatsek, 1999). As with readers in earlier phases of development, intermediate/advanced spellers with AAC needs may benefit from auditory feedback during spelling instruction. For example, an AAC device page can be programmed with a variety of root or base words, prefixes (e.g., *un-, re-, in-*), and suffixes (e.g., *-er, -tion, -sion*) to support exploration of multisyllable words. Students in this phase can learn to spell longer words by combining these chunks rather than processing letter by letter. Foley and Staples (2003) hypothesized that this type of instruction may enable students who use AAC to establish more stable visual and auditory images for targeted morphemes and more efficiently retrieve the spelling of longer words. Students in this phase of literacy development continue to benefit from the spell check and word prediction functions in their AAC devices and word processing programs.

Case Example: Intermediate/Advanced Phase   Beth Anne is a college student who uses a DynaVox for communication and academic participation. She is majoring in creative writing at a small university close to her home. Beth Anne has advanced literacy skills but is challenged by the pace of her university courses. In a webcast (Luciani, Horochak, & McNaughton, 2008), she described several strategies she has used effectively to address the literacy demands of college:

Preparing Well for Postsecondary Education During the Transition Years   School personnel, Beth Anne, and her family anticipated her need for the advanced literacy and study skills required at the college level. She focused on developing these skills during her transition years by participating in the general education curriculum and identifying the AT and AAC supports and other accommodations she would need to be successful in college-level coursework.

Identifying and Obtaining Needed Supports   Beth Anne selected a university that offered comprehensive support services for students with disabilities. Personnel in the Office for Students with Disabilities assist her in choosing classes and instructors and in arranging support services and accommodations such as notetakers and accessible computers.

Reducing the Quantity of Literacy Demands (to Ensure the Quality of Literacy Performance)   Instead of the typical four to five courses, Beth Anne takes two courses per semester. Because she accesses her AAC device with a head switch, she finds that writing assignments can be mentally and physically draining. Even using the rate enhancement features of her AAC device (e.g., word prediction), it takes Beth Anne about 2 hours to type a page of text. As a result, she typically requests take-home rather than in-class exams when extended writing is required. Having extended time to complete tests and assignments enables Beth Anne to produce her best work rather than be limited to the amount she can produce during a single class period. Although Beth Anne is significantly extending the time it will take for her to obtain a degree, her reduced course load enables her to maximize her academic achievement, as evidenced by an overall grade point average of 3.69.

Working Strategically to Meet the Communication and Literacy Demands of New Environments   Once she makes them aware of her need for extra response time, Beth

Anne finds that most of her instructors are quite willing to accommodate her participation needs in the classroom. In addition, Beth Anne requests that instructors provide her with reading lists and assignments well in advance so that she has extra time to prepare for class.

Beth Anne's story illustrates that with access to the general education curriculum, as well as appropriate AT, AAC, instructional, and social supports, adolescents and young adults with AAC needs have the same opportunities for educational growth and achievement as their peers without disabilities. As Beth Anne noted,

> I hope [my story] has encouraged and given hope to some people. College was always a dream of mine. . . . I am living that dream and I couldn't be happier. My mom is the driving force to my success, but my dream also wouldn't be coming true if it weren't for the wonderful people at California University. As my mom said, if it is possible, do it. I am doing it with one of the best support teams ever! (Luciani et al., 2008)

Summary

Evidence-based literacy instructional practices for students without disabilities can be used as a guide for providing literacy instruction for transition-age youth who use AAC. Instructional practices that are effective in improving phonemic awareness, phonics, fluency, vocabulary, text comprehension, and writing can all be adapted to fit the needs of individual students who use AAC, no matter their literacy level or phase of development. By adapting practices to each individual, and by considering related factors such as motivation and level of engagement, teachers can provide high-quality literacy instruction for students of all abilities.

UNANSWERED QUESTIONS

Although the instructional strategies presented in the previous section are promising, their effectiveness has yet to be determined empirically. Many questions remain as to how we as educators can best support literacy development in transition-age youth who use AAC, and there is a critical need for research that can help to answer them. Some questions of interest related to issues addressed in this chapter include the following:

1. How well does literacy intervention research on younger learners apply to adolescents who use AAC? For example, how do priorities for instruction, and instructional strategies, change as students grow older?

2. What strategies are most effective for teaching phonemic awareness and phonics skills to students with severe speech and physical impairments at different stages of literacy development? For example, what is the role of text-to-speech speech synthesis in the development of phonemic awareness and phonics skills in these students?

3. What are the roles and relationships of key literacy components (phonemic awareness, phonics, vocabulary, and fluency) in the development of text comprehension in students who use AAC? For example, how should vocabulary instruction be integrated with comprehension instruction?

4. What are the roles and relationships of key literacy components in the development of writing ability in students who use AAC?

5. Which strategies are effective for improving comprehension of specific kinds of text (e.g., narrative text, expository text using compare/contrast structures)?

6. How do alternative modes of input and output affect comprehension and/or composition of text?

7. How will opportunities for digital access to reading materials affect the literacy performance of individuals with complex communication needs?

8. What is the link between motivation and literacy levels in adolescents who use AAC? What structural elements (e.g., scheduling, grouping configurations, level of teacher support) in middle and high school settings support the successful implementation of reading and writing strategies among students who use AAC?

CONCLUSION

I am thankful for one other gift I received early on in life which most people can take for granted: the gift of literacy—of reading and writing, of making sense out of the world and having the reciprocal ability of letting the world make sense out of you and come to respect you for all that you have to offer and contribute. This to me is the true gift and power of literacy in each of our lives. (Williams, 2000, p. 247)

Literacy is a complex set of skills that includes the interrelated processes of reading and writing within varied communicative contexts. Significant numbers of transition-age youth who use AAC do not achieve literacy levels sufficient to meet the demands of middle school, high school, or adult life. Many do not receive appropriate literacy instruction early in their educational careers. Because their opportunities for literacy intervention decrease markedly when they exit the public school system, it is imperative that educators provide transition-age students who use AAC with the literacy skills they need to succeed in middle school, high school, and beyond.

Although the instructional strategies suggested in this chapter are not yet routinely offered to transition-age youth who use AAC in either segregated or inclusive settings, they should be. We cannot afford to wait for a critical mass of literacy research to accumulate when the results of such research may not be available for several years. The cost of such inaction to students who use AAC is already too high. Everyone involved in educating adolescents who use AAC is challenged to envision the possibilities that exist for improving the literacy lives of such individuals and to help turn these possibilities into realities.

REFERENCES

Alverman, D.E., & Eakle, A.J. (2003). Comprehension instruction: Adolescents and their multiple literacies. In A.P. Sweet & C.E. Snow (Eds.), *Rethinking reading comprehension* (pp. 12–29). New York: Guilford Press.

Atanasoff, L.M., McNaughton, D., Wolfe, P.S., & Light, J. (1998). Communication demands of university settings for students using augmentative and alternative communication. *Journal of Postsecondary Education and Disability, 13*(3), 32–47.

Barrs, M., Ellis, S., Hester, H., & Thomas, A. (1989). *The primary language record.* Portsmouth, NH: Heinemann.

Bear, D., & Barone, D. (1998). *Developing literacy: An integrated approach to assessment and instruction.* Boston: Houghton Mifflin.

Bear, D.R., Invernizzi, M., Templeton, S., & Johnston, F. (2000). *Words their way: Word study for phonics, vocabulary, and spelling instruction* (2nd ed.). Upper Saddle River, NJ: Prentice Hall.

Bear, D.R., Invernizzi, M., Templeton, S., & Johnston, F. (2008). *Words their way: Word study for phonics, vocabulary, and spelling instruction* (4th ed.). Upper Saddle River, NJ: Pearson.

Bedrosian, J., Lasker, J., Speidel, K., & Politsch, A. (2003). Enhancing the written narrative skills of an AAC student with autism: Evidence-based research issues. *Topics in Language Disorders, 2,* 305–324.

Berninger, V., & Gans, B.M. (1986a). Assessing word processing capability of the nonvocal, nonwriting. *Augmentative and Alternative Communication, 2,* 56–63.

Berninger, V., & Gans, B.M. (1986b). Language profiles in nonspeaking individuals of normal intelligence with severe cerebral palsy. *Augmentative and Alternative Communication, 2,* 45–50.

Binger, C., & Light, J. (2008). The morphology and syntax of individuals who use AAC: Research review and implications for effective practice. *Augmentative and Alternative Communication, 24,* 123–138.

Bishop, D.V.M., & Robson, J. (1989a). Accurate non-word spelling despite congenital inability to speak: Phoneme-grapheme conversion does not require subvocal articulation. *British Journal of Psychology, 80,* 1–13.

Bishop, D.V.M., & Robson, J. (1989b). Unimpaired short-term memory and rhyme judgment in congenitally speechless individuals: Implications for the notion of "articulatory coding." *Quarterly Journal of Experimental Psychology, 41A,* 124–140.

Blevins, W. (2001). *Teaching phonics and word study in the intermediate grades.* New York: Scholastic.

Blishak, D.M., Shah, S.D., Lombradino, L.J., & Chiarella, K. (2004). Effects of phonemic awareness instruction on the encoding skills of children with severe speech impairment. *Disability and Rehabilitation, 26,* 1295–1304.

Blockberger, S., & Johnston, J.R. (2003). Grammatical morphology acquisition by children with complex communication needs. *Augmentative and Alternative Communications, 19,* 207–221.

Bopp, K., Brown, K., & Mirenda, P. (2004). Speech-language pathologists' roles in the delivery of positive behavior support for individuals with developmental disabilities. *American Journal of Speech-Language Pathology, 13,* 5–19.

Browder, D.M., Wakeman, S.Y., Spooner, F., Ahlgrim-Delzell, L., & Algozzine, B. (2006). Research on reading instruction for individuals with significant cognitive disabilities. *Exceptional Children, 72,* 392–408.

Browder, D.M. & Xin, Y.P. (1998). A meta-analysis and review of sight word research and its implications for teaching functional reading to individuals with moderate and severe disabilities. *The Journal of Special Education, 32,* 130–153.

Bryant, D.P., Goodwin, M., Bryant, B.R., & Higgins, K. (2003). Vocabulary instruction for students with learning disabilities: A review of the research [Electronic version]. *Learning Disabilities Quarterly, 26,* 117–128.

Bryen, D.N., Carey, A., & Potts, B. (2006). Technology and job-related social networks. *Augmentative and Alternative Communication, 22,* 1–9.

Bryen, D.N., Potts, B.B., & Carey, A.C. (2007). So you want to work? What employers say about job skills, recruitment and hiring employees who rely on AAC. *Augmentative and Alternative Communication, 23,* 126–139.

Carey, A.C., Potts, B., Bryen, D.N., & Shankar, J.A. (2004). Networking towards employment: Experiences of people who use augmentative and alternative communication. *Research and Practice for Persons with Severe Disabilities, 29,* 40–52.

Coleman-Martin, M.B., Heller, K.W., Cihak, D.F., & Irvine, K.L. (2005). Using computer-assisted instruction and the nonverbal reading approach to teach word identification. *Focus on Autism and Other Developmental Disabilities, 20,* 80–90.

Cooper, D.H., Roth, F.P., Speece, D.L., & Schatschneider, C. (2002). The contribution of oral language skills to the development of phonological awareness. *Applied Psycholinguistics, 23,* 399–416.

Cunningham, P.M. (2002). *Systematic sequential phonics and spelling: Learning phonics and spelling through Word Wall and Making Words.* Greensboro, NC: Carson-Dellosa.

Cunningham, P., & Cunningham, J. (1992). Making words: Enhancing the invented spelling-decoding connection. *The Reading Teacher, 46,* 106–115.

Cunningham, P.M., Hall, D.P., & Sigmon, C.M. (1999). *The teacher's guide to the four blocks: A multimethod, multilevel framework for grades 1–3.* Greensboro, NC: Carson-Dellosa.

Cunningham, P.M., Moore, S.A., Cunningham, J.W., & Moore, D.W. (2004). *Reading and writing in elementary classrooms: Research-based K–4 instruction* (5th ed.). Boston: Allyn & Bacon.

Curtis, M. (2004). Adolescents who struggle with word identification: Research and practice. In T. Jetton & J. Dole (Eds.), *Adolescent literacy research and practice* (pp. 119–134). New York: Guilford Press.

Curtis, M.E., & Longo, A.M. (1999). *When adolescents can't read: Methods and materials that work.* Cambridge, MA: Brookline.

Dahlgren Sandberg, A.D. (2001). Reading and spelling, phonological awareness, and working memory in children with severe speech impairments: A longitudinal study. *Augmentative and Alternative Communication, 17,* 11–26.

Dahlgren Sandberg, A.D. (2006). Reading and spelling abilities in children with severe speech impairments and cerebral palsy at 6, 9, and 12 years of age in relation to cognitive development: A longitudinal study. *Developmental Medicine and Child Neurology, 48,* 629–634.

Dahlgren Sandberg, A., & Hjelmquist, E. (1996a). A comparative, descriptive study of reading and writing skills among nonspeaking children: A preliminary study. *European Journal of Disorders of Communication, 31,* 289–308.

Dahlgren Sandberg, A., & Hjelmquist, E. (1996b). Phonological awareness and literacy abilities in nonspeaking preschool children with cerebral palsy. *Augmentative and Alternative Communication, 12,* 138–154.

Dahlgren Sandberg, A., & Hjelmquist, E. (2002). Phonological recoding problems in children with cerebral palsy: The importance of productive speech. In A.F.E. Witruk & T. Lachmann (Eds.), *Basic mechanisms of language and language disorders* (pp. 315–327). Dordrecht, The Netherlands: Kluwer Academic.

Dattilo, J., Estrella, G., Estrella, L.J., Light, J., McNaughton, D., & Seabury, M. (2007). "I have chosen to live life abundantly": Perceptions of leisure by adults who use augmentative and alternative communication. *Augmentative and Alternative Communication, 2*(1), 16–28.

De La Paz, S., & Graham, S. (2002). Explicitly teaching strategies, skills and knowledge: Writing instruction in middle school classrooms. *Journal of Educational Psychology, 94,* 687–698.

Eikeseth, S., & Jahr, E. (2001). The UCLA reading and writing program: An evaluation of the beginning stages. *Research in Developmental Disabilities, 22,* 289–307.

Erickson, K. (2003). Reading comprehension in AAC. *The ASHA Leader, 8*(12), 6–9.

Erickson, K.A., & Clendon, S.A. (2009). Addressing the literacy demands of the curriculum for beginning readers and writers. In G. Soto & C. Zangari (Eds.), *Practically speaking: Language, literacy, and academic development for students with AAC needs* (pp. 195–215). Baltimore: Paul H. Brookes Publishing Co.

Erickson, K., & Koppenhaver, D. (2007). *Children with disabilities: Reading and writing the four blocks way.* Greensboro, NC: Carson-Dellosa.

Erickson, K.A., Koppenhaver, D.A., & Yoder, D.E. (1994). *Literacy and adults with developmental disabilities.* Philadelphia: National Center on Adult Literacy.

Erickson, K.A., Koppenhaver, D.A., Yoder, D.E., & Nance, J. (1997). Integrated communication and literacy instruction for a child with multiple disabilities. *Focus on Autism and Other Developmental Disabilities, 12,* 142–150.

Fallon, K.A., Light, J., McNaughton, D., Drager, K., & Hammer, C. (2004). The effects of direct instruction on the single-word reading skills of children who require augmentative and alternative communication. *Journal of Speech Language Hearing Research, 47,* 1424–1439.

Foley, B.E. (1993). The development of literacy in individuals with severe congenital speech and motor impairments. *Topics in Language Disorders, 13,* 16–32.

Foley, B. (2007). Integrating process writing and self-regulatory strategy development within a written narrative intervention. In D. Lage (Ed.), *Communicative competence and participation over the lifespan: Theoretical and methodological issues in research on augmentative and alternative communication.* Proceedings of the Ninth Biennial Research Symposium of the International Society for Augmentative and Alternative Communication (pp. 138–155), Dusseldorf-Kaiserswerth, Germany, August 2006. Toronto, Ontario: ISAAC.

Foley, B., Koppenhaver, D., & Williams, A. (2009). Writing assessment for students with augmentative and alternative communication needs. In G. Soto & C. Zangari (Eds.), *Practically speaking: Language, literacy, and academic development for students with AAC needs* (pp. 93–128). Baltimore: Paul H. Brookes Publishing Co.

Foley, B., & Pollatsek, A. (1999). Phonological processing and reading abilities in adolescents and adults with severe congenital speech impairments. *Augmentative and Alternative Communication, 15,* 156–173.

Foley, B.E., & Staples, A. (2003). Developing augmentative and alternative communication and literacy interventions in a supported employment setting. *Topics in Language Disorders, 23,* 325–343.

Foley, B.E., & Staples, A. (2006). Assistive technology supports for literacy instruction. *Perspectives on Augmentative and Alternative Communication, 15,* 15–21.

Foley, B., & Staples, A. (2007). Supporting literacy development with assistive technology. In S.R. Copeland & E.B. Keefe (Eds.), *Effective literacy instruction for students with moderate or severe disabilities* (pp. 127–148). Baltimore: Paul H. Brookes Publishing Co.

Ford, A., Davern, L., & Schnorr, R. (2001). Learners with significant disabilities: Curricular relevance in an era of standards-based reform. *Remedial and Special Education, 22,* 214–222.

Fossett, B., & Mirenda, P. (2006). Sight word reading in children with developmental disabilities: A comparison of paired associate and picture-to-text matching instruction. *Research in Developmental Disabilities, 27*(4), 411–429.

Fountas, I.C., & Pinnell, G.S. (2001). *Guiding readers and writers, grades 3–6: Teaching comprehension, genre, and content literacy.* Westport, CT: Heinemann.

Fuchs, L.S., Fuchs, D., Hosp, M., & Jenkins, J.R. (2001). Oral reading fluency as an indicator of reading competence: A theoretical, empirical, and historical analysis. *Scientific Studies of Reading, 5,* 239–256.

Graves, D. (1994). *A fresh look at writing.* Portsmouth, NH: Heinemann.

Guthrie, J.T., & Davis, M.H. (2003). Motivating struggling readers in middle school through an engagement model of classroom practice. *Reading and Writing Quarterly, 19*(1), 59–85.

Hanser, G., & Erickson. K.A. (2007). Integrated word identification and communication instruction for students with complex communication instruction needs: Preliminary results. *Focus on Autism and Developmental Disabilities, 22*(4), 268–278.

Hart, P. (2006). Spelling considerations for AAC intervention. *Perspectives on Augmentative and Alternative Communication, 15,* 12–14.

Houston, D., & Torgesen, J. (2004). *Teaching students with moderate disabilities to read: Insights from research.* Tallahassee: Florida Department of Education, Bureau of Instructional Support and Community Services. Retrieved April 10, 2007, from www.cpt.fsu.edu/ESE/pdf/ESE_Read.pdf#search=%22teaching%students%20moderate%2disabilities%20read%20Florida%22

Iacono, T., Balandin, S., & Cupples, L. (2001). Focus group discussions of literacy assessment and World Wide Web-based reading intervention. *Augmentative and Alternative Communication, 17,* 27–36.

Individuals with Disabilities Education Act Amendments (IDEA) of 1997, PL 105-17, 20 U.S.C. §§ 1400 *et seq.*

Individuals with Disabilities Education Improvement Act (IDEA) of 2004, PL 108-446, 20 U.S.C. §§ 1400 *et seq.*

Juel, C. (1991). Beginning reading. In B. Barr, M.L. Kamil, P. Mosenthal, & P.D. Pearson (Eds.), *Handbook of reading research* (Vol. 2, pp. 759–788). New York: Longman.

Juel, C., & Minden-Cupp, C. (2000). Learning to read words: Linguistic units and instructional strategies. *Reading Research Quarterly, 35,* 458–492.

Kamil, M.L. (2003). *Adolescents and literacy: Reading for the 21st Century.* Washington, DC: Alliance for Excellent Education.

Katims, D.S. (2000a). Literacy instruction for people with mental retardation: Historical highlights and contemporary analysis. *Education and Training in Mental Retardation and Developmental Disabilities, 35,* 3–15.

Katims, D.S. (2000b). *The quest for literacy: Curriculum and instructional procedures for teaching reading and writing to students with mental retardation and developmental disabilities* (MRDD Prism Series, Vol. 2). Reston, VA: Council for Exceptional Children. (ERIC Document Reproduction Service No. ED445454)

Kent-Walsh, J., & Binger, C. (2009). Addressing the communication demands of the classroom for beginning communicators and early language users. In G. Soto & C. Zangari (Eds.), *Practically speaking: Language, literacy, and academic development for students with AAC needs* (pp. 143–172). Baltimore: Paul H. Brookes Publishing Co.

Kent-Walsh, J., & McNaughton, D. (2005). Communication partner instruction in AAC: Present practices and future directions. *Augmentative and Alternative Communication, 21,* 195–204.

Kim, A., Vaughn, S., Wanzek, J., & Wei, S. (2004). Graphic organizers and their effects on reading comprehension of students with LD: A synthesis of research. *Journal of Learning Disabilities, 37*(2), 105–118.

Kinney, E.M., Vedora, J., & Stromer, R. (2003). Computer-presented video models to teach generative spelling to a child with an autism spectrum disorder. *Journal of Positive Behavior Interventions, 5,* 22–29.

Kliewer, C. (1999). Individualizing literacy instruction for young children with moderate to severe disabilities. *Exceptional Children, 66,* 85–100.

Kliewer, C., & Biklen, D. (2001). "School's not really a place for reading": A research synthesis of the literate lives of students with severe disabilities. *Journal of The Association for Persons with Severe Handicaps, 26,* 1–12.

Koppenhaver, D.A. (2000). Literacy in AAC: What should be written on the envelope we push? *Augmentative and Alternative Communication, 16,* 270–279.

Koppenhaver, D.A., & Erickson, K.A. (2003). Natural emergent literacy supports for preschoolers with autism and severe communication impairments. *Topics in Language Disorders, 23,* 283–292.

Koppenhaver, D.A., Evans, D.A., & Yoder, D.E. (1991). Childhood reading and writing experiences of literate adults with severe speech and motor impairments. *Augmentative and Alternative Communication, 7,* 20–33.

Koppenhaver, D., & Yoder, D. (1992). Literacy issues in persons with severe speech and physical impairments. In R. Gaylord-Ross (Ed.), *Issues and research in special education* (Vol. 2., pp. 156–201). New York: Columbia University Teachers College.

Koppenhaver, D.A., & Yoder, D.E. (1993). Classroom literacy instruction for children with severe speech and physical impairments (SSPI): What is and what might be. *Topics in Language Disorders, 13(2),* 1–15.

Light, J., & Kelford Smith, A. (1993). Home literacy experiences of preschoolers who use AAC systems and of their nondisabled peers. *Augmentative and Alternative Communication, 9,* 10–25.

Light, J.C., & McNaughton, D. (2007, November). *Evidence-based literacy intervention for individuals who require AAC.* Seminar presented at the annual convention of the American Speech-Language-Hearing Association, Boston.

Light, J.C., & McNaughton, D. (2009). Addressing the literacy demands of the curriculum for conventional and more advanced readers and writers who require AAC. In G. Soto & C. Zangari (Eds.), *Practically speaking: Language, literacy, and academic development for students with AAC needs* (pp. 217–246). Baltimore: Paul H. Brookes Publishing Co.

Light, J., McNaughton, D., Weyer, M., & Karg, L. (2008). Evidence-based literacy instruction for individuals who require augmentative and alternative communication: A case study of a student with multiple disabilities. *Seminars in Speech and Language, 29,* 120–132.

Light, J., Stoltz, B., & McNaughton, D. (1996). Community-based employment: Experiences of adults who use AAC. *Augmentative and Alternative Communication, 12,* 215–228.

Luciani, B.A., Horochak, S., & McNaughton, D. (2008). *College life and AAC: Just do it!* [Webcast]. Retrieved April 3, 2008, from http://mcn.ed.psu.edu/dbm/bal_cal/index.htm

McCardle, P., & Chhabra, V. (Eds.). (2004). *The voice of evidence in reading research.* Baltimore: Paul H. Brookes Publishing Co.

McNaughton, D., Light, J., & Arnold, K.B. (2002). "Getting your wheel in the door": Successful full-time employment experiences of individuals with cerebral palsy who use augmentative and alternative communication. *Augmentative and Alternative Communication, 18,* 59–76.

McNaughton, D., Symons, G., Light, J., & Parsons, A. (2006). My dream was to pay taxes. *Journal of Vocational Rehabilitation, 25,* 181–196.

McNaughton, D., & Tawney, J. (1993). Spelling instruction for adults who use augmentative and alternative communication. *Augmentative and Alternative Communication, 9,* 72–82.

Meyer, M.S., & Felton, R.H. (1999). Repeated reading to enhance fluency: Old approaches and new directions. *Annals of Dyslexia, 49,* 283–306.

Mike, D.G. (1995). Literacy and cerebral palsy: Factors influencing literacy learning in a self-contained setting. *Journal of Reading Behavior, 27,* 627–642.

Millar, D.C., & Light, J. (2001). *Exemplary practices in writing instruction for young children who use augmentative and alternative communication.* Grant report to the U.S. Department of Education (ERIC Document Reproduction Service No. ED463614).

Millar, D.C., Light, J.C., & Schlosser, R.W. (2004). The impact of augmentative and alternative communication intervention on the speech production of individuals with developmental disabilities: A research review. *Journal of Speech, Language, and Hearing Research, 49,* 248–264.

Mirenda, P., & Erickson, K.A. (2000). Augmentative communication and literacy. In S.F. Warren & J. Reichle (Series Eds.) & A.M. Wetherby & B.M. Prizant (Vol. Eds.), *Communication and language intervention series: Vol. 9. Autism spectrum disorders: A transactional developmental perspective* (pp. 333–367). Baltimore: Paul H. Brookes Publishing Co.

Moats, L.C. (2001). When older students can't read. *Educational Leadership, 58*(6), 36–40.

Moore, D.W., Bean, T.W., Birdyshaw, D., & Rycik, J.A. (1999). *Adolescent literacy: a position statement for the Commission on Adolescent Literacy of the International Reading Association.* Newark, DE: International Reading Association.

National Center for Education Statistics. (2009). *Table 48. Percentage distribution of students with disabilities 6 to 21 years old receiving education services for the disabled, by educational environment and type of disability: Selected years, fall 1989 through fall 2005.* Retrieved February 20, 2009, from http://nces.ed.gov/programs/digest/d07/tables/dt07_048.asp

National Reading Panel. (2000). *Teaching children to read: An evidence-based assessment of the scientific research literature on reading and its implications for reading instruction* (National Institutes of Health Publication No. 00-4754). Washington, DC: U.S. Department of Health and Human Services.

Nelson, N.N., & Calfee, R.C. (Eds.). (1998). *The reading-writing connection: The yearbook of the National Society for the Study of Education.* Chicago: University of Chicago Press.

Newman, L. (2005, April). Postsecondary education participation of youth with disabilities. In M. Wagner, L. Newman, R. Cameto, N. Garza, & P. Levine (Eds.), *After high school: A first look at the postschool experiences of youth with disabilities* (pp. 4-1–4-17). Menlo Park, CA: SRI International. Retrieved June 6, 2009, from www.nlts2.org/reports/2005_04/nlts2_report_2005_04_complete.pdf

No Child Left Behind Act of 2001, PL 107-110, 115 Stat. 1425, 20 U.S.C. §§ 6301 *et seq.*

Nokes, J.D., & Dole, J.A. (2004). Helping adolescent readers through explicit strategy instruction. In T.L. Jetton & J.A. Dole (Eds.), *Adolescent literacy research and practice* (pp. 162–182). New York: Guilford Press.

Pierce, P.L., & Porter, P.B. (1996). Helping persons with disabilities to become literate using assistive technology: Practice and policy suggestions. *Focus on Autism and Other Developmental Disabilities, 11,* 142–146.

Rackensperger, T., Krezman, C., McNaughton, D., Williams, M.B., & D'Silva, K. (2005). "When I first got it, I wanted to throw it off a cliff": The challenges and benefits of learning AAC technologies as described by adults who use AAC. *Augmentative and Alternative Communication, 21,* 165–186.

Resta, P., Bryant, P., Lock, R., & Allan, J. (1998). Infusing a teacher preparation program in learning disabilities with assistive technology. *Journal of Learning Disabilities, 31,* 55–66.

Routman, R. (1988). *Transitions: From literature to literacy.* Portsmouth, NH: Heinemann.

Ryndak, D.L., Morrison, A.P., & Sommerstein, L. (1999). Literacy before and after inclusion in general education settings: A case study. *Journal of The Association for Persons with Severe Handicaps, 24,* 5–22.

Schlagel, B. (2007). Best practices in spelling and handwriting. In S. Graham, C. MacArthur, & J. Fitzgerald (Eds.), *Best practices in writing instruction* (pp. 179–201). New York: Guilford Press.

Singer, A.S., & Bashir, A.S. (2004). Developmental variations in writing composition. In C.A. Stone, E.R. Silliman, B.J. Ehren, & K. Apel (Eds.), *Handbook of language and literacy: Development and disorders* (pp. 559–582). New York: Guilford Press.

Smith, M.M. (1989). Reading without speech: A study of children with cerebral palsy. *Irish Journal of Psychology, 10,* 601–614.

Smith, M.M. (2005). *Literacy and augmentative and alternative communication.* Burlington, MA: Elsevier Academic.

Soto, G., & Hartmann, E. (2006). Analysis of narratives produced by four children who use augmentative and alternative communication. *Journal of Communication Disorders, 39,* 456–480.

Soto, G., Yu, B., & Henneberry, S. (2007). Supporting the development of narrative skills of an 8-year-old child who uses an augmentative and alternative communication device: Case study. *Child Language Teaching and Therapy, 23,* 27–45.

Soto, G., Yu, B., & Kelso, J. (2008). Effectiveness of multifaceted narrative intervention on the stories told by a 12 year old girl who uses AAC. *Augmentative and Alternative Communication, 24,* 76–87.

Stahl, S.A., Duffy-Hester, A.M., & Stahl, K.A.L. (1998). Everything you wanted to know about phonics (but were afraid to ask). *Reading Research Quarterly, 33,* 338–355.

Steelman, J.D., Pierce, P.L., & Koppenhaver, D.A. (1993). The role of computers in promoting literacy in children with severe speech and physical impairments. *Topics in Language Disorders, 13,* 76–88.

Sturm, J. (1998). Literacy development of AAC users. In D. Beukelman & P. Mirenda (Eds.), *Augmentative and alternative communication* (pp. 355–390). Baltimore: Paul H. Brookes Publishing Co.

Sturm, J., & Clendon, S. (2004). AAC, language and literacy. *Topics in Language Disorders, 24,* 76–91.

Sturm, J., & Koppenhaver, D.A. (2000). Supporting writing development in adolescents with developmental disabilities. *Topics in Language Disorders, 20,* 73–92.

Sulzby, E. (1990). Assessment of emergent writing and children's language while writing. In L.M. Morrow & J.K. Smith (Eds.), *Assessment for instruction in early literacy* (pp. 83–109). Englewood Cliffs, NJ: Prentice Hall.

Sutton, A., Soto, G., & Blockberger, S. (2002). Grammatical issues in graphic symbol communication. *Augmentative and Alternative Communication, 18,* 192–204.

Teale, W.H., & Sulzby, E. (Eds.) (1986). Emergent literacy as a perspective for examining how young children become writers and readers. In *Emergent literacy: Writing and reading* (pp. 111–138). Baltimore: Paul H. Brookes Publishing Co.

Templeton, S. (1995). *Children's literacy: Contexts for meaningful learning.* Boston: Houghton Mifflin.

Torgesen, J.K. (2004). Lessons learned from the last 20 years of research on interventions for students who experience difficulty learning to read. In P. McCardle & V. Chhabra (Eds.), *The voice of evidence in reading research* (pp. 355–382). Baltimore: Paul H. Brookes Publishing Co.

Truxler, J., & O'Keefe, B.M. (2007). The effects of phonological awareness instruction on beginning word recognition and spelling. *Augmentative and Alternative Communication, 23,* 164–176.

Underwood, T., & Pearson, P.D. (2004). Teaching struggling adolescent readers to comprehend what they read. In T.L. Jetton & J.A. Dole (Eds.), *Adolescent literacy research and practice* (pp. 135–161). New York: Guilford Press.

Vandervelden, M., & Siegel, L. (1999). Phonological processing and literacy in AAC users and students with motor speech impairments. *Augmentative and Alternative Communication, 15,* 191–211.

Vandervelden, M., & Siegel, L. (2001). Phonological processing in written word learning: Assessment for children who use augmentative and alternative communication. *Augmentative and Alternative Communication, 17,* 11–26.

Wehman, P. (1992). Transition for young people with disabilities: Challenges for the 1990s. *Education and Training in Mental Retardation, 27,* 112–118.

Williams, M.B. (2000). Aging and AAC. *Alternatively Speaking, 4*(3), 5–8.

Zascavage, V.T., & Keefe, C.H. (2004). Students with severe speech and physical impairments: Opportunity barriers to literacy. *Focus on Autism and Other Developmental Disorders, 19,* 223–234.

4

·············

Making School Matter

Supporting Meaningful Secondary Experiences for Adolescents Who Use AAC

Erik W. Carter[1] and John Draper

Middle and high school represents a time of excitement, opportunity, growth, and challenge for many adolescents. Throughout their secondary years, youth encounter new opportunities to develop and deepen their strengths, interests, talents, and aspirations; explore a wide array of classes, extracurricular programs, community-based experiences, and after-school activities; and acquire the skills, knowledge, attitudes, relationships, and supports that will help them transition to adulthood. Adolescence also is a time of emerging independence, when youth become more self-determined and peer relationships assume greater prominence. There is little doubt that the experiences students have during middle and high school play a prominent role in shaping the outcomes they encounter early in and throughout adulthood.

IMPORTANCE OF HIGH-QUALITY SECONDARY SCHOOL EXPERIENCES

For youth with significant disabilities who use or would benefit from augmentative and alternative communication (AAC), these adolescent experiences are equally important as they are for youth without disabilities. Since the emergence of transition initiatives in the mid-1980s (Will, 1984), research, policy, and legislative initiatives have emphasized the importance of equipping youth with disabilities with the instruction, opportunities, services, and supports that will prepare them to transition successfully and seamlessly to life after high school (Johnson, Stodden, Emanuel, Luecking, & Mack, 2002; Rusch, Hughes, Agran, Martin, & Johnson, 2009). Indeed, every prominent secondary transition framework centers on ensuring that youth with disabilities benefit from key experiences during middle and high school that will elevate their future aspirations and shape their postschool outcomes (Kohler & Field, 2003; National Alliance for Secondary Education and Transition, 2005).

A CRITICAL JUNCTURE FOR YOUTH WITH DISABILITIES

The disappointing in- and postschool outcomes reported by many transition-age youth with disabilities who use AAC and their families underscore the considerable need for intentional, research-based efforts to connect these youth to—and to support their participation in—high-quality secondary experiences. Although increasing numbers of youth with disabilities graduate from high school equipped with the skills, experiences, supports, and connections that enable them to attain

[1]Support for preparation of this chapter was provided by a grant from the Centers for Medicare and Medicaid Servies, Medicaid Infrastructure Grant to the Wisconsin Department of Health Services (CFDA No. 93.768).

their goals for adulthood, for many other youth, aspirations go unfulfilled and postschool plans never materialize (Wagner, Newman, & Cameto, 2004). Findings from the National Longitudinal Transition Study-2 indicated that most youth with significant disabilities leave high school without the necessary coursework, academic preparation, instructional supports, and encouragement to pursue further education. As a result, fewer than one sixth of young adults with intellectual disabilities, multiple disabilities, or deafblindness enroll in any type of postsecondary education within 2 years of leaving high school (Wagner, Newman, Cameto, Garza, & Levine, 2005). Many youth also leave high school without the early work, volunteer, and community experiences that can elevate their occupational aspirations and prepare them for the world of work. Consequently, less than one third of young adults with intellectual disabilities, multiple disabilities, or autism are employed 2 years after leaving high school. And far too many youth leave school without the supportive relationships, durable friendships, and sense of belonging that create connections in the community and make life rich and satisfying. It is disappointing that less than one third of young adults with intellectual disabilities, multiple disabilities, or autism see friends weekly outside of school or work 2 years after leaving high school. Such outcomes can have a profound impact on students' overall quality of life (Hamm & Mirenda, 2006; Lund & Light, 2006).

Awareness of the persistence and pervasiveness of these outcomes reinforces and heightens calls to improve the quality of the secondary experiences of youth with significant disabilities (Carter, Ditchman, et al., in press; Rusch et al., 2009). Middle and high school represents an opportune time to provide youth with the learning opportunities, experiences, and relationships that can prepare them for adulthood. Although considerable progress has been made in identifying recommended elements of high-quality secondary educational experiences for youth with disabilities, the field of transition is still fairly young. Despite the emergence of recommended practices in transition, the evidence base for these practices still remains quite uneven—deep in some areas and thin or altogether absent in many others. And for youth with disabilities who use AAC, there is still much the field needs to know.

ORGANIZING FRAMEWORK FOR QUALITY SECONDARY EDUCATIONAL EXPERIENCES

Given the importance and necessity of strengthening the quality of secondary education for *all* students, efforts are under way to align secondary education around the broad themes of rigor, relevance, and relationships (McNulty & Quaglia, 2007). First, all students should access *rigorous* learning opportunities that are challenging, reflect high expectations, and help youth reach their potential. Second, all students should participate in educational experiences that have clear *relevance* for their lives—both now and in the future—and instruction should promote authentic learning. Third, school staff must be intentional about fostering valued *relationships* by providing meaningful opportunities for all youth to know and be known by their peers and school staff, to experience a sense of belonging, and to contribute in valued ways to their school and community. Although these themes have not often focused specifically on the needs of youth with disabilities, the central message of this chapter is that rigor, relevance, and relationships must also characterize the middle and high school experiences of youth who use AAC (McNaughton & Bryen, 2007). Secondary and transition education that attends to *all three* of these areas holds promise for improving postschool outcomes and the quality of life for youth and young adults with disabilities (see Figure 4.1).

How might schools and communities ensure that youth and young adults with disabilities who use AAC participate in experiences defined by rigor, relevance, and relationships? The remainder of this chapter reviews recommended and evidence-based practices for promoting full and meaningful participation of youth with significant disabilities in everyday middle and high school life. Each section addresses the connections among rigor, relevance, and relationships and im-

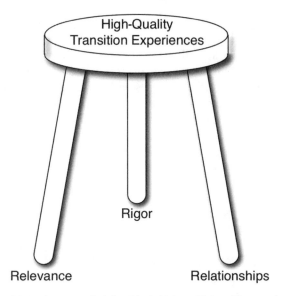

Figure 4.1.   The importance of rigor, relevance, and relationships to high-quality transition experiences.

proved outcomes, barriers to providing these experiences, and recommended and/or research-based strategies for promoting these principles. It is a formidable challenge to address in a single chapter all of the intervention and support strategies needed to ensure that youth both participate fully in the life of their school and leave school well prepared for adulthood. Thus, this chapter highlights just some of the most promising practices and their relevance to youth who use AAC.

It is prudent to begin by emphasizing the considerable diversity among youth with disabilities who use—or would benefit from—AAC. For some students, complex needs in the area of receptive and/or expressive communication represent the primary or exclusive challenge to meaningful school and community participation. Many other youth with significant disabilities, however, have co-occurring disabilities that further increase the complexity of their educational and transition needs. This heterogeneity in strengths, needs, and interests increases the challenges associated with identifying evidence-based practices for transition-age youth who use AAC. As with all aspects of special education and transition services, individualization should be the guiding principle when providing assessment, planning, services, and supports to ensure that the unique needs of every student are addressed.

In writing this chapter, we drew upon both the published research and our own life experiences. Erik, a graduate of Vanderbilt University, is a university-based researcher and teacher educator with a special interest in supporting school-to-work transitions. He summarized the available research, including his own ongoing work, and provided the organizational framework for this chapter. John has a journalism degree from Durham College and is the director of Together We Rock!, a company that provides educational presentations to schools and businesses to promote the inclusion and meaningful participation of people with disabilities. John's experiences as an individual who uses AAC are integrated into this chapter to provide a personal perspective on the research trends identified by Erik (see Box 4.1).

Promoting Rigor

Rigor is evidenced when teachers hold high expectations for every student, design learning experiences that stretch students to realize their potential, provide the individualized supports students will need to succeed, and remove barriers to learning and achievement. For youth with disabilities,

BOX 4.1.   John's Story

My educational journey during middle school and high school was within an inclusive context. As a student with a physical disability and as an augmentative communication user, I experienced both successes and challenges in my academic pursuits. My successes were aided by the presence in my life of visionary parents, open-minded educators, dedicated paraprofessionals, and an exemplary team of communication specialists who were committed to working together to explore possibilities and find solutions. The efforts of these individuals and my own eagerness culminated in my acceptance into a college journalism program.

With my love of writing and passion for the culinary arts, my career goal was to be a restaurant critic for a local newspaper. But as the iconic John Lennon once said, "Life is what happens to you while you're busy making other plans." My experiences at college led me in a different career direction than the one I had planned. While at college, I began to understand that the world is not as accessible to and inclusive of people who have disabilities as I had been led to believe. My efforts to increase accessibility on campus were recognized and honored by my college community. Their encouragement led me, after graduation, to establish a business called Together We Rock!® This entrepreneurial endeavor provides leadership and learning opportunities to community members, employers, media representatives, and students of all ages to build communities that are accessible to and inclusive of people who have a disability.

discussions about rigor increasingly occur within conversations about access to the general education curriculum. Standards-based reform efforts—spurred by an array of legislative, policy, and research initiatives—are challenging schools to ensure that *every* student receives and makes progress within a rigorous academic curriculum addressing a shared set of learning standards. It is widely held that secondary education must focus on promoting high expectations for student learning while simultaneously ensuring that youth receive the quality instruction and individualized supports needed to meet those expectations (Johnson et al., 2002).

Although early efforts to promote inclusion were spurred by philosophical, values-based, and legislative arguments, empirical evidence of the academic, economic, and social benefits associated with the participation in general education of students with significant disabilities—many of whom have AAC-related needs—has steadily accrued (e.g., Cole, Waldron, & Majd, 2004; Hunt & Goetz, 1997; Koppenhaver, Evans, & Yoder, 1991; McNaughton, Light, & Arnold, 2002; Ryndak & Fisher, 2003). Indeed, participation in general education is associated with an array of academic, social, behavioral, and other advantages for students with disabilities. Moreover, general and special educators who have included students who use AAC in their classrooms speak to numerous additional yet less tangible benefits of inclusive education for the students, for peers, and for themselves (Carter & Hughes, 2006; Kent-Walsh & Light, 2003).

Yet inclusive education still remains elusive for most middle and high school students with significant disabilities. Although national educational placement data are not disaggregated based upon whether students use AAC, most students with intellectual disabilities (57%), multiple disabilities (70%), deafblindness (66%), and autism (53%) spend most of their school day outside of general education classrooms (U.S. Department of Education, 2009). Moreover, access to core academic classes such as language arts, math, science, and social studies remains especially limited for these youth during middle and high school (Wagner, Newman, et al., 2004). A central tenet of recommended practices in secondary education is that students have the opportunities and supports needed to access rigorous, relevant, and inclusive learning experiences during adolescence (see Box 4.2).

BOX 4.2. Rigor

Being in an inclusive school environment, I was able to learn from the same range of accomplishments and setbacks as my peers did. I was able to reach my full personal and academic potential as a result of taking challenging classes and attempting a curriculum that many thought I couldn't complete. It is true that taking some advanced courses proved especially difficult. I struggled particularly with the Shakespeare unit of my English course in my final year of high school. As an augmentative and alternative communication user with a conceptual learning disability, I found it very difficult to understand the concepts of theme, character development, plot, and stylistic devices. At the halfway point of the semester, it became clear that despite all of my hard work, and the best efforts of my teacher, I was not going to pass. As a diligent student, I was devastated, but I also gained a tremendous amount of respect for my teacher in treating me the same way he was treating my peers and in having the courage to fail me. At the same time, it proved to be a crucial learning experience, as I gained a better understanding of my strengths and weaknesses. Without participating fully in an inclusive school that had the same expectations of me as of my peers, I doubt that I would have learned that important lesson.

My success in meeting the rigors of the school curriculum depended in large part on the extent to which my educational team worked collaboratively. It was not uncommon for more than 30 professionals to be involved in my life at any one time. It was a constant struggle to get everyone to work together effectively and not to become distracted by their individual mandates, policies, and turfs. It took time for everyone to realize that true collaboration could be achieved only when the team understood everyone's individual roles, clarified expectations in writing, and established communication guidelines.

Also critical to ensuring that I achieved stated academic expectations was the creation of an individualized plan for me. Initially, my individualized education program was characterized by very broad goals that were so vague and generic that it was impossible to measure my progress. It was when the plan featured specific goals and outcomes that we were able to focus on priorities and not get caught up in insignificant details.

Important Elements of Inclusive Education   Although it matters *where* middle and high school students with disabilities who use AAC receive their instruction, it is equally important to attend to *how* youth are supported within these settings. Merely attending a general education class does not automatically confer access to rigorous learning opportunities (Carter, Sisco, Brown, Brickham, & Al-Khabbaz, 2008; Wehmeyer, Lattin, Lapp-Rincker, & Agran, 2003). Research involving students who use AAC has suggested that several elements contribute to high-quality learning experiences within inclusive classrooms (Calculator, 2009; McSheehan, Sonnenmeier, & Jorgensen, 2009). These elements include 1) collaborative teaming, 2) comprehensive and individualized planning, 3) high-quality instruction, 4) appropriate modifications and curricular accommodations, and 5) individualized communication supports.

Collaborative Teaming   A crucial component of quality inclusive education for youth who use AAC is collaborative teaming (Hunt, Soto, Maier, Muller, & Goetz, 2002; Snell & Janney, 2005; Soto, Muller, Hunt, & Goetz, 2001). Meeting the multifaceted needs of youth who use AAC requires the active involvement of multiple individuals with diverse knowledge, expertise, and experience, including general and special educators, related service providers, paraprofessionals, parents, and—particularly during secondary school—youth themselves. These individuals should work collaboratively to identify and work toward a set of shared, individually defined educational and communication goals for a student. Recommended practices indicate that effective teams collectively 1) share a common vision and framework (e.g., beliefs, values, assumptions) for inclusive education; 2) hold regular planning meetings; 3) clarify each member's roles and responsibilities related to service and support delivery; 4) establish a defined process for arriving at consensus decisions; 5) collaboratively develop, prioritize, and implement effective instructional approaches, accommodations, and modifications based on students' goals; and 6) regularly assess the quality and efficacy of the instruction and supports youth receive, problem-solving any issues that arise (Giangreco, 2000; Giangreco, Cloninger, Dennis, & Edelman, 2002; Hunt, Soto, Maier, & Doering, 2003).

Comprehensive and Individualized Planning   Individualized planning involves determining and detailing how students will participate in the full range of instructional, social, and other experiences that take place within inclusive classrooms. For youth who use AAC, attention must be directed toward addressing social, communication, and language needs within the classroom. At the same time, students' academic-related support needs should be given similar attention (see Chapter 3). Several individualized planning models—including the Instructional Activities Assessment (Cushing, Clark, Carter, & Kennedy, 2005), the Beyond Access model (Jorgensen, McSheehan, & Sonnenmeier, 2010; Sonnenmeier, McSheehan, & Jorgensen, 2005), and the Vermont Interdependent Services Team Approach (VISTA; Giangreco, 2000)—have demonstrated promise for children and youth with significant disabilities as part of multicomponent support packages. For example, Hunt, Doering, Hirose-Hatae, Maier, and Goetz (2001), Hunt et al. (2003), and Hunt et al. (2002) evaluated the efficacy of Unified Plans of Support for including students with AAC needs in general education classrooms. These plans were designed by collaborative, interdisciplinary teams within a process that involved 1) assessing the current academic and social needs of the student; 2) determining curricular, communication, and participation support needs; 3) delineating which team member(s) would deliver each support; 4) implementing supports with consistency and fidelity; and 5) continuously evaluating the student's academic and social progress. Students for whom this planning was conducted evidenced improvements in academic skills, class participation, and peer interactions. Although primarily evaluated in elementary classrooms, this planning approach aligns well with secondary classrooms.

High-Quality Instruction   Successful academic learning is predicated on having high expectations for youth with disabilities and a presumption that all students can benefit from strong instruction. Meta-analyses have provided ample evidence that students with significant learning and communication needs can learn core academic skills when provided with systematic instruction (e.g., Browder, Ahlgrim-Delzell, Spooner, Mims, & Baker, 2009; Browder, Spooner, Ahlgrim-Delzell, Harris, & Wakeman, 2008). In addition, innovations in the areas of universal design for learning (Dymond et al., 2006), embedded instruction (Jameson, McDonnell, Polychronis, & Riesen, 2008), differentiated instruction (Lawrence-Brown, 2004), and authentic instruction (Phelps, 2003) hold promise for helping educational teams more effectively meet the needs of all students within inclusive classrooms (see Table 4.1). In other words, curricular materials and instructional approaches should be designed from the outset to meet the educational needs of a heterogeneous classroom, with additional instructional supports provided to address the individualized goals of students who use AAC.

Appropriate Modifications and Curricular Accommodations   Although students who use AAC should be working toward similar learning standards as their same-age peers, they may demonstrate progress on those standards in somewhat different ways. Educational teams must

Table 4.1.   Some elements of high-quality instruction

Approach	Definition
Universal design for learning	The designing of curricula and instruction so that, from the outset, it is accessible to a wide range of learners. Universal design for learning principles call for "multiple means of representation...multiple means of action and expression...and multiple means of engagement" (Center for Applied Special Technology, 2008, pp. 2–3).
Embedded instruction	Systematic instruction within the ongoing and natural opportunities that exist within inclusive classrooms and other settings. Unlike massed practice teaching formats, instruction occurs within the context of typical routines, activities, and transitions.
Differentiated instruction	The process of "ensuring that what a student learns, how he/she learns it, and how the student demonstrates what he/she has learned is a match for that student's readiness level, interests, and preferred mode of learning" (Tomlinson, 2004, p. 188).
Authentic instruction	Instruction that promotes higher order thinking, depth of knowledge, connectedness to the world beyond the classroom, substantive conversation, and social support for student achievement (Newman & Wehlage, 1993).

identify and develop the modifications and accommodations youth will need to participate fully in all aspects of classroom activities and to demonstrate their academic learning (Calculator, 2009). These accommodations and modifications should be identified during the planning process but continuously evaluated to determine their relevance and effectiveness.

Individualized Communication Supports   The quality and extent of AAC services provided during adolescence can influence the outcomes youth attain upon leaving high school (Lund & Light, 2007). Education teams must "understand what AAC means for individual students, [understand] how to identify learning opportunities for communication development, understand their individual roles in teaching communication skills, and learn specific strategies for teaching those skills" (Downing, 2005, p. 134). Team members should carefully assess students' communication needs within the classroom 1) to ensure that students can actively participate in and contribute to the full range of instructional and learning activities and 2) to address communication-related barriers that could impede participation.

Individually Designed Natural Supports   Careful consideration should be given to the specific approaches used to support youth who use AAC within general education classrooms. Schools rely heavily or exclusively on adults—such as paraprofessionals, special educators, or related service providers—individually assigned to support the inclusion of a particular middle or high school student with significant disabilities in classrooms and school activities (Suter & Giangreco, 2009). At the same time, available research suggests that there may be distinct advantages to relying on more natural avenues of support within inclusive classrooms.

Peer Supports   The capacity of youth to naturally and effectively provide support to their classmates is substantial, yet youth are rarely drawn upon to support inclusive educational experiences. An array of peer-mediated intervention strategies, including cooperative learning groups, peer tutoring, and peer-assisted learning strategies (e.g., Jameson et al., 2008; Stenhoff & Lingugaris, 2007), have been evaluated in the literature. Peer support strategies hold particular promise within secondary classrooms given their flexibility and feasibility. Peer support arrangements typically involve one or more students without disabilities providing academic, social, and other supports to classmates with disabilities while receiving guidance and feedback from educators and/or paraprofessionals (Carter & Kennedy, 2006). For example, students might support goals related to academics (e.g., working together on assignments, providing feedback on performance, highlighting key concepts, reviewing course content), classroom participation (e.g., demonstrating self-management strategies, sharing class materials), communication (e.g., reinforcing communication attempts, modeling social skills), and/or peer interaction (e.g., exchanging social and emotional support, conversing about shared interests, making introductions to classmates).

Research suggests that when provided with initial information, basic strategies, and ongoing support from paraprofessionals and other educators, peers can effectively support the academic and social participation of youth who use AAC in inclusive classrooms. Specifically, for students with significant disabilities, peer support interventions have been associated with increased engagement in ongoing instruction, access to curricular content, academic achievement, and attainment of individually determined goals (Carter, Cushing, Clark, & Kennedy, 2005; Carter, Sisco, Melekoglu, & Kurkowski, 2007; Gilberts, Agran, Hughes, & Wehmeyer, 2001; Jameson et al., 2008). At the same time, peers who have the opportunity to work with and get to know their classmates with disabilities also receive substantive benefits, including increased academic engagement, greater advocacy skills, deeper understanding of diversity, personal growth, and the opportunity to develop new friendships (Copeland et al., 2004; Cushing & Kennedy, 1997; Shukla, Kennedy, & Cushing, 1998). Collectively, these findings call into question the extensive reliance on adults as the exclusive or dominant avenue of support in many secondary classrooms.

Paraprofessional Supports   The influence of paraprofessionals on the academic and social participation of youth with disabilities is fairly complex and multifaceted. During adolescence, the manner in which adults provide support to youth can either foster or inadvertently stifle academic engagement and peer interactions (Carter, Sisco, et al., 2008; Giangreco, Edelman, MacFarland, & Luiselli, 1997; Shukla et al., 1998; Simpson, Beukelman, & Sharpe, 2000). As peers become more actively involved and confident in supporting the academic and social participation of their classmates with significant disabilities, paraprofessionals should typically begin fading their close proximity and assuming other responsibilities within the classroom (e.g., supporting the classroom teacher in meeting the needs of all students, collecting data on individualized education program progress). However, the facilitative efforts of paraprofessionals can still serve to promote collaborative work and create important social connections among students with and without disabilities (Causton-Theoharis & Malmgren, 2005). To foster these outcomes, paraprofessionals will likely need training on strategies for identifying, creating, and reinforcing opportunities for students to use AAC during interactions with peers and educators (Bingham, Spooner, & Browder, 2007).

General Educator Supports   The attitudes and knowledge general educators hold related to inclusion and to the specific needs of youth with disabilities who use AAC are often cited as potential barriers to access to general education (Carter & Hughes, 2006; Giangreco et al., 1997; Kent-Walsh & Light, 2003). Recommended practices emphasize the importance of general educators holding high expectations for all students in their classroom and assuming primary instructional responsibilities for students with disabilities rather than deferring to paraprofessionals or special educators. Including general educators—who possess content and pedagogical expertise—as active members of collaborative educational teams is an important aspect of promoting rigor. When it comes to assuming these roles, general educators have articulated a need for high-quality professional development, coaching, and/or other learning opportunities that will encourage and equip them to adopt and integrate effective support and instructional practices into their classroom instruction (Beck et al., 2001; Kent-Walsh & Light, 2003; Soto et al., 2001).

Related Services Provider Supports   Trends toward inclusive education are also challenging related services providers (e.g., speech-language pathologists, occupational therapists, physical therapists, assistive technology specialists) to reconsider where and how they provide support services to AAC users. Pull-out approaches have been replaced by inclusive models in which needed services and supports are delivered and integrated within the ongoing routines of the classroom (Giangreco et al., 1997; Giangreco, Prelock, Reid, Dennis, & Edelman, 2000). Given the shifting role adults play in the lives of adolescents, one salient concern involves finding avenues for delivering these supports in ways that do not stigmatize or draw undue attention to specific youth. Interviews with and surveys of related service providers have also suggested a continued need for both innovation and research to 1) ensure that related service providers maintain appropriately sized caseloads to allow for active contributions to the educational team; 2) provide adequate time to plan, coordinate, and/or deliver support within the classroom; and 3) deliver preservice and professional development training that builds expertise and confidence in areas such as literacy, language, and curricular access (Beck et al., 2001; Dowden et al., 2006).

Self-Directed Supports   The emphasis on promoting self-determination and independence among middle and high school students with disabilities has spurred the development of an array of student-directed learning strategies (see Chapter 2). These strategies are designed to provide instruction on self-determination skills (e.g., choice making, goal setting, self-management, and self-evaluation) with the aim of involving youth more actively in their own learning and in recruiting needed supports. Such strategies increase the independence of youth who use AAC within inclusive classrooms, promote acquisition of academic skills, elevate expectations for what youth with significant disabilities can accomplish, and decrease students' extensive or exclusive reliance on educators for ongoing or constant support (e.g., Agran, Cavin, Wehmeyer, & Palmer, 2006; Hughes et al., 2002; Palmer, Wehmeyer, Gipson, & Agran, 2004). For example, Gilberts and colleagues (2001) involved peers in teaching five middle school students with significant disabilities to self-monitor their use of 11 academic survival skills (e.g., bringing appropriate materials to class, greeting peers and teachers, asking questions). All of the students readily learned to self-manage their own behavior, evidenced increased participation in classroom activities, and interacted more with teachers and peers.

Ensuring Relevance

Accessing a rigorous academic curriculum ensures that youth who use AAC have opportunities to learn important skills and knowledge as well as opens doors to new postsecondary educational and employment opportunities. At the same time, youth should experience a broad range of learning opportunities that extend beyond the academic domain and that have relevance for other aspects of their lives during and after leaving school (Bassett & Kochhar-Bryant, 2006). Relevance is evidenced when learning opportunities are engaging, build upon and expand students' interests and strengths, offer a blend of personal experiences in and linkages to the community, and equip youth with the skills and knowledge they will need to be active citizens and participate meaningfully in the life of their community. Although most middle and high schools are rich with opportunities to gain these experiences, youth with disabilities often are not active participants in these activities (Kleinert, Miracle, & Sheppard-Jones, 2007; Wagner, Cadwallader, Garza, & Cameto, 2004). This participation gap—which remains sizable in most secondary schools—must be addressed through intentional planning and well-designed supports. This section highlights three avenues through which all middle and high school students—and particularly students who use AAC—might access experiences that provide contextualized learning, offer opportunities to develop interests, and address real-life issues: 1) extracurricular and after-school activities; 2) work-based learning and career development experiences; and 3) service-learning, community service, and volunteering (see Box 4.3).

Extracurricular and After-School Activities   Involvement in extracurricular activities has been associated with a number of substantial benefits for youth (Mahoney, Harris, & Eccles, 2006; McGuire & McDonnell, 2008). Such experiences can provide students with enjoyable and

BOX 4.3.   Relevance

In my educational experience, *relevance* simply meant that what I was learning would have benefit for my current or future life. Like most typical middle and high school students, I did not appreciate the value of some of the things I studied until much later in life; however, there were circumstances in which the relevance of a subject to my life was simply not there. For example, as a student in Ontario, Canada, I was required to take French as part of the middle school curriculum. Within the context of providing an inclusive educational environment, my communication display board was translated, and specialized French software was purchased for my communication technology. Suddenly, a second language was introduced into my life when I was having enough trouble mastering English. After a few weeks, I was totally frustrated, and my progress was dismal. In a school meeting, I questioned the relevance of having to learn to communicate in French when I couldn't effectively communicate in my primary language of English. Eventually, after several meetings, the school board granted me an exemption from the subject of French, and I pursued another academic subject in its place.

As I entered high school, I began a dialogue with family, friends, and professionals regarding my future. Basically, I wanted an immediate answer to the question "What am I going to do with the rest of my life?" But I was only really able to answer that question after participating in various learning opportunities that helped me to begin to understand my strengths, limitations, and interests. For example, I took optional subjects, such as entrepreneurial studies—and an independent class project that focused on creating a business—that provided valuable information relevant to my future as an entrepreneur. There was also a work-based learning opportunity at a local community newspaper that proved to be a win–win situation for both my employer and me. My assignments enabled me to improve my writing skills, and my employer learned firsthand about the need and requirement to have a workplace that is accessible to and inclusive of people who have a disability.

motivating contexts for discovering and deepening their interests, strengths, and preferences; create new opportunities to affiliate with peers and teachers, develop friendships, and access social support; foster a sense of belonging and value within the school community; and promote acquisition of important recreational, social, self-determination, academic, and everyday life skills that prepare youth for adulthood and provide lifelong enjoyment. A well-rounded secondary education should provide opportunities for youth who use AAC to participate in inclusive extracurricular activities that bring satisfaction, build skills, and enhance relationships.

However, research suggests that the extracurricular involvement of youth with significant disabilities is strikingly limited. Parent interview findings from the National Longitudinal Transition Study-2 indicated that only 33% of youth with intellectual disabilities, 30% of youth with autism, and 37% of youth with multiple disabilities participated in any organized school activities outside of class during the previous year (Wagner, Cadwallader, et al., 2004). Such involvement appears to be particularly limited for youth who use assistive technology and/or who have more significant disabilities (Kleinert et al., 2007). Similarly, empirical studies have identified a number of salient barriers to extracurricular involvement, including the attitudes of activity sponsors, low expectations among educators and/or parents, limited opportunities for youth to make choices about desired involvement, insufficient social and personal supports, inadequate instruction on relevant skills, absence of flexible communication devices and assistive technology, limited transportation, and inaccessible activities (e.g., Dattilo et al., 2008; Powers et al., 2005).

Although no experimental studies have focused on increasing extracurricular involvement for youth who use AAC, available research suggests promising steps. Consistent with directives contained within the Individuals with Disabilities Education Improvement Act (IDEA) of 2004 (PL 108-446), educational teams should intentionally address the services and supports youth with disabilities who use AAC need to "participate in extracurricular and other nonacademic activities" (§300.320[a][4][ii]). Carter, Swedeen, Moss, and Pesko (in press) identified a series of steps educational teams might take to foster broader school and community involvement, including 1) assessing extracurricular opportunities and barriers that exist in a school; 2) actively engaging youth in identifying opportunities that build upon their interests; 3) equipping youth with the skills and communication supports needed to participate meaningfully in desired activities; 4) preparing educators, activity sponsors, and/or peers to provide needed supports and accommodations; 5) keeping families informed about and involved in supporting extracurricular opportunities; and 6) expanding the roles and experiences youth have over time. To increase such participation, educators and service providers should be encouraged to prioritize extracurricular involvement as a domain within transition planning; to ensure that the recreation and leisure activities of youth who use AAC are not characterized as solitary, stereotypical, sedentary, or segregated; and to secure the active support of family members, as extracurricular activities often extend beyond the school day and necessitate parental support (Carter, Ditchman, et al., in press; Rose, McDonnell, & Ellis, 2007).

Work-Based Learning and Career Development Experiences

Adolescence is a time when most youth participate in school- or community-based work experiences that can equip them with important occupational skills and values, inform their career decision making, and shape their aspirations for the future (Vondracek & Porfeli, 2003). Recognizing these valuable benefits, secondary educators have long played a role in designing, offering, or sponsoring experiences that further the preparation of youth for the world of work (Phelps & Hanley-Maxwell, 1997; Will, 1984). Such work experiences may be especially important for youth who use AAC, providing a meaningful context for learning functional and social skills, informing future career plans, expanding social networks, and promoting self-determination skills. At the same time, successful high school work experiences can raise the career-related expectations of youth, their parents, employers, and community members. Involvement in work experiences during middle and high school not only is a normative adolescent experience (Zimmer-Gembeck & Mortimer, 2006), but it also represents one of the most consistent predictors of favorable postschool employment outcomes for youth with disabilities (e.g., Benz, Lindstrom, & Yovanoff, 2000).

Research describing the early work and career development experiences of youth with significant disabilities has clearly emphasized the need for intentional efforts to increase access to these experiences for youth who use AAC (Carter, Ditchman, et al., in press; Estrada-Hernandez, Wadsworth, Nietupski, Warth, & Winslow, 2008). Yet findings from Wave 1 of the National Longitudinal Transition Study-2 indicated that fewer than one third of youth with intellectual disabilities, autism, or multiple disabilities were involved in school-sponsored work experiences or held a paid after-school and/or summer job (Wagner, Cadwallader, & Marder, 2003). Too many youth with disabilities are exiting school without the skills, attitudes, experiences, and linkages that will launch them successfully into the world of work and/or inform their career paths.

Although numerous model demonstration projects, research studies, and policy initiatives have coalesced into a set of recommended guidelines for high-quality, early work experiences, there have been few rigorous evaluations of—and limited involvement of AAC users in—these intervention efforts. Carter, Trainor, Ditchman, Swedeen, and Owens (in press) examined the efficacy of a multicomponent intervention package to increase the summer employment experiences of youth with significant disabilities. Youth who participated in intentional planning efforts and accessed support from identified school staff and employer liaisons were 4 times more likely to obtain paid, community-based jobs during the summer than youth who did not access these strategies. Quality indicators articulated by the National Alliance for Secondary Education and Transition (2005) highlight the importance of ensuring that all youth 1) participate in career awareness, exploration, and preparatory activities; 2) enroll in courses and programs that integrate career development activities; 3) receive instruction that promotes the acquisition of employment and technical skills, knowledge, and behaviors; and 4) have opportunities to participate in meaningful school- and community-based work experiences of their choosing.

At the same time, several prominent barriers to meaningful involvement in these activities for youth who use AAC must be addressed. Research has suggested that more concerted efforts may be needed to assist youth in developing needed employment and collateral skills, expanding their social networks (Carey, Potts, Bryen, & Shankar, 2004), strengthening their literacy skills (Foley & Staples, 2003), and increasing their access to and fluency with communication systems aligned with the range of social- and work-related interactions that take place in the workplace and during the interview process (McNaughton & Bryen, 2002). Concurrently, steps must be taken to dispel myths and attitudinal barriers evidenced among employers; increase access to transportation and worksite accessibility; develop natural supports that enhance workplace performance, status, and relationships; and equip special educators and job coaches to collaborate effectively with coworkers and supervisors (Bryen, Potts, & Carey, 2007; Luecking, 2008; McNaughton et al., 2002).

Service-Learning, Community Service, and Volunteering   Conversations about school reform efforts increasingly highlight the importance of promoting civic engagement and community involvement as integral elements of rigorous, relevant secondary educational experiences. Service-learning and volunteer experiences are both advocated as promising avenues for helping middle and high school students recognize the relevance of what they learn in school to the world outside of the classroom and to their future goals (Dymond, Renzaglia, & Chun, 2008b). Hands-on service experiences have the potential to benefit youth by promoting school and community engagement, instilling a sense of civic pride, enhancing self-esteem and motivation, teaching academic and life skills in applied contexts, developing leadership skills, and expanding awareness of career and community opportunities (Brill, 1994; Miller et al., 2002). At the same time, well-designed service activities place youth with disabilities in valued roles in which they have meaningful opportunities to contribute to their school and community, work alongside their peers, and gain community-based experiences.

Although substantial numbers of middle and high schools offer service-learning or community service experiences as part of their curricular offerings, youth with significant disabilities either have had limited participation in these experiences (Wagner, Newman, et al., 2004) or have been the focus of such service efforts (Gurecka & Gent, 2001). Efforts to expand access to meaningful, inclusive service opportunities during secondary school have the potential to foster skills, attitudes, and experiences that promote civic engagement; they may also shift societal perspectives about the contributions that youth who use AAC might make to their communities and dispel myths that people with disabilities should be the designated beneficiaries of service endeavors.

Although these experiences are widely advocated, research addressing service-learning and volunteer experiences for adolescents with significant disabilities is still emerging (Brill, 1994; Trembath, Balandin, & Togher, 2009). Dymond, Renzaglia, and Chun (2007, 2008b) examined key elements characterizing high-quality service-learning programs. Their research suggests that service-learning projects should occur within an authentic context (i.e., meet real needs within the actual settings), link directly with the academic curriculum and with state standards, involve sustained school–community–home partnerships, receive sufficient administrative and resource support, include extended service engagement, address several programmatic components (i.e., learning, service, reflection, celebration, program evaluation), and promote active student and teacher/

adult participation. However, additional research is needed to identify how these elements can best be implemented within inclusive experiences (Dymond, Renzaglia, & Chun, 2008a; Gent & Gurecka, 1998).

As with the other out-of-the-classroom experiences described in this section, several barriers must be addressed to ensure that youth with significant disabilities who use AAC can participate meaningfully (Miller, Schleien, & Bellini, 2003). For example, secondary educators and program coordinators will need to ensure that volunteer sites are accessible, youth are involved in selecting and directing service activities, appropriate modifications and adaptations are established, high expectations for participation are held for all youth, peers and adults are equipped with adequate information and skills to support students with disabilities, students' communication-related needs are continually assessed and addressed, and activities are aligned with students' individualized education program goals. As within inclusive classrooms, peer support strategies represent a promising approach for promoting active participation, learning, and social relationships within service-learning and volunteer activities (Hughes & Carter, 2008).

Fostering Relationships

When most youth talk about school, conversations turn quickly to their friendships and activities they share with their peers. It is through their interactions and relationships with peers that adolescents develop a sense of self; exchange social, emotional, and other support systems; learn peer norms and values; and acquire social, academic, self-determination, and other valuable life skills (Brown & Klute, 2003; Gifford-Smith & Brownell, 2003). Most important, peer relationships can provide a sense of enjoyment, promote engagement in school, and influence one's quality of life. It is clear that relationships can have a profound impact on the lives of students. Put simply, every middle and high school student should experience a sense of belonging, be recognized, and know—and be known by—their peers.

For youth and young adults who use AAC, these relationships are *no less* important (Schnorr, 1997). Peer relationships have been linked to numerous benefits for youth with significant disabilities, including social, academic, and functional skill development; improved social competence; broader school inclusion; enhanced social networks; and increased school engagement (Carter & Hughes, 2005; Hunt & Goetz, 1997). At the same time, such relationships become increasingly elusive during adolescence. Throughout middle and high school, peer group affiliations assume greater importance, interactions shift away from the presence of adults, and the ways and contexts in which students interact increase in complexity. When students with significant disabilities have limited involvement in general education classes and extracurricular activities, as well as rely extensively or exclusively on adults for direct support, their opportunities to develop and maintain relationships may be severely curtailed.

The previous sections on rigor and relevance addressed the range of locations and contexts within which youth should spend their school day. However, the quality of these learning experiences is clearly influenced by the interactions and relationships that youth have—or do not have—with their peers in these settings. This section addresses 1) critical elements for supporting peer relationships, 2) promising strategies for use within and beyond the classroom, and 3) the importance of supportive relationships with adults (see Box 4.4).

Critical Elements for Supporting Peer Relationships   Numerous studies have suggested that relationships among students with and without significant disabilities are unlikely to occur apart from intentional efforts (Carter & Hughes, 2005; Carter, Sisco, et al., 2008; Snell, Chen, & Hoover, 2006). At the same time, myriad qualitative, descriptive, and intervention studies have identified important elements that may set the occasion for interactions to occur and may

BOX 4.4.   Relationships

Of utmost importance to me was having a sense of belonging in my school community. By virtue of my physical and communication challenges, I didn't readily fit into the social circles of high school. This reality, combined with the lack of knowledge on the part of many school personnel on how to promote disability awareness or foster peer relationships, resulted in many missed opportunities. One example in high school was how lockers of students who had a disability were grouped in a separate location rather than integrated into the alphabetical order of the rest of the student population. Another example was the practice of having students who had a disability work with paraprofessionals in a segregated resource room during free periods rather than allowing us to interact with our peers in the school library. These practices limited my chances of connecting with my peers, and I was successful in my efforts to persuade school officials to change them. My involvement in extracurricular activities such as the Yearbook Club, social justice events, and school dances proved to be a valuable way for my peers to get to know me. I even ran for Student Council one year to increase my profile. But it was a struggle to be accepted. Eventually I did experience true friendship. Although I was not the most popular student at high school, I did have friends with whom I went to school sports events, skipped school (only once!), and went to the senior prom. I have often wondered how much more rewarding my high school experiences would have been had more of the teachers and paraprofessionals in my life understood the critical connection between fostering relationships and achieving educational success.

encourage relationships to develop among youth with and without significant disabilities. The following sections address some of these elements as they relate to youth who use AAC.

Flexible and Relevant Communication Systems   The quantity and quality of students' interactions will be enhanced by the availability and accessibility of communication systems that are contextually relevant to the types and range of interactions adolescents have with their peers and others (Williams, Krezman, & McNaughton, 2008). The diversity, complexity, and nuance of adolescent interactions and relationships mean that careful attention must be given to ensuring the relevance, flexibility, and acceptability of students' communication systems (Smith, 2005). The instruction youth receive and the communication systems they use should allow for more than simply making basic requests and discrete choices. In other words, youth need the flexibility to greet someone they pass in the hallway, engage in social conversation over lunch, offer and receive assistance during small-group activities, and invite a classmate to hang out together after school. Youth should also be given opportunities to contribute meaningfully to decisions about the communication systems and devices they prefer using in different contexts.

Instruction in Social and Communication Skills   The social and communication skills students possess can also influence the quality and range of interactions they have with their peers. Several systematic reviews have identified evidence-based instructional strategies for building social and communication skills among middle and high school students who use AAC (Carter & Hughes, 2005; Snell et al., 2006). For example, successful intervention efforts have focused on teaching discrete social skills (e.g., initiations, social amenities, conversational turn taking), communication device use (e.g., communication books, speech-generating devices), self-management skills (e.g., self-prompting, self-monitoring, and self-instructing interactions), and collateral skills (e.g., leisure and related skills that provide a context for interactions). These intervention efforts typically are individualized, systematic, and sustained, and usually involve peers in delivering instruction or serving as conversational partners.

Meaningful and Regular Opportunities   In many middle and high schools, opportunities for students with and without disabilities to interact with one another are either uneven or altogether unavailable. Although having reliable means of communication and the requisite skills to interact is essential, youth also need meaningful and regular interaction opportunities. Educational teams should ensure that youth who use AAC have sustained and recurring opportunities to engage in shared learning and social activities together with their classmates—whether in the classroom, at lunch, during breaks, or in extracurricular and after-school activities (Carter, Swedeen, & Kurkowski, 2008). Moreover, these should be high-interest activities that engage youth with disabilities in valued roles.

Relevant Information   Some peers may evidence uncertainty or hesitation about interacting with a classmate who uses AAC, particularly if they have had few prior opportunities to get to know one another (Siperstein, Parker, Bardon, & Widaman, 2007). Youth are likely to benefit—at least initially—from additional information and guidance on how to interact with and support one another (Copeland et al., 2004; Kent-Walsh & McNaughton, 2005). This information often is quite targeted, focusing on helping peers learn about a student's interests, as well as the ways in which he or she communicates, benefits from specific supports, or participates in typical activities (Carter & Kennedy, 2006; Haring & Breen, 1992). Although the focus of communication partner–directed interventions efforts should be individually determined, several example issues highlighted in the literature include 1) recognizing and responding to naturally occurring communicative opportunities or events, 2) learning how to interact with someone using a specific approach or device, 3) identifying and interpreting more subtle or idiosyncratic communicative behaviors, 4) implementing effective facilitation strategies, and 5) fostering interactions with other peers (e.g., Carter et al., 2007; Kent-Walsh, 2008; Sigafoos, 1999). As much as possible, youth should be involved in determining what information is shared, how, and by whom—an important aspect of fostering self-determination.

Supporting Interactions in the Classroom   Although middle and high school students may spend 6 hours or more per day in classrooms, these learning contexts are still replete with opportunities to interact and establish relationships with classmates. The peer support strategies discussed previously represent one evidence-based approach for promoting social interaction skill acquisition, expanding students' social networks, and promoting new friendships. These arrangements provide teacher-sanctioned interaction opportunities, involve peers in modeling and reinforcing communication skills, and reduce the ongoing need for adult presence. At the same time, the manner in which instruction is delivered and supports provided also influences the opportunities youth have to work and interact together. Although didactic, lecture-based instructional approaches dominate many secondary classrooms, cooperative grouping arrangements hold considerable promise for promoting both peer interaction and academic engagement (Jacques, Wilton, & Townsend, 1998). Finally, students who use AAC should be explicitly taught the social, communication, and literacy skills needed to participate fully in, and contribute meaningfully to, the life of the classroom (Downing, 2005).

Promoting Relationships Outside of the Classroom   Attention should also be directed toward the range of noninstructional times (e.g., lunch, breaks, homeroom, before and after school) during which friendships form and deepen. There is some empirical support that peer network interventions address the social-related needs of youth that extend beyond the classroom and school day (Haring & Breen, 1992; Hughes & Carter, 2008). These strategies typically involve identifying a small group of peers who are interested in getting to know their schoolmate with significant disabilities, providing initial orientation regarding the roles peers should and should not assume, and meeting periodically to problem-solve challenges and expand the network. In addition, logistical issues related to transportation, safety, accessibility, scheduling, and costs may need to be addressed when activities and interactions extend off campus.

The advent and rapid proliferation of technological innovations is also transforming how and where youth interact with one another, the avenues through which they remain connected, and the contexts in which friendship take place. Web-based social networking sites (e.g., Facebook, My-Space) and online communities are emerging as primary contexts through which youth exchange information and make social plans. Similarly, e-mail, text messaging, and instant messaging technologies are redefining the ways in which youth communicate and interact with one another outside of the school day. Although such innovations have great potential for expanding communication access for youth who use AAC, many challenges to access remain, and little research is available to guide these efforts. Youth—as well as their teachers and parents—may benefit from instruction in the use of the social-related technologies, appropriate adaptations to ensure that these technologies are accessible, seamless integration between communication systems and these technologies, and sufficient opportunities to use them.

Importance of Supportive Relationships with Adults   Although the primary emphasis in this section has been on fostering relationships with peers, it is important to acknowledge the influential role that adult–youth relationships can play in promoting school engagement, learning, and quality of life. Ensuring that every youth—especially youth with significant disabilities—has a caring and supportive relationship with an adult (e.g., special educator, extracurricular sponsor, guidance counselor, general educator) is a recommended component of both dropout prevention and school engagement efforts (Sinclair, Christenson, & Thurlow, 2005). Although most youth with AAC often have an abundance of adults and professionals in their daily lives, it is important that they feel assured that the adults in their lives are focused on their well-being and educational success.

RESEARCH RECOMMENDATIONS

As noted throughout this chapter, there is much still to learn about how best to design secondary educational and transition experiences that enhance learning, relationships, quality of life, and other valued outcomes for youth and young adults who use AAC. The following research areas hold promise for filling critical gaps in the evidence base.

First, although individualized educational and transition planning is specifically mandated in IDEA 2004 (PL 108-446), there is little empirical guidance addressing the most effective approaches for actively involving youth who use AAC in these critical conversations about their plans for life during and after high school (Lohrmann-O'Rourke & Gomez, 2001; Test et al., 2004). Sorely needed are evidence-based models for supporting youth with significant communication disabilities in making meaningful contributions to both assessment and planning efforts.

Second, self-determination has emerged as a central concept within the field of transition, and adolescence represents an opportune time to foster the attitudes, behaviors, knowledge, and experiences that enhance self-determination. Research should explore the ways in which the various educational experiences described in this chapter might be designed and aligned to promote self-determination among youth who use AAC. Previous studies have focused largely on the self-determination needs of youth with less extensive support needs.

Third, to enhance the acceptability, relevance, and sustainability of recommended secondary education and transition practices for youth who use AAC, additional efforts should be made to incorporate into research endeavors the perspectives of youth themselves on their experiences during high school, their perceptions of their own support and service needs, and their recommendations for the ways in which educators and related service providers should address these needs

(Broer, Doyle, & Giangreco, 2005; Clarke, McConachie, Price, & Wood, 2001). However, capturing the perspectives of youth with significant communication challenges will require innovative and alternative approaches for conducting social validity assessments.

Fourth, the increasing cultural and linguistic diversity among students in the United States is mirrored among youth who use AAC and their families. As the secondary and transition evidence base both broadens and deepens, attention must be given to ensuring that those practices validated in the literature reflect the values, expectations, resources, and circumstances of diverse youth and their families; are responsive to the varied ways in which youth and their families communicate; and are effective for the broad range of students with disabilities served in U.S. schools (Huer, Parette, & Saenz, 2001).

Fifth, the fields of secondary transition and AAC are rapidly evolving, and it is essential that educators and service providers remain on the cusp of emerging developments in evidence-based practices. Future research should explore the efficacy of preservice training and professional development opportunities for equipping general and special educators, paraprofessionals, and related service providers with the attitudes, knowledge, strategies, and initiative to design instruction and supports that enhance the school and community participation of adolescents who use AAC (Kent-Walsh & Light, 2003; Soto et al., 2001). In particular, research exploring the integration of emerging AAC technologies with developments in inclusive instructional strategies is needed.

Sixth, an understanding of the complexity and scope of secondary education and transition services for youth with significant disabilities will require the application of a constellation of research designs, interpretive strategies, and measures. The identification of evidence-based practices will likely be enhanced when multiple methodologies (e.g., experimental, single case, qualitative, survey) can be carefully and thoughtfully integrated to illuminate which educational practices work best for which students under which conditions.

CONCLUSION

The experiences and opportunities youth with significant disabilities have during middle and high school really do matter. Access to a rigorous curriculum can raise expectations and lead youth to perform to their potential. Relevant educational opportunities can enable youth to make meaningful connections between learning and life. And the relationships youth develop can make the journey through middle and high school an enjoyable one. Although youth who use AAC may require more intentional and individualized services and supports to participate fully in the life of their school, rigor, relevance, and relationships are still critically important. If secondary schools are intentional about addressing these three elements for youth with and without significant disabilities, will it elevate achievement, promote belonging, and better prepare them for life high school? The best evidence suggests yes. However, systematic and sustained efforts are needed to develop a strong and broad evidence base focused on improving the quality of educational and transition services for youth who use or would benefit from AAC.

REFERENCES

Agran, M., Cavin, M., Wehmeyer, M., & Palmer, S. (2006). Participation of students with moderate to severe disabilities in the general curriculum: The effects of the self-determined learning model of instruction. *Research and Practice for Persons with Severe Disabilities, 31,* 230–241.

Bassett, D.S., & Kochhar-Bryant, C.A. (2006). Strategies for aligning standards-based education and transition. *Focus on Exceptional Children, 39*(2), 1–19.

Beck, A.R., Thompson, J.R., Clay, S.I., Hutchins, M., Vogt, W.P., Romaniak, B., et al. (2001). Preservice professionals' attitudes toward children who use augmentative/alternative communication. *Education and Training in Mental Retardation and Developmental Disabilities, 36,* 255–271.

Benz, M.R., Lindstrom, L., & Yovanoff, P. (2000). Improving graduation and employment outcomes of students with disabilities: Predictive factors and student perspectives. *Exceptional Children, 66,* 509–529.

Bingham, M.A., Spooner, F., & Browder, D. (2007). Training paraeducators to promote the use of augmentative and alternative communication by students with significant disabilities. *Education and Training in Developmental Disabilities, 42,* 339–352.

Brill, C.R. (1994). The effects of participation in service-learning on adolescents with disabilities. *Journal of Adolescence, 17,* 369–380.

Broer, S.M., Doyle, M.B., & Giangreco, M.F. (2005). Perspectives of students with intellectual disabilities about their experiences with paraprofessional support. *Exceptional Children, 71,* 415–430.

Browder, D., Ahlgrim-Delzell, L., Spooner, F., Mims, P.J., & Baker, J.N. (2009). Using time delay to teach literacy to students with severe developmental disabilities. *Exceptional Children, 75,* 343–364.

Browder, D.M., Spooner, F., Ahlgrim-Delzell, L., Harris, A., & Wakeman, S. (2008). A meta-analysis on teaching mathematics to students with significant disabilities. *Exceptional Children, 74,* 407–432.

Brown, B.B., & Klute, C. (2003). Friendships, cliques, and crowds. In G.R. Adams & M.D. Berzonsky (Eds.), *Blackwell handbook of adolescence* (pp. 330–348). Malden, MA: Blackwell.

Bryen, D.N., Potts, B., & Carey, A. (2007). So you want to work? What employers say about needed skills, job search, and hiring. *Augmentative and Alternative Communication, 22,* 1–9.

Calculator, S.N. (2009). Augmentative and alternative communication (AAC) and inclusive education for students with the most severe disabilities. *International Journal of Inclusive Education, 13,* 93–113.

Carey, A.C., Potts, B., Bryen, D.N., & Shankar, J.A. (2004). Networking towards employment: Experiences of people who use augmentative and alternative communication. *Research and Practice for Persons with Severe Disabilities, 29,* 40–52.

Carter, E.W., Cushing, L.S., Clark, N.M., & Kennedy, C.H. (2005). Effects of peer support interventions on students' access to the general curriculum and social interactions. *Research and Practice for Persons with Severe Disabilities, 30,* 15–25.

Carter, E.W., Ditchman, N., Sun, Y., Trainor, A.A., Swedeen, B., & Owens, L. (in press). Summer employment and community experiences of transition-age youth with severe disabilities. *Exceptional Children.*

Carter, E.W., & Hughes, C. (2005). Increasing social interaction among adolescents with intellectual disabilities and their general education peers: Effective interventions. *Research and Practice for Persons with Severe Disabilities, 30,* 179–193.

Carter, E.W., & Hughes, C. (2006). Including high school students with severe disabilities in general education classes: Perspectives of general and special educators, paraprofessionals, and administrators. *Research and Practice for Persons with Severe Disabilities, 31,* 174–185.

Carter, E.W., & Kennedy, C.H. (2006). Promoting access to the general curriculum using peer support strategies. *Research and Practice for Persons with Severe Disabilities, 31,* 284–292.

Carter, E.W., Sisco, L.G., Brown, L., Brickham, D., & Al-Khabbaz, Z.A. (2008). Peer interactions and academic engagement of youth with developmental disabilities in inclusive middle and high school classrooms. *American Journal on Mental Retardation, 113,* 479–494.

Carter, E.W., Sisco, L.G., Melekoglu, M., & Kurkowski, C. (2007). Peer supports as an alternative to individually assigned paraprofessionals in inclusive high school classrooms. *Research and Practice for Persons with Severe Disabilities, 32,* 213–227.

Carter, E.W., Swedeen, B., & Kurkowski, C. (2008). Friendship matters: Fostering social relationships in secondary schools. *TASH Connections, 34*(6), 9–12, 14.

Carter, E.W., Swedeen, B., Moss, C.K., & Pesko, M.J. (in press). "What are you doing after school?" Promoting extracurricular involvement for transition-age youth with disabilities. *Intervention in School and Clinic.*

Carter, E.W., Trainor, A.A., Ditchman, N., Swedeen, B., & Owens, L. (in press). Evaluation of a multicomponent intervention package to increase summer work experiences for transition-age youth with severe disabilities. *Research and Practice for Persons with Severe Disabilities.*

Causton-Theoharis, J.N., & Malmgren, K.W. (2005). Increasing peer interactions for students with severe disabilities via paraprofessional training. *Exceptional Children, 71,* 431–444.

Center for Applied Special Technology. (2008). *Universal design for learning guidelines.* Wakefield, MA: Author.

Clarke, M., McConachie, H., Price, K., & Wood, P.J. (2001). Views of young people using alternative and augmentative communication systems. *International Journal of Language and Communication Disorders, 36,* 107–115.

Cole, C.M., Waldron, N., & Majd, N. (2004). Academic progress of students across inclusive and traditional settings. *Mental Retardation, 42,* 136–144.

Copeland, S.R., Hughes, C., Carter, E.W., Guth, C., Presley, J., Williams, C.R., et al. (2004). Increasing access to general education: Perspectives of participants in a high school peer support program. *Remedial and Special Education, 26,* 342–352.

Cushing, L., Clark, N., Carter, E.W., & Kennedy, C. (2005). Access to the general education curriculum for students with cognitive disabilities. *TEACHING Exceptional Children, 38,* 6–13.

Cushing, L.S., & Kennedy, C.H. (1997). Academic effects on students without disabilities who serve as peer supports for students with disabilities in general education classrooms. *Journal of Applied Behavior Analysis, 30,* 139–152.

Dattilo, J., Estrella, G., Estrella, L.J., Light, J., McNaughton, D., & Seabury, M. (2008). "I have chosen to live life abundantly": Perceptions of leisure by adults who use augmentative and alternative communication. *Augmentative and Alternative Communication, 24,* 16–28.

Dowden, P., Alarcon, N., Vollan, T., Cumley, G., Kuehn, C., & Amtmann, D. (2006). Survey of SLP caseloads in Washington State schools: Implications and strategies for action. *Language, Speech, and Hearing Services in Schools, 37,* 200–208.

Downing, J.E. (2005). Inclusive education for high school students with severe intellectual disabilities: Supporting communication. *Augmentative and Alternative Communication, 21,* 132–148.

Dymond, S.K., Renzaglia, A., & Chun, E. (2007). Elements of effective high school service learning programs that include students with and without disabilities. *Remedial and Special Education, 28,* 227–243.

Dymond, S.K., Renzaglia, A., & Chun, E. (2008a). Elements of high school service learning programs. *Career Development for Exceptional Individuals, 31,* 37–47.

Dymond, S.K., Renzaglia, A., & Chun, E. (2008b). Inclusive high school service learning programs: Methods and barriers to including students with disabilities. *Education and Training in Developmental Disabilities, 43,* 20–36.

Dymond, S.K., Renzaglia, A., Rosenstein, A., Chun, E.J., Banks, R.A., Niswander, V., et al. (2006). Using a participatory action research approach to create a universally designed inclusive high school science course: A case study. *Research and Practice for Persons with Severe Disabilities, 31,* 293–308.

Estrada-Hernandez, N., Wadsworth, J.S., Nietupski, J.A., Warth, J., & Winslow, A. (2008). Employment or economic success: The experience of individuals with disabilities in transition from school to work. *Journal of Employment Counseling, 45,* 14–24.

Foley, B.E., & Staples, A.H. (2003). Developing augmentative and alternative communication and literacy interventions in a supported employment setting. *Topics in Language Disorders, 23,* 325–343.

Gent, P.J., & Gurecka, L.E. (1998). Service learning: A creative strategy for inclusive classrooms. *Journal of the Association for Persons with Severe Handicaps, 23,* 261–271.

Giangreco, M.F. (2000). Related service research for students with low-incidence disabilities: Implications for speech-language pathologists in inclusive classrooms. *Language, Speech, and Hearing Services in Schools, 31,* 230–239.

Giangreco, M.F., Cloninger, C.J., Dennis, R.E., & Edelman, S.W. (2002). Problem-solving methods to facilitate inclusive education. In J.S. Thousand, R.A. Villa, & A.I. Nevin (Eds.), *Creativity and collaborative learning: The practical guide to empowering students, teachers, and families* (2nd ed., pp. 111–134). Baltimore: Paul H. Brookes Publishing Co.

Giangreco, M.F., Edelman, S.W., MacFarland, S., & Luiselli, T.E. (1997). Attitudes about educational and related service provision for students with deaf-blindness and multiple disabilities. *Exceptional Children, 63,* 329–342.

Giangreco, M.F., Prelock, P.A., Reid, R.R., Dennis, R.E., & Edelman, S.W. (2000). Roles of related service personnel in inclusive schools. In R.A. Villa & J.S. Thousand (Eds.), *Restructuring for caring and effective education: Piecing the puzzle together* (2nd ed., pp. 360–388). Baltimore: Paul H. Brookes Publishing Co.

Gifford-Smith, M.E., & Brownell, C.A. (2003). Childhood peer relationships: Social acceptance, friendships, and peer networks. *Journal of School Psychology, 41,* 235–284.

Gilberts, G.H., Agran, M., Hughes, C., & Wehmeyer, M. (2001). The effects of peer delivered self-monitoring strategies on the participation of students with severe disabilities in general education classrooms. *Journal of The Association for Persons with Severe Handicaps, 26,* 25–36.

Gurecka, L.E., & Gent, P.J. (2001). Service-learning: A disservice to people with disabilities? *Michigan Journal of Community Service Learning, 8,* 36–43.

Hamm, B., & Mirenda, P. (2006). Post-school quality of life for individuals with developmental disabilities who use AAC. *Augmentative and Alternative Communication, 22,* 134–147.

Haring, T.G., & Breen, C.G. (1992). A peer-mediated social network intervention to enhance the social integration of persons with moderate and severe disabilities. *Journal of Applied Behavior Analysis, 25,* 319–333.

Huer, M.B., Parette, H.P., & Saenz, T.I. (2001). Conversations with Mexican Americans regarding children with disabilities and augmentative and alternative communication. *Communication Disorders Quarterly, 22,* 197–206.

Hughes, C., & Carter, E.W. (2008). *Peer buddy programs for successful secondary school inclusion.* Baltimore: Paul H. Brookes Publishing Co.

Hughes, C., Copeland, S.R., Agran, M., Wehmeyer, M.L., Rodi, M.S., & Presley, J.A. (2002). Using self-monitoring to improve performance in general education high school classes. *Education and Training in Mental Retardation and Developmental Disabilities, 37,* 262–272.

Hunt, P., Doering, K., Hirose-Hatae, A., Maier, J., & Goetz, L. (2001). Across-program collaboration to support students with and without disabilities in a general education classroom. *Journal of The Association for Persons with Severe Handicaps, 26,* 240–256.

Hunt, P., & Goetz, L. (1997). Research on inclusive educational programs, practices, and outcomes for students with severe disabilities. *Journal of Special Education, 31,* 3–29.

Hunt, P., Soto, G., Maier, J., & Doering, K. (2003). Collaborative teaming to support students at risk and students with severe disabilities in general education classrooms. *Exceptional Children, 69,* 315–332.

Hunt, P., Soto, G., Maier, J., Muller, E., & Goetz, L. (2002). Collaborative teaming to support students with augmentative and alternative communication needs in general education classrooms. *Augmentative and Alternative Communication, 18,* 20–35.

Individuals with Disabilities Education Improvement Act (IDEA) of 2004, PL 108-446, 20 U.S.C. §§ 1400 *et seq.*

Jacques, N., Wilton, K., & Townsend, M. (1998). Cooperative learning and social acceptance of children with mild intellectual disability. *Journal of Intellectual Disability Research, 42,* 29–36.

Jameson, J.M., McDonnell, J., Polychronis, S., & Riesen, T. (2008). Embedded, constant time delay instruction by peers without disabilities in general education classrooms. *Intellectual and Developmental Disabilities, 46,* 346–363.

Johnson, D.R., Stodden, R.A., Emanuel, E.J., Luecking, R., & Mack, M. (2002). Current challenges facing secondary education and transition services: What research tells us. *Exceptional Children, 68,* 519–531.

Jorgensen, C.M., McSheehan, M., & Sonnenmeier, R.M. (2010). *The Beyond Access Model: Promoting membership, participation, and learning for students with disabilities in the general education classroom.* Baltimore: Paul H. Brookes Publishing Co.

Kent-Walsh, J. (2008). Communication partner interventions for students who use AAC. *Perspectives on Augmentative and Alternative Communication, 17,* 27–32.

Kent-Walsh, J., & Light, J. (2003). General education teachers' experiences with inclusion of students who use augmentative and alternative communication. *Augmentative and Alternative Communication, 19,* 104–124.

Kent-Walsh, J., & McNaughton, D. (2005). Communication partner instruction in AAC: Present practices and future directions. *Augmentative and Alternative Communication, 21,* 195–204.

Kleinert, H.L., Miracle, S., & Sheppard-Jones, K. (2007). Including students with moderate and severe intellectual disabilities in school extracurricular and community recreation activities. *Intellectual and Developmental Disabilities, 45,* 46–55.

Kohler, P.D., & Field, S. (2003). Transition-focused education: Foundation for the future. *Journal of Special Education, 37,* 174–183.

Koppenhaver, D., Evans, D., & Yoder, D. (1991). Childhood reading and writing experiences of literate adults with severe speech and motor impairments. *Augmentative and Alternative Communication, 7,* 20–33.

Lawrence-Brown, D. (2004). Differentiated instruction: Inclusive strategies for standards-based learning that benefit the whole class. *American Secondary Education, 32,* 34–62.

Lohrmann-O'Rourke, S., & Gomez, O. (2001). Integrating preference assessment within the transition process to create meaningful school to life outcomes. *Exceptionality, 9,* 157–174.

Luecking, R.G. (2008). Emerging employer views of people with disabilities and the future of job development. *Journal of Vocational Rehabilitation, 29,* 3–13.

Lund, S.K., & Light, J. (2006). Long-term outcomes for individuals who use augmentative and alternative communication: Part I—What is a "good" outcome? *Augmentative and Alternative Communication, 22,* 284–299.

Lund, S.K., & Light, J. (2007). Long-term outcomes for individuals who use augmentative and alternative communication: Part III—Contributing factors. *Augmentative and Alternative Communication, 23,* 323–335.

Mahoney, J.L., Harris, A.L., & Eccles, J.S. (2006). Organized activity participation, positive youth development, and the over-scheduling hypothesis. *Social Policy Report, 20*(4), 3–32.

McGuire, J., & McDonnell, J. (2008). Relationships between recreation and levels of self-determination for adolescents and young adults with disabilities. *Career Development for Exceptional Individuals, 31,* 154–163.

McNaughton, D., & Bryen, D.N. (2002). Enhancing participation in employment through AAC technologies. *Assistive Technology, 14,* 58–70.

McNaughton, D., & Bryen, D.N. (2007). AAC technologies to enhance participation and access to meaningful societal roles for adolescents and adults with developmental disabilities who require AAC. *Augmentative and Alternative Communication, 23,* 217–229.

McNaughton, D., Light, J., & Arnold, K.B. (2002). "Getting your wheel in the door": Successful full-time employment experiences of individuals with cerebral palsy who use augmentative and alternative communication. *Augmentative and Alternative Communication, 18,* 59–76.

McNulty, R.J., & Quaglia, R.J. (2007). Rigor, relevance, and relationships. *The School Administrator, 64*(8), 18–23.

McSheehan, M., Sonnenmeier, R.M., & Jorgensen, C.M. (2009). Membership, participation, and learning in general education classrooms for students with autism spectrum disorders who use AAC. In P. Mirenda & T. Iacono (Eds.), *Autism spectrum disorders and AAC* (pp. 413–439). Baltimore: Paul H. Brookes Publishing Co.

Miller, K.D., Schleien, S.J., & Bellini, L.A. (2003). Barriers to the inclusion of volunteers with developmental disabilities. *Journal of Volunteer Administration, 21,* 25–30.

Miller, K.D., Schleien, S.J., Rider, C., Hall, C., Roche, M., & Worsley, J. (2002). Inclusive volunteering: Benefits to participants and community. *Therapeutic Recreation Journal, 36,* 247–259.

National Alliance for Secondary Education and Transition. (2005). *National standards and quality indicators: Transition toolkit for systems improvement.* Minneapolis: University of Minnesota, National Center on Secondary Education and Transition.

Newman, F.M., & Wehlage, G.G. (1993). Five standards of authentic learning. *Educational Leadership, 50*(7), 8–12.

Palmer, S.B., Wehmeyer, M.L., Gipson, K., & Agran, M. (2004). Promoting access to the general curriculum by teaching self-determination skills. *Exceptional Children, 70,* 427–439.

Phelps, L.A. (2003). High schools with authentic and inclusive learning practices: Selected features and findings. *NCSET Research to Practice Brief, 2*(2), 1–4.

Phelps, L.A., & Hanley-Maxwell, C. (1997). School-to-work transitions for youth with disabilities: A review of outcomes and practices. *Review of Educational Research, 67,* 197–226.

Powers, K.M., Gil-Kashiwabara, E., Geenan, S.J., Powers, L., Balandran, J., & Palmer, C. (2005). Mandates and effective transition planning practices reflected in IEPs. *Career Development for Exceptional Individuals, 28,* 47–59.

Rose, T.E., McDonnell, J., & Ellis, G. (2007). The impact of teacher beliefs on the provision of leisure and physical activity education curriculum decisions. *Teacher Education and Special Education, 30,* 183–190.

Rusch, F.R., Hughes, C., Agran, M., Martin, J.E., & Johnson, J.R. (2009). Toward self-directed learning, post-high school placement, and coordinated support: Constructing new transition bridges to adult life. *Career Development for Exceptional Individuals, 32,* 53–59.

Ryndak, D., & Fisher, D. (Eds.). (2003). *The foundations of inclusive education: A compendium of articles on effective strategies to achieve inclusive education* (2nd ed.). Baltimore: TASH.

Schnorr, R.F. (1997). From enrollment to membership: "Belonging" in middle and high school classes. *Journal of The Association for Persons with Severe Handicaps, 22,* 1–15.

Shukla, S., Kennedy, C.H., & Cushing, L.S. (1998). Component analysis of peer support strategies: Adult influence on the participation of peers without disabilities. *Journal of Behavioral Education, 8,* 397–413.

Sigafoos, J. (1999). Creating opportunities for augmentative and alternative communication: Strategies for involving people with developmental disabilities. *Augmentative and Alternative Communication, 15,* 183–190.

Simpson, K., Beukelman, D., & Sharpe, T. (2000). An elementary student with severe expressive communication impairment in a general education classroom: Sequential analysis of interactions. *Augmentative and Alternative Communication, 16,* 107–121.

Sinclair, M.F., Christenson, S.L., & Thurlow, M.L. (2005). Promoting school completion of urban secondary youth with emotional or behavioral disabilities. *Exceptional Children, 71,* 465–482.

Siperstein, G.N., Parker, R.C., Bardon, J.N., & Widaman, K.F. (2007). A national study of youth attitudes toward the inclusion of students with intellectual disabilities. *Exceptional Children, 73,* 435–455.

Smith, M.M. (2005). The dual challenges of aided communication and adolescence. *Augmentative and Alternative Communication, 21,* 67–79.

Snell, M., Chen, L., & Hoover, K. (2006). Teaching augmentative and alternative communication to students with severe disabilities: A review of intervention research 1997-2003. *Research and Practice for Persons with Severe Disabilities, 31,* 203–214.

Snell, M.E., & Janney, R. (2005). *Collaborative teaming* (2nd ed.). Baltimore: Paul H. Brookes Publishing Co.

Sonnenmeier, R.M., McSheehan, M., & Jorgensen, C.M. (2005). A case study of team supports for a student with autism's communication and engagement within the general education curriculum: Preliminary report of the Beyond Access model. *Augmentative and Alternative Communication, 21,* 101–115.

Soto, G., Muller, E., Hunt, P., & Goetz, P. (2001). Critical issues in the inclusion of students who use augmentative and alternative communication: An educational team perspective. *Augmentative and Alternative Communication, 17,* 62–72.

Stenhoff, D.M., & Lignugaris, B. (2007). A review of the effects of peer tutoring on students with mild disabilities in secondary settings. *Exceptional Children, 74,* 8–30.

Suter, J.C., & Giangreco, M.F. (2009). Numbers that count: Exploring special education and paraprofessional service delivery in inclusion-oriented schools. *Journal of Special Education, 43,* 81–93.

Test, D.W., Mason, C., Hughes, C., Konrad, M., Neale, M., & Wood, W.M. (2004). Student involvement in individualized education program meetings. *Exceptional Children, 70,* 391–412.

Tomlinson, C.A. (2004). Sharing responsibility for differentiating instruction. *Roeper Review, 26,* 188–189.

Trembath, D., Balandin, S., & Togher, L. (2009). Volunteering amongst persons who use augmentative and alternative communication. *Journal of Intellectual & Developmental Disability, 34,* 87–88.

U.S. Department of Education. (2009). *28th annual report to Congress on the implementation of the Individuals with Disabilities Education Act, 2006.* Washington, DC: Author.

Vondracek, F.W., & Porfeli, E.J. (2003). The world of work and careers. In G.R. Adams & M.D. Berzonsky (Eds.), *Blackwell handbook of adolescence* (pp. 109–128). Malden, MA: Blackwell.

Wagner, M., Cadwallader, T.W., Garza, N., & Cameto, R. (2004). Social activities of youth with disabilities. *NLTS2 Data Brief, 3*(1), 1–4.

Wagner, M., Cadwallader, T., & Marder, C. (2003). *Life outside of the classroom for youth with disabilities.* Menlo Park, CA: SRI International.

Wagner, M., Newman, L., & Cameto, R. (2004). *Changes over time in the secondary school experiences of students with disabilities.* Menlo Park, CA: SRI International.

Wagner, M., Newman, L., Cameto, R., Garza, N., & Levine, P. (2005). *After high school: A first look at the postschool experiences of youth with disabilities.* Menlo Park, CA: SRI International.

Wehmeyer, M.L., Lattin, D.L., Lapp-Rincker, G., & Agran, M. (2003). Access to the general curriculum of middle school students with mental retardation: An observational study. *Remedial and Special Education, 24,* 262–272.

Will, M. (1984). *OSERS programming for the transition of youth with disabilities: Bridges from school to working life.* Washington, DC: Office of Special Education and Rehabilitative Services.

Williams, M.B., Krezman, C., & McNaughton, D. (2008). "Reach for the stars": Five principles for the next 25 years of AAC. *Augmentative and Alternative Communication, 24,* 194–206.

Zimmer-Gembeck, M.J., & Mortimer, J.T. (2006). Adolescent work, vocational development, and education. *Review of Educational Research, 76,* 537–566.

III

Employment and Volunteer Programs

5

Post–High School Transition Supports and Programs in Postsecondary Education for Young Adults Who Use AAC

Christy A. Horn and Randy Joe May

In the summer of 1987, Randy Joe May came to our campus riding a cart that his grandfather had made and communicating with a board with letters carved into the wood. When Randy graduated in May 1993 with a degree in political science, he traveled across the stage in his "Husker" red wheelchair with an augmentative and alternative communication (AAC) system in addition to his updated letterboard. I (Christy) was a new director of services for students with disabilities, and in the 6 years that Randy attended the University of Nebraska–Lincoln (UNL), we worked together through all of the challenges inherent in being a student with cerebral palsy who relies on AAC and is determined to fully participate in the college experience. Randy has since passed away, but as I thought and wrote about the challenges of succeeding in postsecondary education as a student who relies on AAC, it became clear to me that so much of what I know I learned from him. Therefore, I have named him as my coauthor. Many of the stories in this chapter are "Randy" stories. He was not the first student to rely on AAC at UNL, as he was preceded by Bill Rush, and he certainly has not been the last, but he was the one who had the most impact on how UNL views accommodation for students with complex communication needs. What we learned as Randy encountered each new environment within the institution led to many of the supports still in place, and his legacy has facilitated the success of many students who followed.

Having education beyond high school is essential to being competitive in today's labor market. Whether the postsecondary environment is college, adult and continuing education, or technical preparation, education beyond a high school diploma is an important step toward career opportunities and financial independence for all people, but particularly for people with disabilities (Gajar, Goodman, & McAfee, 1995; Getzel, Stodden, & Briel, 2001). Stodden (1998) found that the relationship between level of education and rate of employment is more strongly positive for people with disabilities than for the general population. In other words, it is even more important for people with disabilities to obtain a post–high school education than it is for the general population. Although barriers do exist to employment, there are success stories among people who use AAC, and their numbers are increasing (McNaughton, Light, & Arnold, 2002; McNaughton, Light, & Groszyk, 2001). There are important skills and abilities to be learned by engaging in post-secondary education. Some skills that are important in securing successful employment are appropriate educational preparation; skills in using assistive technology; and an understanding of *work culture,* or "acceptable standards relating to actions, etiquette, and appropriate dress" (McNaughton, Light, & Gulla, 2003, p. 244).

Strategies and programs that are successful for students in postsecondary educational environments who rely on AAC are not well documented. In fact, students with complex communication needs are often excluded from research studies, particularly those using interviews (e.g., Williams-Diehm & Lynch, 2007), leaving researchers and practitioners with little knowledge about what leads to success for these young adults. The number of students who use AAC in postsecondary education is unknown. Blackstone (1990) suggested that 0.2% to 0.6% of school-age students worldwide have a severe speech limitation. As students with disabilities receive better services as a result of the Individuals with Disabilities Education Improvement Act (IDEA) of 2004 (PL 108-446), more will successfully complete secondary education and move into postsecondary education.

The information provided in this chapter is based on more than the available literature about transition into postsecondary education for students with disabilities. It is also based on 25 years of experience working with students with disabilities, including those who rely on AAC, at a public university with both undergraduate and graduate programs. Students who rely on AAC face many of the same issues that other students with disabilities encounter, but they have a special set of issues that need to be addressed if they are to participate fully in the postsecondary environment. Although very little information beyond personal accounts has been collected specific to postsecondary students who rely on AAC (e.g., Creech, 1992; Rush, 1986), what has been learned about transitioning other students with disabilities can be of assistance to students who use AAC, their parents, and teachers in planning for the transition into postsecondary education.

SECONDARY VERSUS POSTSECONDARY EDUCATION

It is important for students with disabilities and their parents to have relevant knowledge about regulatory and service differences between secondary and postsecondary educational environments. Many times students and their parents only become aware of the differences when the services they have become accustomed to receiving are not automatically provided in the postsecondary environment (Stodden, Conway, & Chang, 2003). This lack of awareness can be a result of misunderstandings about the differences that exist in the rights, services, and funding of the two educational environments. Parents have reported not knowing where to seek information about available service providers, students' rights, and community resources (U.S. General Accounting Office, 2003). In addition, there is a general lack of awareness on the part of parents and teachers, even those very well versed in the regulations under IDEA, about the differences in policy and services between IDEA and the Americans with Disabilities Act (ADA) of 1990 (PL 101-336) and Section 504 of the Rehabilitation Act of 1973 (PL 93-112). Briefly, IDEA governs policy at the secondary level, whereas ADA and Section 504 underlie service provision and accommodation at the postsecondary level (Getzel & Wehman, 2005; Stodden, Galloway, & Stodden, 2003).

IDEA (2004) mandates that all students in secondary education programs have the right to a "free appropriate public education." This means that students with disabilities will sometimes receive substantially modified instruction (e.g., one-to-one instruction in a resource room), changes in instructional content (e.g., a teacher may decide to reduce the amount of instructional materials covered in order to pursue mastery of a small set of key academic content), or alternative assessment activities (e.g., the student may be allowed to take a test with extended time). These are appropriate for the secondary environment, as the school has a responsibility to provide remediation, but they are very different from what is called for under the ADA in a postsecondary education environment. The only services provided in secondary schools that would be the equivalent to the accommodations offered in the postsecondary environment include strategies such as extra time to complete assignments or exams, provision of a quiet working environment, access to tutors, readers for tests, and seating in the front of the classroom. However, Sharpe, Johnson, Izzo, and Murray (2005) found that even the accommodation most commonly provided at the secondary level (i.e., extra time) is used by only 28% of students with disabilities. This means that students entering postsecondary education likely have little experience with many of the accommodations that they will need to be competitive (extra time is used by 83% of postsecondary students with disabilities). These researchers also found that only 1% of students with disabilities communicated with teachers about accommodations in the secondary environment—a percentage that rises to 50% at

Table 5.1.   Comparison of supports and services under IDEA and ADA

Issue	IDEA	ADA
How is disability defined?	Individuals ages 3–21 who are determined by a multidisciplinary team to need special education and related services	Individuals regardless of age who have a physical or mental impairment that substantially limits one or more life activities
Who is responsible for evaluating eligibility for services?	The school is responsible for identifying and evaluating students	The student must provide documentation of disability according to the institution's documentation guidelines.
Who determines what accommodations are needed?	A multidisciplinary team creates an individualized education program in consultation with parents and the student	Accommodation plans are developed by the student and the disability service provider at the student's request.
Who provides services or accommodations?	The school identifies students with disabilities and develops an individualized education program (with input from parents and the student)	The student must request accommodation and provide documentation through the office that serves students with disabilities.
What services are provided?	Remedial services and accommodations are provided	Accommodations are provided to eliminate barriers to educational access.
Who pays for accommodations?	The school	The postsecondary educational institution.
Who provides funding?	Schools receive federal funding	ADA is an unfunded mandate.

Key: ADA, Americans with Disabilities Act of 1990; IDEA, Individuals with Disabilities Education Improvement Act of 2004

the postsecondary level. Students' lack of experience with and understanding of the importance of communicating with their instructors can significantly affect their success in postsecondary education. Faculty at the postsecondary level report that a major factor in their willingness to work with a student with a disability is directly related to their knowledge and understanding of the student's needs (e.g., Rao, 2004). Postsecondary students who use AAC need to initiate discussion with their instructors so that faculty can become familiar with the students' AAC technology and the impact it will have on class participation and assessment activities.

Some of the primary contextual differences between secondary and postsecondary education are time in class, class size, time spent preparing for class, frequency and type of tests, minimum grades required, teaching practices, and the amount of discretionary time students have (Brincker-hoff, 1996). These are challenges experienced by all students making the transition from secondary to postsecondary school. Students with disabilities have added challenges because they have the responsibility of managing their accommodations while experiencing a decrease in teacher–student contact, an increase in academic competition, a change in personal support networks, and the loss of a protective school environment (Gartin, Rumrill, & Serebreni, 1996; Getzel, 2008).

Table 5.1 outlines some of the differences between IDEA and ADA in terms of what services are provided and who is responsible for providing them. It is clear that the transition to postsecondary education means that students will need to be ready to take on new responsibilities in managing their educational programs and accommodations.

POSTSECONDARY EDUCATION

One thing that all the participants agreed on was that, in order to successfully transition to and succeed in college, they need certain skills, abilities, and knowledge, as well as an affective component that facilitates a better understanding of self and others. These skills, abilities, knowledge, and empowering emotions [equip] them with the necessary tools to better understand themselves and others and deal with all the ups and downs life brings. How each individual student uses and combines these "ingredients" is what makes them, as all individuals, unique. (Webster, 2004, p. 167)

When students with disabilities graduate from secondary school, they move from a protective environment in which school personnel are required by law to identify their needs and provide the services that fulfill those needs to an environment in which they are expected to self-identify as having a disability and be able to articulate what accommodations they need under ADA and Section 504 of the Rehabilitation Act (Gartin et al., 1996). Students with disabilities who rely on AAC not only need to be prepared academically and socially to transition into postsecondary education, but they also need to effectively communicate their needs to many individuals who have little or no experience interacting with individuals with complex communication needs. Students in postsecondary education have to independently operate in environments ranging from communicating with a clerk in the bookstore to engaging in a classroom discussion. The communication skills needed in the postsecondary environment are very different than those used in high school (McKeachie, 2006) and are even more challenging for students who use AAC. This is because these students are generally accustomed to interacting with people who have knowledge of AAC systems and who understand their individual needs and communication styles.

As students arrive in the postsecondary environment, their goals must include attaining the supports necessary to be able to fully participate in the learning experience. Students who use AAC will require more classroom support than is commonly provided to students with disabilities. Addressing issues concerning performance, persistence, and retention is critical to the success of students with disabilities in postsecondary education; however, most service providers at this level are concerned primarily with providing basic accommodations (e.g., arranging extended time for tests) that are often not sufficient to support students with significant disabilities. The resources available to support students in postsecondary education are generally inadequate, leaving service providers able to provide only basic services (National Center for the Study of Postsecondary Educational Supports, 2000). Under ADA, students must have access to the same educational opportunities as their peers without disabilities, so buildings must be physically accessible and educational materials must be available in alternative formats. However, although these broad principles are acknowledged, there are no mandates regarding the accommodations that have to be provided and no minimum standards of accommodation. If a student can read and can physically turn pages but prefers books on tape, the university is not required to provide this service without documentation of a disability-related need. If the student can type but takes a long time to generate text, faculty are required to allow more time to generate the text but are not required to reduce expectations regarding the length of the assignment. This leaves the student in the position of negotiating accommodations while adapting to a new environment and lifestyle.

Simply being present in the classroom is not sufficient to be successful in postsecondary education. Students need to be able to ask questions, discuss ideas and misconceptions, seek assistance from professors, explore the library, collaborate on research projects, and take part in social and cultural events. It is critical for students with disabilities to receive support both inside and outside the classroom so they can engage in the developmental process that will allow them to become independent and successful. Postsecondary education is about broadening knowledge and experience both inside and outside the classroom. Critical to this process is communication, and for students who rely on AAC, this is perhaps one of the most difficult challenges.

Communication

> The usual reaction to communicating with a speech-impaired person is nervous anxiety. Some people will avoid contact with an augmented speaker because they cannot overcome their anxiety, or should I say, fear. Most of my friends confessed to being anxious, afraid or scared stiff when they first met me. (Creech, 1992, p. 35)

In a study by Atanasoff, McNaughton, Wolfe, and Light (1998), college students who used AAC reported that they were involved in face-to-face communication, written communication, and distance communication (e.g., telephone, e-mail). One of the students interviewed used a social conversation strategy to introduce others to his system and relieve some of their anxieties:

> In order to make them feel comfortable when they see me with a communicator (AAC device), I usually try to start a conversation with them. I may also say "Good Morning/Good Afternoon" or say "How's it going". Or, I may after greeting them tell them a joke that I heard (this generally loosens everyone up). (Larry, as quoted in Atanasoff et al., 1998, p. 37)

The students in this study talked about some strategies they used to make communication easier, including "using preprogrammed vocabulary in their computer-based device (n = 4), repeating their message (n = 2), and using alternate modes (e.g., directing communication partners to look at the screen on their computer-based device if the computer-generated speech is not understood (n = 2))" (pp. 36–37). Isaac reported using a place-holding strategy: "Sometimes I will tell them 'I have an idea about that, give me a minute to put it together' or 'Hang in there a minute, I need to spell a few words'" (p. 37). Students offered a number of suggestions for how to best communicate with individuals who rely on AAC. Their suggestions were summarized in a statement by Fiona:

> The biggest thing people can do is to be honest when they don't understand me. It is extremely frustrating for me when people pretend to understand me. The other thing people can do is try to be patient and concentrate on what is being said. (p. 37)

As the only study conducted to date with postsecondary students about how they use their AAC (Atanasoff et al., 1998), this work offers some important suggestions concerning interactions with faculty. Students indicated that they spoke to faculty to

- Initiate communication at the beginning of a semester
- Ask for a course syllabus or notes
- Schedule a meeting with the professor
- Discuss accommodations
- Discuss alternative assignments
- Discuss communication strategies.

Table 5.2 lists some AAC supports for communicating in the postsecondary environment. The table is adapted from suggestions provided by McNaughton and colleagues (2003) for the work environment.

Writing

Writing is another significant component of communication in the postsecondary environment, particularly because e-mail has become one of the most efficient mechanisms for communicating with faculty. Writing is also often one of the most difficult skills to develop, as it requires significant feedback. Many students with significant disabilities who use augmented writing systems initially receive little critical feedback on their writing, as the focus is primarily on using the system for face-to-face interaction. When these students enroll in writing courses at the postsecondary level, they are often frustrated by the amount of feedback they receive. Moreover, their professors are frustrated with the lack of sophistication they see in the students' writing.

One of the drawbacks of technology is that there is sometimes the perception on the part of faculty that the technology removes the impact of the disability on the student's performance. Postsecondary faculty may assume that students with severe disabilities have had the same educational experiences as students without disabilities, and these faculty may have little understanding of what

Table 5.2.   AAC supports for communication in the postsecondary education environment

Support	Examples
Communication	Use of a high-tech AAC device
	Use of preprogrammed phrases and acceleration techniques in high-tech AAC devices
	Communication skills of the person who uses AAC (e.g., being witty, articulate)
	Faculty and staff knowledge of appropriate response to AAC
Accessing traditional academic tasks and activities	Alternative access to computers
	Ability of the person who uses AAC to be "tech savvy" and to have AAC resources
	Faculty's willingness to modify tasks and activities
Academic and vocational skill levels	Literacy skills and supports for the postsecondary environment
	Specific training in the use of the AAC device
Personal care assistance	Personal care attendant
	Institutional support with activities of daily living
	Family support with activities of daily living
Accessibility	Inclusion of the individual who uses AAC in making housing arrangements
	Use of telecommunications in residence halls
Personal commitment of faculty and staff	Faculty and staff's willingness to work with and commitment to people with disabilities

Source: McNaughton et al. (2003).

gaps in knowledge may exist for students with severe disabilities. Sometimes students with severe disabilities have not had an opportunity to participate in challenging coursework in their high school programs (Luciani, Horochak, & McNaughton, 2008) and hence are at a substantial disadvantage in postsecondary environments. For example, when Randy took a course in economics, he discovered that somehow in his academic career he had missed learning how to figure percentages from fractions. It was causing him great confusion until it was identified and remedied. It was a gap easily fixed, but others we encountered over the years were not.

Some universities have gone beyond reducing architectural barriers and assessment modifications to consider the skills students will need to be independent learners in a postsecondary environment. UNL provides the course College Survival Skills to transition students with severe disabilities into postsecondary education. One student in this course who used an augmented writing system with word prediction arrived at the postsecondary level with inadequate experience in writing. His first semester he was given an assignment to write a persuasive argument on a controversial subject. The professor gave feedback to all of the students focusing on their construction of a coherent and logical argument supporting their position. Because of his lack of experience dealing with feedback on the ideas expressed in his writing, the student became very distressed and misunderstood the professor's intent. He came to the study skills class in a highly agitated state because he had chosen a religious topic, and he interpreted the professor's feedback as a criticism of his faith. The study skills class provided an opportunity for the student to better understand the professor's concerns on this particular essay (and how to address them), as well as the more general issue of how to deal with critical feedback in any academic activity.

Another challenge in this situation was that the student was not accustomed to having his grammar and spelling graded. In a writing course at the postsecondary level, papers have to be correctly spelled, and grammar has to be correct. This has been an issue with many students with disabilities who were allowed in secondary school to disregard spelling and grammar but found to their surprise that, with the exception of in-class writing, this was not an accepted accommodation in postsecondary education. Postsecondary institutions need to hold students with disabilities to the same academic standards as other students, because they will be held to those standards in the workplace (McNaughton et al., 2003).

Accommodation Services

When accommodation services are not sufficient, students with disabilities are either unable to participate or discouraged from engaging in postsecondary education. A national survey developed and distributed to postsecondary students with disabilities by the National Center for the Study of Postsecondary Educational Supports (2000) found that although supports such as testing accommodations, notetakers, personal counseling, and advocacy assistance were commonly provided to students with disabilities, disability-specific scholarships and assessments/evaluations, real-time captioning, assistive technology, and study abroad opportunities were rarely offered (Stodden, Whelley, Chang, & Harding, 2001). Another finding of this study was that 50% of institutions did not offer accessible transportation, and many institutions still had physical barriers problematic for students in wheelchairs or those with mobility impairments. The survey furthermore found that equal access and reasonable accommodations are still a significant issue for students who require more than notetakers or extended time. One example is the lack of residential housing to accommodate students who require more than just accessible doorways. Another significant problem is the lack of sufficient staffing in the offices that serve students with disabilities. Most Services for Students with Disabilities offices are not staffed to provide the kind of individualized instructional support students received in high school—rather, they are organized to confirm disability status, provide a statement concerning eligibility for assessment accommodations, and arrange some academic supports as required (e.g., note-taking services, books on tape/CD). A broad range of students are served by what is typically a very lightly staffed office (e.g., students with learning disabilities, attention-deficit/hyperactivity disorder, traumatic brain injury, mental health issues, visual impairments, hearing impairments, physical disabilities), and this makes specialization in any one area difficult. These conditions make providing the kind of educational supports and specialized services needed by students who use AAC a significant challenge.

Table 5.3 provides a basic list of indicators of the level of commitment a postsecondary institution has to accessibility and to the provision of services to students with disabilities. Again, it should be noted that the emphasis of these accommodations is on *access* to educational activities—there is the expectation that once barriers are removed, students will be able to benefit from the same academic content as their peers, delivered with the same instructional procedures.

Faculty Attitudes

Positive attitudes and the support of faculty members are critical to the success of students in postsecondary education (Luciani et al., 2008). It is not that faculty do not provide instructional and testing accommodations. They simply do not know what they are responsible for under the disability laws, and they have no familiarity with accommodation strategies. They are also unaware of what disability support services exist to assist them in the accommodation process (Bourke, Strehorn, & Silver, 1997; Burgstahler, 2002; Wilson, Getzel, & Brown, 2000), and they are unsure about what they can do to change their teaching (Leyser, Vogel, Brulle, & Wyland, 1998; Thompson, Bethea, & Turner, 1997). Students are responsible for explaining which accommodations they need to faculty who often do not understand how a particular disability affects a student's academic performance or how to provide accommodations. Some institutions send out letters to faculty members telling them that they will have a student in their course who uses AAC, but it is also important that the student interact with the faculty member before classes start, if possible, so that the faculty member can become familiar with how to most effectively facilitate communication.

Table 5.3.   AAC college accessibility checklist

Visibility of services for students with disabilities	The services office should be advertised on the web site and highlighted in admissions and student information. Services should be reasonably staffed with a director with the appropriate training and expertise.
Program access	All event announcements (e.g., study abroad, field trips, athletic events) should include information about how accommodations can be made.
Physical access	There should be curb cuts, a lack of obstacles on sidewalks, automatic doors, accessible residence hall rooms, classrooms with accessible seating, and so forth.
Signs	There should be directional signs indicating accessible entrances and elevators. Room number signage should be high contrast and in braille.
Safety	There should be visible information about emergency evacuation.
Computer access	In public areas, computers should be physically accessible and equipped with screen enlargement software and text-to-speech software.
Web pages	Distance education and web-based classes should be accessible and compatible with assistive technology.
Alternative formats	There should be a procedure in place for students to get e-text, taped textbooks, and braille.
Events	Interpreters and auxiliary aids should be readily available for all events.
ADA coordinator	There should be a visible ADA coordinator with the authority to ensure reasonable accommodation.
Transportation	Transportation services provided for the general student population should also be offered to individuals with disabilities.
Parking	Accessible parking should be provided as close as possible to accessible entrances to buildings.

Key: ADA, Americans with Disabilities Act of 1990.

The first day of class is always hectic for faculty and students and is not the best time for a faculty member, who may have a number of students with questions, to explore how to communicate with a student who relies on AAC. Students have found it useful to either write a letter or e-mail their professor before class begins as an introduction and as an opportunity to initiate conversation about accommodations.

Faculty participation in and support of classroom accommodations is critical for all students with disabilities but is particularly important for students who rely on AAC. As described by Harris, Horn, and McCarthy, "Ideally an accommodation results from collaborative effort among the students, faculty, and the student affairs professional designated to assist in this individualized process" (1995, p. 40). Faculty have reported that the more resources, guidance, and support they are given, the more they are willing to accommodate students with disabilities (Bourke et al., 1997). However, Leyser et al. (1998) found that 83.5% of faculty members in their study reported having limited contact with students with disabilities, 40% felt they had limited knowledge and skills to make accommodations, and 55% reported being unfamiliar with campus resources and services that might help students with disabilities. In short, students with disabilities need to have the skills to advocate for themselves, to clearly articulate their needs, and to be able to direct faculty to resources (e.g., services offices, information online) that can be of assistance in the accommodation process. This requires that students have a clear understanding of both their needs and available resources.

Social Involvement

Campus involvement has a positive impact on a student's college experience (Astin, 1993). In a survey of 251 college and university students with disabilities, 84% reported that they were not at all involved in extracurricular campus activities (Johnson et al., 1998). A student's ability to engage in social relationships is a critical aspect of the college experience, and an inability to engage in positive social interactions can result in alienation and academic failure (Kupersmidt, Coie, & Dodge, 1990; Miller, Lane, & Wehby, 2005). Students who rely on AAC have some challenges communicating in social situations—especially on a college campus, where students often interact in between classes or in the student union. McNaughton and colleagues (2003) outlined some challenges that apply to the workplace but that can also be extended to postsecondary environments: 1) the increased time required for communication exchanges; 2) the inability of others to understand gesture, speech approximations, or low-tech means of communication (e.g., communication boards); 3) difficulty speaking in noisy places; 4) difficulty with people unfamiliar with AAC strategies; 5) the reluctance of others to socialize; and 6) the challenge of communication technology not working when needed. "I have a hard time keeping the person's attention until I finish what I have to say. They usually don't hang around to [*sic*] long for me to complete my conversation" (Isaac, as quoted in Atanasoff et al., 1998, p. 36).

Students who have enjoyed both the academic and social sides of postsecondary education have spoken of the need to find a balance. Rick Creech, who used a head pointer and a Liberator (Liberator Ltd) to communicate while completing an undergraduate degree at East Carolina University, wrote the following:

> During my first years, I concentrated on my studies so much that I neglected my social life. On weekdays, I would go to my classes, go back to my room and study, go to dinner and go back to my room and study. On weekends, I might take a half-day break from studying. The second year, I got better, and by my fourth year in college, I was a good student. I mean that I had learned to balance my academic and my social life so I excelled in both. A person does not attend college just to get an education. People who attend college just for the education are as wrong as people who attend college just to party. Both are failures as students. I had to learn this, and I did. (1992, p. 25)

Independent Living

Hiring and supervising personal attendants is generally a new experience for students with significant disabilities and can be a considerable challenge for a student who has never had to supervise anyone. One student in a study conducted by Webster had the following insight:

> I really never thought of myself having leadership skills. When I really think about it, I suppose I have some leadership type skills when I explain to my attendants who help me, how they can help me, train them, and answer any questions they might have. . . . When and if I notice a problem with one of them I need to resolve it, or if they need to quit helping, it's my job to find myself a new attendant and train them. (Webster, 2004, p. 160)

Postsecondary institutions are not responsible for hiring or supervising attendants. Although accommodations should be made for parking and access to the residence halls for the attendants, the student is responsible for the attendants' interaction with the institution and their adherence to the residence hall rules.

Financial Aid

For all students, the cost of postsecondary education can be a major barrier. But cost is even more of an issue for students with disabilities—especially for students with complex medical and technology needs. Time is one factor, as students with disabilities often take longer to complete a college degree. The increased time also affects eligibility for many federally funded scholarships, loans, work-study awards, and grants; many times students are unable to have a part-time job because of the time they must spend on their academic work.

Guidelines for federal funding are often rigid and present yet another barrier for students with disabilities. According to a National Postsecondary Student Aid Study conducted by the National Center for Education Statistics in 1995–1996, only 48% of students with disabilities received financial aid, compared with 59% of students without disabilities. When students with disabilities did obtain aid, the amount was lower than that of their peers without disabilities despite the fact that their costs were higher. Two promising resources for many students are government benefits programs (e.g., Social Security) and vocational rehabilitation funding.

Social Security   The majority of students who use AAC are eligible for Supplemental Security Income (SSI), Social Security Disability Insurance, and the Plan to Achieve Self-Support program. SSI supplements a person's income up to a certain level that varies from state to state. Parent income and assets are considered when deciding if a child younger than 18 qualifies for SSI. Individual state tax-free college savings plans (509 plans) are considered resources under SSI, and students who have such plans are ineligible for SSI. It is best to check state rules as early as possible to avoid making mistakes that will cost a student the financial support that will allow him or her to obtain a postsecondary education.

Vocational Rehabilitation   Vocational rehabilitation is another source of funds and support. Typically a vocational rehabilitation counselor considers a person eligible for services if he or she meets the following three conditions:

1. The person has a physical or mental disability that is documented by medical records or through testing that verifies the disability.

2. The person is unable to get or keep a job.

3. The person requires vocational rehabilitation services to get or keep a job that matches his or her strengths, resources, priorities, interests, and choice.

Vocational rehabilitation agencies vary from state to state in the types of services they provide and in the number of clients they serve. Again, it is best for students who rely on AAC and their families to become familiar with individual state requirements, the level of support that will be provided for the student, and what the application process is to obtain that support.

Specific Financial Obligations Associated with Disabilities

Students who use AAC will most likely have financial obligations associated with their disability. These students and their families are likely responsible for acquiring and maintaining motorized wheelchairs, communication systems, computers with special software and assistive technology, medical expenses not covered by insurance, transportation, and personal attendants. None of the assistive or AAC technology or personal care services that students have for personal use is the responsibility of the postsecondary institution. The institution is responsible for providing assistive technology in general computer facilities or for the purpose of taking exams, but no equipment used in students' residence hall rooms is the responsibility of the college.

Ultimately, it is the students' responsibility to find and coordinate resources with the college, Vocational Rehabilitation Services, Health and Human Services, or other resources. Postsecondary financial aid offices generally do not have expertise in providing assistance with SSI and vocational rehabilitation to students with disabilities. Because of differences in state policies (particularly state vocational rehabilitation policies) and the lack of experience in college financial aid offices, postsecondary students and their families must develop some level of expertise in coordinating funding agencies to ensure that students receive all appropriate assistance. Many federal loan and grant programs require students to be enrolled in school full time. It has become more common for universities to grant an accommodation that allows a person to be considered a full-time student when he or she is taking less than a full load. If the accommodation is granted by the postsecondary institution, allowances can be made in the financial aid policy.

Interagency Coordination

The number of opportunities in postsecondary education for students with disabilities has greatly increased through the efforts of students, parents, and service providers. However, there are still many challenges to successful participation in postsecondary education, particularly for students who use AAC. One of those challenges revolves around the lack of coordination among various agencies and funding sources, resulting in the need for students to spend substantial amounts of time dealing with the provision of the educational and related services and supports necessary for them to participate in postsecondary education.

Although there have been many efforts to improve the quality of postsecondary educational outcomes for students with disabilities, accessing service systems remains difficult at best. Often, students are put in the position of choosing from an array of services that can be contradictory and that restrict their freedom of choice. Whether a student with a disability will receive support often depends on decisions that are agency driven or based on available funding rather than what would be best for the student or what the student would choose. Agencies may have a particular philosophy concerning what program of studies is appropriate for a student with a given disability or may only be willing to support students in certain majors. These decisions can be appealed successfully, but the process of working with the agencies and finding out their processes and rules should begin when the student is in secondary school. This way, if there is a need for an appeal, it can happen before the student enters postsecondary education.

Internships and Field Experiences

A study on postsecondary internships found that 86% of students complete one or more internships by graduation and 69% complete two or more (Briel & Getzel, 2005). Employers, faculty, and students have realized that internships are an excellent way to develop employment skills and abilities and to be able to apply knowledge gained in classes (Reardon, Lenz, & Folsom, 1998).

Secondary students with disabilities generally have limited career development activities in high school, have little or no work experience, and, therefore, have difficulty evaluating the impact their disability will have on a career choice (Hitchings et al., 2001). Having internships during postsecondary education allows students the opportunity to experience how the accommodations they are currently receiving will need to be adapted to support them in a work environment. These experiences allow students to begin developing the support networks that they will need as they move into their careers while they still have the support of their college services personnel. If the internship or field placement is connected to academic credit hours, the postsecondary institution has some responsibility for accommodation support in conjunction with vocational rehabilitation. Vocational rehabilitation will often provide support in this area, as internships and field placements are considered part of students' vocational training. Accommodations for internships and field placements are generally different and more extensive than those provided in the academic environment, so having the expertise and support of the postsecondary service provider and vocational rehabilitation counselors is of great help in facilitating success in this new environment.

Preparations need to be made to ensure that internships and field placements are successful. Field liaisons, site supervisors, and advisors may be unclear about how to interact with students who rely on AAC. McNaughton et al. (2003) made the following recommendations to those who used AAC in the employment environment:

- Ensure that relevant employment vocabulary is prestored in the AAC device.

- Develop good skills with the AAC device.

- Make sure employers and coworkers are made aware of the presence and role of a personal care attendant, if one is needed.

- Have a plan for breakdowns of technology, personal care assistance, or transportation.

Internships and other career-related experiences are an important link enabling students with disabilities to apply the knowledge and skills they acquire in college to a work environment. These experiences can also provide motivation as they give students the opportunity to see where their hard work will lead (Getzel, 2008).

PREPARATION FOR POSTSECONDARY EDUCATION

One of the most critical parts of choosing a postsecondary institution is finding the right environment. The right postsecondary institution is the one that fits the student's needs in terms of career goals, accommodation, and support. For students who need a significant amount of support to be successful in the postsecondary environment, it is never too early to start the search process. Students who rely on AAC should be particularly concerned about finding an institution that has established support services for students with disabilities, preferably staff who have worked in the past with students who use AAC. When Randy came to UNL, he had access to the expertise of David Beukelman and the AAC laboratory at Barkley Memorial Center. Dr. Beukelman was able to assist us in evaluating and supporting an AAC system and work with us on accommodation and writing supports for Randy. UNL students with complex communication needs continue to receive support from the Barkley Memorial Center. Generally, even if the postsecondary institution has an assistive technology center (something that has become reasonably common), the technicians who are responsible for those facilities have little expertise in AAC and will not be able to provide other sophisticated technological supports without assistance from someone with such expertise. AAC devices themselves are considered personal equipment and therefore not the responsibility of the postsecondary institution.

When students who use AAC look for a postsecondary institution, it is critical that they consider what resources are available to provide technical support, what resources will be needed to secure that support, and how long it would take to receive technical support and/or repairs. Because students may have to move from building to building in all types of weather, there are challenges related to the environment. Over the years, UNL has had to find resources to create "raincoats" for AAC devices, customized trays or supports to hold the devices, and back-up plans to keep students going when the system goes down. We have found that many students, especially those who have had their communication devices from an early age, rely almost exclusively on these devices and are not comfortable with some of the low-tech forms of communicating, such as letterboards. This is sometimes problematic in an environment in which a student encounters dozens of people every day who are not familiar with AAC and who often do not have the time or opportunity to familiarize themselves with a more sophisticated device. Knowing when to be flexible is critical for successful communication. One of the students who knew him described how Randy initiated communication:

> Randy used two different types of communication boards to communicate during the time that I knew him. Both were made especially for him by friends who attended the same church he did. They were customized for Randy and the way he spoke. Each board had the alphabet and numbers as well as several frequently used words around the outside. On the back of the board it said "Hi, my name is Randy" in big bold letters. That, along with a big smile, was the only introduction Randy needed to meet someone. (Jill, personal communication, June 2, 2009)

Randy's board also included some short phrases such as HOW ARE YOU and THANK YOU. These phrases were on his board long before an official analysis was done of his communication needs at UNL; they had been part of his method of communicating during his entire school career.

When students who rely on AAC are in secondary school, the school is responsible for identifying them, assessing their needs, and developing an individualized education program that outlines their need for assistance. The level of engagement these students have in educational activities—especially the core curriculum—in secondary education has a significant impact on their preparation for the postsecondary environment. Beukelman and Mirenda (2005) suggested that three levels (i.e., competitive, active, and involved) characterize the educational participation of students who use AAC and that students' level of participation determines their opportunity to build the same skills and abilities as their peers who are preparing for postsecondary education. Students who are *competitive* participate in the same educational activities and assignments as their peers and are held to the same standard. However, usually some accommodations need to be made, as students who use AAC may not be able to write or communicate as quickly. These accommodations are necessary, but care should be taken to ensure that the academic standard is the same as for other students. Students who are *active* also participate in the same activities as their peers, but their expected learning outcomes are not the same, and they are evaluated according to individualized goals and standards. *Involved* students participate in the same educational activities as their peers but are generally expected to learn communication, social, and motor skills rather than academic skills. Students who use AAC and who have the intellectual capacity and the desire to pursue postsecondary education are advised to follow the competitive model, as this type of preparation will assist them in building the academic skills that will be needed to move into an environment that will necessitate independent functioning and the ability to be academically competitive.

Being academically prepared is critical to the success of students with disabilities in postsecondary education. Unfortunately, it is still common for some secondary schools to place students with disabilities in separate classrooms in which they may receive curricular content that does not prepare them academically to be competitive in the postsecondary environment (Stodden, Conway, et al., 2003; Stodden, Galloway, et al., 2003). This is done to provide the students with specialized services and supports but can lead students to be much less proactive about learning. Unfortunately, these placements may result from teachers, career counselors, administrators, and family members having low expectations and a limited sense of the opportunities available in the postsecondary educational environment (Stodden, Jones, & Chang, 2002). These placements generally do not adequately prepare students for the demands that will be placed on them in postsecondary education. In addition, sometimes there is a belief on the part of the secondary school and parents that postsecondary education will continue the level of service provided at the secondary level. Neither of these beliefs is useful in preparing students for postsecondary education, as they are not based on the realities of the postsecondary environment.

Another problem that exists in secondary environments is the lack of experience that students have with accommodation. Services that are provided in the secondary environment are often determined by professionals, teachers, and parents, with students in attendance but not active in the process. Therefore, students are not given an opportunity to develop and practice the self-advocacy and self-determination skills that they will need as in college (Izzo & Lamb, 2002). This leads to students graduating from high school without the necessary knowledge about how their disability affects their learning, which thereby limits their ability to appropriately advocate for themselves in the postsecondary environment (National Center for the Study of Postsecondary Educational Supports, 2000; Stodden, Conway, et al., 2003).

Careful planning needs to take place to ensure that students not only are prepared academically but also can handle all other aspects of life as a college student. Table 5.4 outlines many of the planning activities that have been found to be important preparation for postsecondary education. The planning process needs to begin as early as the student's freshman year in secondary school so

Table 5.4.   Suggested activities to assist secondary students who rely on AAC in preparing for college

Year	Activities
Freshman	Understand and be able to explain how your disability affects your learning.
	Actively participate in individualized education program meetings with a focus on assistive technology that can support writing and study skills (e.g., WYNN [NanoPac, Inc.], Inspiration [Inspiration Software, Inc.], CoWriter [Don Johnston Incorporated]).
	Work with a guidance counselor to make sure that you are on track to meet college requirements.
	Learn what accommodations you need and how they can support your learning.
	Take advantage of school and community activities to practice your AAC skills.
Sophomore	Continue to be an active member of your individualized education program meeting with a focus on developing writing, mathematics, and study skills.
	Begin exploring agencies such as those that provide vocational rehabilitation; explore how you can involve these agencies in your future plans.
	Begin to explore career interests by volunteering or job shadowing.
	Develop communication skills by interacting with people who are not familiar with AAC.
	Begin preparations to take the SAT or ACT exam; know what accommodations you should request.
Junior	Increase your focus on possible career goals, and seek out opportunities to learn more.
	Practice initiating conversations with your AAC system and with other forms of communication (e.g., letterboards, index cards with key phrases).
	Begin to look at postsecondary institutions that meet your interests and can support your accommodation needs.
	Register to take the SAT or ACT with accommodation.
	Explore summer employment through the Summer Youth Job Training Partnership Act program.
	Learn about college financial aid opportunities and available scholarships.
	Apply for vocational rehabilitation services and Supplemental Security Income.
Senior	Prepare questions for offices that serve students with disabilities.
	Contact colleges of interest, apply for scholarships and financial aid, and visit campuses, if possible.
	Open a bank account and manage your application fees for college.
	Obtain a list of providers of vocational rehabilitation who conduct person-centered planning for careers.
	Explore service agencies, transportation services, and community resources.

that the appropriate academic courses can be taken. Many postsecondary institutions have core course requirements and do not admit students who have not met those requirements.

"Students with significant disabilities can and do access the core curriculum with appropriate accommodations and modifications" (Fisher & Frey, 2001, p. 155). In both 1997 and 2004, IDEA emphasized the critical need to make sure students with disabilities have access to the general education curriculum. Instructional and assistive technology has been used in secondary classrooms to increase the participation of students both with and without disabilities, help students find connections among curriculum areas, and facilitate students' ability to communicate (Fisher, Frey, & Sax, 1999). Ensuring that students with disabilities are actively engaged in learning, are exposed to the same content as their peers, and are learning the study strategies and the self-discipline that will allow them to be competitive at the postsecondary level is critical to their success as they move from one educational environment to another.

Providing services such as taped texts and test accommodations, and teaching skills such as notetaking or writing, is important at the secondary level to assist students in learning the academic skills necessary to succeed in postsecondary education. However, postsecondary educational institutions are not required to provide many of the adjustments made in the secondary schools (e.g., modified instruction, alternative testing formats or assignments), which means that many students are not knowledgeable about what accommodations or alterations can be provided as they enter the postsecondary environment. Yet it is in this environment that students with disabilities are expected to self-advocate, to be responsible for requesting the accommodations they need, and to be able to describe to service providers and faculty members why they need such accommodations.

Students who rely on AAC many times are not mainstreamed in all of their secondary education classes, but accommodations can and should be made to allow these students to participate in the general classroom—especially in core courses. When students who use AAC participate in a mainstream classroom, there needs to be a balance between helping these students participate in the public school environment and preparing them for the postsecondary environment. For example, as described by Fisher and Frey, an instructional accommodation for a student who relied on AAC required substantial work on the part of the teacher:

> The teacher consistently asked Marshawn questions in a yes/no format that he could independently answer with his eyes. The teacher also required students to respond to a number of questions related to the class topic at the end of each day. Marshawn's (assignment) had fewer questions, with fewer possible choices (same, only less). These questions were asked aloud by a peer or teacher's assistant (accommodation). Marshawn was provided with a number of pictures from which to choose the correct answer. (2001, p. 152)

This teacher provided Marshawn with the opportunity to actively engage in his education, thereby allowing him to develop the knowledge and skills that could someday lead to his being prepared for postsecondary education. He was also provided with the opportunity to communicate in a way that allowed him to be a member of the class in the true sense. However, when Marshawn moves to a postsecondary environment, these instructional accommodations will not be required, and faculty will be unlikely to provide the kind of alterations that were done in this environment. Students in such a situation would need to negotiate this with the instructor and make suggestions as to how they could participate in the classroom.

NEED FOR RESEARCH

Although there is research concerning the effectiveness of available support and services in postsecondary education for people with high-incidence disabilities (Johnson, Sharpe, & Stodden, 2000; Stodden, Stodden, & Gilmore, 2000), there is little research on these issues among people who rely on AAC. There are also very few data on how to prepare students with significant disabilities to transition into postsecondary education and no evidence-based practices to assist in determining how to best coordinate the various agencies that are involved in supporting students who rely on AAC. In addition, there is little information about what accommodations students with severe disabilities receive and how successful they are when used. What we do know is from individuals who succeeded but nothing from the students who were unable to overcome the challenges of postsecondary education.

There have been very few studies involving the voice of the students. Although such studies that have been completed and reported have provided important insight (e.g., U.S. Department of Education, 1999), they are so few in number that it is difficult to make decisions based on what has been learned from them. More information is needed about exactly how students use the accommodations they are given and what impact these accommodations have on student learning. The field also needs studies that evaluate the impact of internships on the employability of students who rely on AAC and, in particular, on the employers and their willingness to employ people who use AAC. There is also a need to follow up to see what happens after graduation in terms of employment, further educational opportunities, adjustment to life in the community, and whether students find employment in the field they studied.

CONCLUSION

For many students, postsecondary education provides an important period of personal and academic growth: Students participate in challenging coursework, interact with peers, and make decisions about long-term vocational goals. But for students who use AAC, postsecondary education poses many challenges—not only in terms of the skills they will need to participate fully, but also sometimes in terms of the negative attitudes they will encounter as they pursue their goals.

In recent years, however, increasing numbers of students who use AAC have demonstrated themselves to be willing to take on that challenge (Atanasoff et al., 1998; Creech, 1992; Rush, 1986). Beth Anne Luciani is one of those young people. As she described in a webcast (Luciani et al., 2008), Beth Anne is pursuing a degree in creative writing at California University of Pennsylvania. She has maintained a strong grade point average (3.7) through her own hard work and with the support of her family, university faculty, and the Office of Disability Services. Clearly there have been challenges—it has been difficult for Beth Anne to keep up with the quantity of writing demanded, so she limits the number of classes she takes each year. Beth Anne has also found that her best friends continue to be those she made during high school—interaction with classmates at college has been limited. At the same time, Beth Anne has participated extensively in class discussions, completed an internship with the college newspaper, and fully enjoyed her college experience. As Beth Anne described, "College was always a dream of mine. I am living that dream and I couldn't be happier."

Over the years, many students who rely on AAC have received their degrees and, in some cases, found their life partners at UNL. Like Beth Anne, each has faced challenges, and each has had a different postsecondary experience. This diversity stems from many factors, but generally these experiences have been influenced less by the severity of the disability and more by each individual's personality and the support systems he or she brings to and builds while at the university. Connections made through religious organizations and family, participation in extracurricular activities, and a willingness to get outside their comfort zones have had much to do with the experiences these students have had in the postsecondary environment.

REFERENCES

Americans with Disabilities Act (ADA) of 1990, PL 101-336, 42 U.S.C. §§ 12101 *et seq.*

Astin, A. (1993). *What matters in college? Four critical years revisited.* San Francisco: Jossey-Bass.

Atanasoff, L., McNaughton, D., Wolfe, P.S., & Light, J. (1998). Communication demands of university settings for augmentative and alternative communication users. *Journal of Postsecondary Education and Disability, 13*(3), 32–47.

Beukelman, D.R., & Mirenda, P. (2005). *Augmentative and alternative communication: Supporting children and adults with complex communication needs* (3rd ed.). Baltimore: Paul H. Brookes Publishing Co.

Blackstone, S. (1990). Populations and practices in AAC. *Augmentative Communication News, 3*(4), 1–3.

Bourke, A.B., Strehorn, K.C., & Silver, P. (1997). Faculty members' provision of instructional accommodations to students with LD. *Journal of Learning Disabilities, 33*(1), 26–32.

Briel, L.W., & Getzel, E.E. (2005). Internships and field experiences. In E.E. Getzel & P. Wehman (Eds.), *Going to college: Expanding opportunities for people with disabilities* (pp. 271–290). Baltimore: Paul H. Brookes Publishing Co.

Brinckerhoff, L. (1996). Making the transition to higher education. *Journal of Learning Disabilities, 29*(2), 118–136.

Burgstahler, S. (2002). Accommodating students with disabilities: Professional development needs of faculty. *To Improve the Academy: Resources for Faculty, Instructional, and Organizational Development, 21,* 151–183.

Creech, R. (1992). *Reflections from a unicorn.* Greenville, NC: R.C. Publishing.

Fisher, D., & Frey, N. (2001). Access to the core curriculum. *Remedial and Special Education, 22*(3), 148–157.

Fisher, D., Frey, N., & Sax, C. (1999). *Inclusive elementary schools: Recipes for success.* Colorado Springs, CO: PEAK.

Gajar, A., Goodman, L., & McAfee, J. (1995). *Secondary school and beyond: Transition of individuals with mild disabilities.* New York: Macmillan.

Gartin, B.C., Rumrill, P., & Serebreni, R. (1996). The higher education transition model: Guidelines for facilitating college transition among college-bound students with disabilities. *TEACHING Exceptional Children, 29*(1), 30–33.

Getzel, E.E. (2008). Addressing the persistence and retention of students with disabilities in higher education: Incorporating key strategies and supports on campus. *Exceptionality, 16,* 207–219.

Getzel, E.E., Stodden, R., & Briel, L.W. (2001). Pursuing postsecondary education opportunities for individuals with disabilities. In P. Wehman (Ed.), *Life beyond the classroom: Transition strategies for young people with disabilities* (3rd ed., pp. 247–259). Baltimore: Paul H. Brookes Publishing Co.

Getzel, E.E., & Wehman, P. (Eds.). (2005). *Going to college: Expanding opportunities for people with disabilities.* Baltimore: Paul H. Brookes Publishing Co.

Harris, R.W., Horn, C.A., & McCarthy, M.A. (1995). Physical and technological access. In D. Ryan & M.A. McCarthy (Eds.), *A student affairs guide to the ADA & disability issues* (Monograph 17, pp. 33–50). Washington, DC: National Association of Student Personnel.

Hitchings, W.E., Lizzo, D.A., Ristow, R., Horvath, M., Tetishe, P., & Tanners, A. (2001). The career development needs of college students with learning disabilities: In their own words. *Learning Disabilities Research & Practice, 16*(1), 8–17.

Individuals with Disabilities Education Act Amendments (IDEA) of 1997, PL 105-17, 20 U.S.C. §§ 1400 *et seq.*

Individuals with Disabilities Education Improvement Act (IDEA) of 2004, PL 108-446, 20 U.S.C. §§ 1400 *et seq.*

Izzo, M., & Lamb, M. (2002). *Self-determination and career development: Skills for successful transition to postsecondary education and employment.* Retrieved September 21, 2009, from http://www.ncset.hawaii.edu/publications/pdf/self_determination.pdf

Johnson, D.R., Sharpe, M.N., & Stodden, R.A. (2000). The transition to postsecondary education for students with disabilities. *Impact, 13*(2), 26.

Johnson, D., Stockdill, S., Chelberg, G., Harbour, W., Egan, E., & Lorsung, T. (1998). *Engage: Disability access to student life. Final report.* Minneapolis: University of Minnesota, Disability Services.

Kupersmidt, J., Coie, J., & Dodge, K. (1990). The role of peer relationships in the development of disorders. In S.R. Asher & J.D. Coie (Eds.), *Peer rejection in childhood* (pp. 274–308). New York: Cambridge University Press.

Leyser, Y., Vogel, S.A., Brulle, A., & Wyland, S. (1998). Faculty attitudes and practices regarding students with disabilities: Two decades after implementation of 504. *Journal of Postsecondary Education and Disability, 13*(2), 1–10.

Luciani, B.A., Horochak, S., & McNaughton, D. (2008). *College life and AAC: Just do it!* [Webcast]. Retrieved April 3, 2008, from http://mcn.ed.psu.edu/dbm/bal_cal/index.htm

McKeachie, W. (2006). *Teaching tips: Strategies, research and theory for college and university teachers.* Boston: Houghton Mifflin.

McNaughton, D., Light, J., & Arnold, K.B. (2002). "Getting your wheel in the door": Successful full-time employment experiences of individuals with cerebral palsy who use augmentative and alternative communication. *Augmentative and Alternative Communication, 18,* 59–76.

McNaughton, D., Light, J., & Groszyk, L. (2001). "Don't give up": Employment experiences of individuals with amyotrophic lateral sclerosis who use augmentative and alternative communication. *Augmentative and Alternative Communication, 17,* 170–195.

McNaughton, D., Light, J., & Gulla, S. (2003). Opening up a "whole new world": Employer and co-worker perspectives on working with individuals who use augmentative and alternative communication. *Augmentative and Alternative Communication, 19,* 235–253.

Miller, M.J., Lane, K.L., & Wehby, J.H. (2005). Social skills instruction for students with high incidence disabilities: An effective, efficient approach for addressing acquisition deficits. *Preventing School Failure, 49,* 27–40.

National Center for the Study of Postsecondary Educational Supports. (2000). *Focus group discussion on supports and barriers in lifelong learning.* Honolulu: University of Hawaii at Manoa, Rehabilitation Research and Training Center.

Rao, S. (2004). Faculty attitudes and students with disabilities in higher education: A literature review. *College Student Journal, 38*(2), 191–198.

Reardon, R., Lenz, R., & Folsom, B. (1998). Employer ratings of student participation in non-classroom-based activities: Findings from a campus survey. *Journal of Career Planning and Employment, 58*(4), 36–39.

Rehabilitation Act of 1973, PL 93-112, 29 U.S.C. §§ 701 *et seq.*

Rush, W. (1986). *Journey out of silence.* Lincoln, NE: Media Productions & Marketing.

Sharpe, M.N., Johnson, D.R., Izzo, M., & Murray, A. (2005). An analysis of instructional accommodations and assistive technologies used by postsecondary graduates with disabilities. *Journal of Vocational Rehabilitation, 22*(10), 3–11.

Stodden, R.A. (1998). School-to-work transition: Overview of disability legislation. In F.R. Rusch & J.G. Chadsey (Eds.), *Beyond high school: Transition for school to work* (pp. 60–76). Belmont, CA: Wadsworth Group.

Stodden, R.A., Conway, M.A., & Chang, K.B.T. (2003). Findings from the study of transition, technology and postsecondary supports for youth with disabilities: Implications for secondary school education. *Journal of Special Education Technology, 18*(4), 29–43.

Stodden, R.A., Galloway, L.M., & Stodden, N.J. (2003). Secondary school curricula issues: Impact on postsecondary students with disabilities. *Exceptional Children, 70*(1), 9–25.

Stodden, R.A., Jones, M.A., & Chang, K.B.T. (2002). *Services, supports and accommodations for individuals with disabilities: An analysis across secondary education, postsecondary education, and employment. A White Paper developed for the National Center for the Study of Postsecondary Supports.* Retrieved September 21, 2009, from http://www.ncset.hawaii.edu/publications/pdf/services_supports.pdf

Stodden, R.A., Stodden, N.J., & Gilmore, S. (2000). *Review of secondary school curricula issues and impact upon access and participation of youth with disabilities in postsecondary education.* Retrieved September 21, 2009, from http://www.rrtc.hawaii.edu/documents/products/phase1/051-H01.pdf

Stodden, R.A., Whelley, T., Chang, C., & Harding, T. (2001). Current status of educational support provisions to students with disabilities in postsecondary education. *Journal of Rehabilitation, 16,* 189–198.

Thompson, A.P., Bethea, L., & Turner, J. (1997). Faculty knowledge of disability laws in higher education: A survey. *Rehabilitation Counseling Bulletin, 40*(3), 166–180.

U.S. Department of Education. (1999). *Twenty-first annual report to Congress on the implementation of the Individuals with Disabilities Act.* Washington, DC: Author.

U.S. General Accounting Office. (2003). *Special education: Federal actions can assist states in improving postsecondary outcomes for youth.* Washington, DC: Author.

Webster, D.D. (2004). Giving voice to students with disabilities who have successfully transitioned to college. *Career Development for Exceptional Individuals, 27*(2), 151–175.

Williams-Diehm, K.L., & Lynch, P.S. (2007). Student knowledge and perceptions of individual transition planning and its process. *Journal for Vocational Special Needs Education, 29*(3), 13–21.

Wilson, K., Getzel, E., & Brown, T. (2000). Enhancing the post-secondary campus climate for students with disabilities. *Journal of Vocational Rehabilitation, 14,* 37–50.

6

Developing Skills, "Making a Match," and Obtaining Needed Supports

Successful Employment for Individuals Who Use AAC

David B. McNaughton, Anthony Arnold, Sam Sennott, and Elizabeth Serpentine

> Having a job may mean you can determine where you live, what you eat, how you spend your leisure time, how you feel about yourself, and how your neighbors and community see you as a person. In short, having a job may mean more control over what you do with your life. (Williams, 1994, p. 1)

Employment is a key issue in the lives of many individuals who use augmentative and alternative communication (AAC). Our job is part of how we define ourselves; for many adults, including individuals with disabilities, what we do is who we are (Rifkin, 1995). Individuals who use AAC and who are employed describe a variety of benefits from employment, including not only the income earned but also the opportunity to interact with others and an enhanced sense of self-esteem from contributing to society (Isakson, Burgstahler, & Arnold, 2006; McNaughton, Light, & Arnold, 2002; McNaughton, Symons, Light, & Parsons, 2006).

However, obtaining and maintaining employment poses many challenges for individuals with complex communication needs. Only a small percentage of individuals who use AAC are employed, despite the efforts of many of these people to obtain and maintain work. For example, a nationwide survey by Light, Stoltz, and McNaughton (1996) identified 25 individuals who used AAC and who worked more than 10 hours per week in community-based employment settings. Attitudinal barriers, inadequate educational preparation, and a lack of appropriate community supports prevent many individuals who use AAC from participating in the workplace (Bryen, Potts, & Carey, 2007; McNaughton, Light, & Groszyk, 2001; McNaughton, Light, & Gulla, 2001).

Although the challenges are significant, employment is an achievable goal for individuals with complex communication needs (Chapple, 2000; McNaughton & Bryen, 2002, 2007). Table 6.1 summarizes some published studies of the work experiences of individuals who use AAC; these studies provide evidence of successful employment for individuals with autism, cerebral palsy, developmental delays, and other disabilities. Individuals with a wide range of skills and abilities participate in the work force, and experts are developing a better understanding of what it takes to "make it work." In this chapter we discuss employment for individuals who use AAC, and how concerned individuals can support positive outcomes for transition-age youth.

EMPLOYMENT AND INDIVIDUALS WHO USE AAC

The evidence from both group and individual research studies suggest that there are three key components for obtaining and maintaining employment:

1. Developing employee knowledge and skills that are valued in the workplace (e.g., communication skills, personal areas of expertise, strong work ethic)

2. Identifying jobs that are a good match for the skills and interests of individuals who use AAC (e.g., fulfilling work activity, appropriate time commitment, committed employer)

3. Ensuring that needed supports are available to maintain employment success (e.g., transportation and personal care assistance, assistive technology, support network).

Although these three components are presented sequentially, they often occur concurrently or in a different order—for example, information about possible jobs and employer expectations is key to developing employee skills, and ongoing supports are important for maintaining positive employer attitudes.

Developing Knowledge and Skills that Are Valued in the Workplace

Individuals who use AAC are employed in a wide variety of full- and part-time jobs, including as clerical staff, laborers, public educators and teachers, technology consultants, policy analysts, counselors, writers, and artists (Light et al., 1996; McNaughton, Light, & Groszyk, 2001; McNaughton, Light, & Gulla, 2001; McNaughton et al., 2002, 2006). Individuals with strong literacy skills and severe physical disabilities are frequently involved in computer-based activities (e.g., research report writing, data entry), whereas individuals without physical disabilities have the additional option of jobs involving manual labor (e.g., gardening, cleaning, delivering messages; Light et al., 1996). Although many individuals work for government or educational institutions, more and more individuals are beginning to work in private industry (McNaughton, Light, & Gulla, 2003; see Box 6.1).

One of the most challenging populations for job development is individuals with both significant physical and cognitive challenges (Wagner, Newman, Cameto, Garza, & Levine, 2005). One promising approach is the use of *job carving,* which involves determining a person's skills and interests and then matching these skills to some portion of duties in an existing job (Griffin & Targett, 2006). For example, "Haylie" is a young woman with developmental delay who communicates using a portable speech-generating device (SGD). She works with support personnel to deliver sandwiches to local businesses (McNeill, McNaughton, & Light, 2008). Box 6.2 describes how even though Haylie cannot complete all aspects of a job independently, she is still able to participate in the work force by completing a portion of identified job activities and working with a support team.

Research by Storey and Provost (1996) and Wolf-Heller et al. (1996) provides additional evidence of how individuals with a wide range of physical and intellectual abilities can enjoy employment success; the research also presents clear alternatives to sheltered workshops (Mirenda, 1996). The greater a person's physical and cognitive challenges, the greater the need for employment support teams to think creatively about how to identify a variety of employment opportunities, how to work with employers to modify job activities, and how to ensure the ongoing provision of supports.

In today's rapidly changing economy, it is difficult to think that an individual will perform the same task throughout his or her work life. Instead, that individual is more likely to have a career—a series of work activities joined by a common interest. Thus, it is inappropriate for an individual to spend an inordinate amount of time in prevocational training for a specific task. Rather, the best place to learn most skills is on the job, where the individual learns to deal with the wide range of work requirements and supports that exist in the real world (Mirenda, 1996; Wehman, Brooke, & West, 2006). However, some skills and knowledge are common to all employment situations and can help smooth the transition to employment: communication skills, personal areas of expertise, and a strong work ethic.

BOX 6.1   Anthony's Story

Anthony Arnold is 33 years old and uses an ECO-14 (Prentke Romich Company) to communicate with others. Anthony works from home and has provided both product testing and customer support for the Prentke Romich Company, a manufacturer of AAC technology. As an individual who uses AAC technology to communicate, Anthony has specialized expertise and a special interest in helping others to use the technology effectively. Some customers who require technical support make a special effort to contact Anthony for assistance because of the respect they have for his skills with the devices.

Anthony credits both his expert use of communication technology as well as high school work experiences for his employment success today.

> I have a brother who is 4 years younger, and John attained a newspaper route at the age of 11. He was earning a paycheck to buy extra things his allowance wouldn't cover, and I think that is when I first began wanting a job so I could buy stuff I couldn't afford on just my allowance. So that following summer I asked my parents to drop me off at Job Services. My parents let me do my own speaking to express what I wanted, and I was then placed in youth job training for a month. They then placed me at a computer store where I did data entry during my junior and senior years of high school. I credit working at this computer store for my current success working in technical service at the Prentke Romich Company because I learned a great deal about software, hardware, and operating systems during those 2 years. Those are the same skills I have to use today when I troubleshoot a person's device. (A. Arnold, personal communication, May 12, 2009)

More information on Anthony's story is available in Isakson et al. (2006).

BOX 6.2   Haylie's Story

Haylie is a 24-year-old with significant cognitive challenges who communicates using a Vantage Plus, speech approximations, and gestures. Working 1 day per week, Haylie takes lunch orders from local businesses and then delivers sandwiches from a local delicatessen.

Haylie's business began while she was in high school and has now been in operation for 3½ years. Her vocational rehabilitation staff and her mother provide support with transportation, money management, collecting orders, and delivering lunches. Haylie is not able to operate her business independently, but with the assistance of others she is able to provide a needed service and earn a little discretionary income. As Haylie's mother wrote,

> Haylie thrives on interaction with people. She likes that what she does has a sense of purpose (helping others). She also likes to be "on the go". She would be miserable idling her time away at home or "killing time" in a segregated setting. (McNeill et al., 2008)

Communication Skills   The ability to communicate effectively in the workplace is frequently described as a key skill by both individuals who use AAC and their employers (Bryen et al., 2007). Individuals with disabilities who are perceived as competent communicators earn on average more than 3 times as much as employed individuals who are only able to participate in limited conversations (Mank, Cioffi, & Yovanoff, 1997). It is inappropriate to think that there is some threshold series of communication skills required for employment. However, compared to their counterparts who can communicate effectively, individuals with limited communication skills are more dependent on the availability of skilled communication partners and more limited in their job options. Adding to the challenge of preparing for communication in the workplace is the fact that whereas some vocabulary is easily anticipated, some is job specific. Rick Creech uses AAC and once worked for a state department of education. He noted, "The workplace requires an expanded vocabulary because in the workplace employees use words they do not use anywhere else" (Creech, 1993, p. 105). Individuals who use AAC have spoken not only of the importance of easy access to a wide variety of vocabulary items, but also the ability to participate in fast-moving conversations and meetings. It is important for these individuals to not only have a way to access vocabulary quickly but also to have additional strategies to ensure that their views are heard. Some individuals speak of the use of a variety of strategies (e.g., pre-programming of frequently used words and phrases, increased use of written communication and e-mail) to address the challenges of face-to-face communication.

Communication in the workplace is about more than negotiating work activities. Many individuals who use AAC have described the challenges of confronting negative societal attitudes in the workplace (McNaughton et al., 2006). It is important that individuals who use AAC are able to participate in the social interactions that maintain a positive work environment (Staw, Sutton, & Pelled, 1994). Jim Prentice worked as a statistical record keeper for the Westinghouse Corporation in Pittsburgh, Pennsylvania, and used a portable SGD in the workplace. He described the importance of establishing a positive social climate:

> When I started to work, I'm sure that all the employees surrounding my workstation probably thought I was someone from Mars. I rode in on my motorized wheelchair and had some sort of device attached to my chair. I rode past them, and they really didn't know whether I was able to talk. If they did talk to me, they weren't sure I was able to answer them. They never saw someone coming to their work with a communicator. I stopped them in their tracks, before they were frozen on the spot, and said, "Good morning, my name is Jim. How are all of you doing today?" Big smiles came on their faces, and they seemed to answer in unison, "We are fine, and it's nice to have you working with us." That sure broke the ice, I felt like one of the team then. I made sure I programmed a few jokes into my communicator so that it would make my conversations more friendly and comfortable for them. It worked! (Prentice, 2000, p. 209)

As Jim's story makes clear, workers need access not only to work-related vocabulary but also to social vocabulary. Storey and Provost (1996) described the positive impact of the introduction of communication skills instruction and communication books featuring social vocabulary (e.g., sports, hobbies) on the social interactions of three workers with complex communication needs. Balandin and Iacono (1999) made clear the importance of considering the specific work environment and typical conversation topics of employees in identifying needed vocabulary. Although some core vocabulary items are common to many workplaces, some fringe vocabulary will be specific to a particular type of conversation. For example, Balandin and Iacono reported that expletives were an important part of social mealtime discussions for some of the conversations they observed, but clearly this vocabulary is not appropriate to all workplaces and settings!

Closely related to communication skills are literacy skills, because an individual has access to any desired vocabulary item only if he or she is able to spell. Literacy should not be considered a prerequisite for employment—48% of the participants in the Light et al. (1996) study (all of whom were employed individuals who used AAC) were unable to read a newspaper and so would be considered to have limited literacy skills. However, participants in the Light et al. study who demonstrated better literacy skills frequently enjoyed jobs with better pay, reported higher levels of satisfaction, and had more opportunities for advancement.

Personal Areas of Expertise   Obtaining employment requires in part that an employee have some unique skill that is of value to an employer. Some individuals who use AAC and who are employed have developed their areas of expertise through traditional education, completing high school and often earning a university degree before entering the workplace. For example, Mc-Naughton et al. (2002) identified eight individuals who used AAC and who were employed full time. All of these individuals had at least some college coursework, and some had successfully completed postgraduate degrees. Solomon Rakhman, a young man with cerebral palsy, communicates using a portable SGD. His experience provides an interesting illustration of using formal education to prepare for the workplace (see Box 6.3).

For those individuals whose educational programs have focused on life skills, some creativity may be needed to think of ways in which they can be employed. However, careful attention to an individual's strengths and available work opportunities can lead to positive outcomes (see Box 6.4).

Strong Work Ethic   Employment, especially full-time employment, presents many challenges for individuals with severe disabilities: scheduling transportation, arranging personal assistance services, and dealing with negative societal attitudes (McNaughton et al., 2002). To obtain and maintain employment requires a strong commitment on the part of the individual who uses AAC.

For many, this drive is closely tied to personal identity. "Michael," an individual who uses AAC and who is employed full time, wrote the following:

> If somebody asks me why I work full time, I would ask him or her the same thing. Why wouldn't I work? I'm not rich. Everybody works. Yes, I have disabilities. However, it does not mean that I'm not a human being. Why did I go to school? Why does anybody go to school? It is to learn. Me, too. If I did not go to school and do not want to work, what is the difference between a dog and me? Last time I checked, I was still a human being. (as quoted in McNaughton et al., 2002, p. 65)

BOX 6.3   Solomon's Story

Solomon is employed as a computer assistant by the Integrated Logistics and Fleet Maintenance Department of the U.S. Navy. Working both at the office and from home (via the Internet), he prepares ship maintenance documents so they can be read in a variety of electronic formats.

Solomon's parents traveled from Russia to America when he was 15, in part to obtain better therapy services for him. Solomon learned English as he attended high school and then graduated *cum laude* from Temple University. As graduation approached, Temple's Office of Disabled Student Services put Solomon in touch with the President's Committee on Employment of People with Disabilities. With the assistance of this federal program, Solomon received an interview with the U.S. Navy, which then led to his job.

Solomon has clearly benefited from a strong family support network—his mother took notes for him while he attended college, his father designed and built Solomon's specialized workstations, and his uncle provides attendant care services at the beginning and end of each day. Equally important has been his strong educational preparation and his systematic pursuit of his personal life goals. As Solomon wrote, "I have achieved my American dream. I am working, earning my living, paying my share of taxes, and saving for my retirement as a majority of my fellow citizens do" (Rakhman, 2003, p. 35). More information on Solomon's story is available in Rakhman (2003) and Rakhman (2005).

> ### BOX 6.4   Paul's Story
>
> Paul is a 31-year-old with autism who communicates using a Hip Talk (Enabling Devices), a dedicated voice output communication device. With the support of his family, his speech-language pathologist, and a parent advocacy group, Paul obtained a job bagging groceries at a local supermarket.
>
> Paul's employer was initially reluctant to hire an individual with autism. A trial employment period demonstrated that not only was Paul able to complete the essential job requirements of bagging groceries in an efficient manner (and to thank shoppers using his Hip Talk), but he also had the best on-time attendance record of any of the baggers. More information on Paul's story is available online (McNaughton, n.d.).

Identifying and Creating Good Job Matches

Individuals who use AAC have the ability to fulfill traditional job requirements in ways that meet and exceed employer expectations (Chapple, 2000). However, the development of an effective job match is key to both employee and employer satisfaction. There are three key components to a good job match: 1) a fulfilling work activity, 2) an appropriate time commitment, and 3) a committed employer.

Fulfilling Work Activity   When discussing the benefits of employment, individuals who use AAC go beyond simply talking about the money (although that is important!). They describe their interest in participating in a fulfilling work activity, contributing to society, and having an opportunity to interact with others (McNaughton et al., 2002).

Some individuals who use AAC have obtained employment by combining the skills they learned in school with a self-developed personal area of expertise and then actively pursuing employment situations that allow them to make use of their unique skills (see Box 6.1). Some individuals with severe disabilities experience difficulty with activities requiring extensive background knowledge and skills. For such individuals, significant support from an employment team may be necessary to ensure ongoing employment success in a fulfilling work activity. McNeill et al. (2008) described the employment activities of Bob, an individual with severe physical disabilities who successfully operates an organic egg farm (see Box 6.5).

Appropriate Time Commitment   Individuals who use AAC experience success in both full- and part-time activities. Individuals engaged in full-time employment speak of their enjoyment of financial independence; however, the physical strain of working a full work week while scheduling and carrying out activities of daily living is an important concern (McNaughton et al., 2002). Individuals who work part time or are self-employed also experience the benefits of income and workplace interactions and enjoy the personal flexibility associated with being their own boss (McNaughton et al., 2006).

Committed Employer   Key to any successful employment match is an employer who has made a decision to invest time and effort into making the situation work. This approach is not specific to the hiring of an individual with complex communication needs—many organizations have come to realize that a committed work force requires ongoing support from the employer (Wiesenfeld, Raghuram, & Garud, 2001). What is unique about the employment of individuals with complex communication needs is both the increased effort that may be necessary at the beginning of the employment process as well as any ongoing needs for assistance with work activities and activities of daily living in the workplace (e.g., setting up assistive technology, assistance with mealtimes).

> ## BOX 6.5   Bob's Story
>
> Bob is a 29-year-old who communicates using a single switch to operate an auditory scanning program on the DynaVox 4 (DynaVox Mayer-Johnson), a dedicated SGD. Bob helps to operate an organic egg farm by assisting with taking care of the chickens, collecting and delivering eggs to local merchants, and keeping the books.
>
> Bob's egg business is an excellent example of a *microenterprise*—a small business in which participating in the community, interacting with others, and gaining a sense of contribution and self-worth are as important (if not more important) than making a profit (McNeill et al., 2008). In a microenterprise, the interests and talents of the individual with a disability drive the business.
>
> Bob has significant physical challenges, but by working with vocational rehabilitation staff and his family, he plays an active role in both caring for the chickens and making decisions associated with the business. In describing his activities in developing his own business, Bob commented, "Be ready to put in a lot of time and effort. Don't be afraid to make your own decisions. Do what you want to do" (McNeill et al., 2008).

Employers who have not had experience with individuals with disabilities typically express concerns about the costs associated with hiring such an individual, the need for additional supervision, and the possibility that the individual might not have the essential job skills (Wehman et al., 2006). Happily, those who have employed individuals with complex communication needs in the past typically describe themselves as interested in doing so again (Bryen et al., 2007; McNaughton et al., 2003). The challenge is to build this network of potential employers over time: The most likely employer of an individual with severe disabilities is someone who has already had personal experience with a person with disabilities (Levy, Jessop, Rimmerman, Francis, & Levy, 1993; Levy, Jessop, Rimmerman, & Levy, 1992; McFarlin, Song, & Sonntag, 1991).

Obtaining Needed Supports

As in any employer–employee relationship, successful employment requires the provision of needed supports. For the individual with complex communication needs, three supports are of especial importance: 1) supports for workplace participation (i.e., transportation and personal care assistance for activities of daily living), 2) supports for completing job duties (i.e., assistive technologies), and 3) supports for developing and maintaining positive coworker relationships.

Transportation and Personal Care Assistance for Activities of Daily Living   Individuals who use AAC and who are employed at traditional worksites frequently describe the daily challenges associated with arranging transportation to work and receiving support for activities of daily living while at the workplace (McNaughton et al., 2002). In this sense, individuals with complex communication needs are in some ways different from many other individuals who make use of vocational rehabilitation services. Whereas many individuals with cognitive disabilities or mild physical disabilities will become more independent at the workplace in time as they learn the essential requirements of the work activity (Mawhood & Howlin, 1999), individuals with more severe physical disabilities may always require significant physical assistance in the workplace (McNaughton et al., 2002). It can be difficult to obtain funding for assistance and even more difficult to obtain reliable and professional care when providing such care often pays little more than minimum wage (Creech, 2001).

The challenges of dealing with transportation and arranging personal care assistance in the workplace have led some individuals who use AAC to consider innovative approaches to employment, such as telework. *Telework* involves engaging in work activities outside the usual work setting; it is made possible by the Internet and telecommunication technologies. Rackensperger, Arnold, McNaughton, Baker, and Dorn (2005) reported on telework activities among nine individuals who used AAC. Employment activities included database management, technical support, and teaching. Concerns included the challenge of staying motivated while working from home, difficulties troubleshooting technical problems, and the implications of reduced social interactions. However, participants reported that the concerns were outweighed by the benefits, which included the efficiency of working at home, the advantages of having a flexible schedule, and the possibility of having positive interactions with coworkers via e-mail.

Assistive Technology   As can be seen in Table 6.1, some individuals who use AAC are employed in jobs that have minimal technology demands (e.g., gardening, bagging groceries, cleaning). However, for many individuals who use AAC, employment is dependent upon assistive technology that allows them to bypass physical constraints and demonstrate their skills (McNaughton & Bryen, 2007). For some, the technology mainly supports the communication needed for their work activity (see Box 6.2). For others, both the expert use of an AAC device for face-to-face communication and the ability to use that device to connect with mainstream office technology are essential requirements (Chapple, 2000).

For many individuals with severe physical disabilities, technology provides a means of engaging in "low-input, high-output activities"—jobs in which a minimal number of movements produces a highly valued outcome. Anthony Arnold's situation provides a good example of this (see Box 6.1): Because of his expert knowledge of AAC systems, with a small number of movements Anthony can quickly compose a solution to a challenging technical problem. An individual without Anthony's expert knowledge, even one who is able-bodied and an expert typist, would need to invest much more time and effort to become an expert in communication technology and to stay current in technical developments.

Giving technology a pivotal role in employment success brings its own rewards and risks. Technology can have a powerful amplifier effect, enabling individuals with significant physical challenges to participate in the workplace (Burgstahler, 2003). However, on days when technology is not working, these individuals may be unable to fulfill essential job requirements (McNaughton et al., 2002). Some have suggested that individuals need a "backup to the backup" in order to ensure that they will be ready to complete work activities. For example, Bob Williams, Commissioner for the Administration on Developmental Disabilities under President Bill Clinton, famously kept two SGDs on hand at all times so a replacement was immediately available (Williams, Krezman, & McNaughton, 2008). At a minimum, individuals need a low-tech communication system (e.g., an alphabet board) that can fulfill critical employment and communication demands.

Support Network   As with any worker, people who use AAC benefit from the availability of a support network to provide both employment-related assistance as well as social support when needed (Wiesenfeld et al., 2001). For individuals with more severe disabilities, this network plays an especially important role. For Larry, a young man with autism (McNaughton, Light, & Gulla, 2001), an extended network of family members, professionals, and friends played an important role in identifying a job placement and supporting a positive work experience (see Box 6.6).

IMPLICATIONS FOR EDUCATIONAL PROGRAMS

Getting ready for the world of work requires a long-term coordinated effort by the individual with complex communication needs, family members, and school personnel. Appropriate educational

Table 6.1.   Employment experiences of individuals who use AAC

Study	Number of participants	Disability	Employment activities	AAC systems used
Isakson et al. (2006)	1	Cerebral palsy	Customer technical support at an AAC company	Liberator TouchTalker, Pathfinder
Light et al. (1996)	25	Cerebral palsy, traumatic brain injury, autism, developmental disabilities	Clerical workers, laborers, public educators and consumer advocates, writer, educational/therapy aides	Voice output communication aids, light-tech alphabet and wordboards, amplification system, speech, gestures, handwriting
McNaughton, Light, & Groszyk (2001)	5	Amyotrophic lateral sclerosis	Pharmacist, school administrator, corporate contract negotiator, organizer for advocacy organization, writer	Link message board, teletype, gestures, text-to-speech software, Madentec ScreenDoors, E-Tran alphabet board, EZ Keys
McNaughton et al. (2002)	8	Cerebral palsy	Teacher, software engineer, database manager, policy analyst, disability advocate, research analyst, editor/researcher, educational consultant/ web specialist	Liberator, EZ Keys, Delta Talker, Speech-to-Speech, speech interpreter
McNaughton et al. (2006)	7	Cerebral palsy	Web site developer, office printer, youth pastor, musician, pottery maker, freelance journalist, artist	Liberator, DynaVox 3100, Vanguard, E-Tran board with letters
Odom & Upthegrove (1997)	1	Cerebral palsy	Data entry	Liberator
Storey & Provost (1996)	2	Developmental disabilities	Employment at a health club and nursery: sweeping, clipping, watering, and moving plants	Light-tech communication books
Wolf-Heller et al. (1996)	3	Deafblindness, hearing loss	Break time communications	Light-tech communication boards

programs, including opportunities to develop valued skills, learn about possible job matches, and manage needed supports, play a key role.

Developing Valued Skills

Preparation for employment needs to be addressed as a long-term goal in educational planning (Trainor, Carter, Owens, & Swedeen, 2008). Too often, however, there is only minimal planning to prepare for life after high school, and the individual who uses AAC is rarely asked to consider his or her career interests (Cohen, Bryen, & Carey, 2003). These low expectations are manifested in high school coursework that does not challenge the student or prepare him or her for employment. Given today's rapidly changing economy, it is clearly difficult to identify the specific job that an individual will obtain. However, three key areas of skill and knowledge can be addressed in educational programs prior to employment: communication skills, personal areas of expertise, and a strong work ethic.

Communication Skills   Although it is often difficult to find appropriate supports for the development of AAC skills while in school (McNaughton et al., 2008), finding such support after school is even more problematic (Hamm & Mirenda, 2006). Therefore, it is important that the

BOX 6.6   Larry's Story

Larry is 37-year-old diagnosed with autism. He communicates using sign language and can also read and write short sentences. As a high school student, he participated in job placements in business offices, where he used his literacy skills to complete simple clerical duties (e.g., filing). As is the case with many others, Larry's family and teachers made use of their social networks to identify possible job opportunities for him. Larry's teacher contacted her brother-in-law, who worked for a television cable company; she then worked with the company to "job carve" a unique employment position for Larry.

The employment team identified a number of activities that were good matches for Larry's skills. At the worksite, he learned to deliver office mail and to complete photocopying work requests. At the same time, he began to learn basic typing skills in anticipation of taking on new office responsibilities. What is interesting is that the office supervisor took a special interest in ensuring that Larry had a positive work experience. As an individual who speaks English as a second language, she was very aware of the challenges of communication in the workplace, and she played an important role in supporting Larry's workplace participation.

school years be productive. Communication involves at least two people, and the skills of both parties are important. However, it is critical that transition programs consider the ability of the individual who uses AAC to become competent at using his or her AAC system prior to leaving the school system (see Chapter 11).

There is not space here for a detailed discussion of all the factors that contribute to communicative competence for an individual who uses AAC (see Beukelman & Mirenda, 2005). Clearly, it is critical that the individual have both the opportunity to participate in a challenging curriculum and access to appropriate AAC technology (Beukelman & Mirenda, 2005). Two closely related areas that are regularly identified as important to employment are literacy and social skills.

Literacy is not a prerequisite for employment. Light et al. (1996) reported that almost half of the individuals in their study who used AAC and who were employed had minimal literacy skills. However, it is important to recognize that many of these individuals were involved in manual labor (e.g., as gardeners or parking lot attendants). Those individuals with the lowest literacy levels were also the least satisfied with their pay and the least satisfied with their jobs in general. Literacy skills provide a way to move between jobs and quickly learn new job activities, a critical skill in today's economy. Chapter 3 provides guidelines for the development of literacy instruction for adolescents with complex communication needs.

Transition teams should also consider the usefulness of organized instruction in social skills and communication strategies for enhancing partners' perceptions of communicative competence. Storey and Provost (1996) described the positive impact of the introduction of simple communication displays and some basic social skills instruction (e.g., how to initiate a conversation) for two adults with complex communication needs in supported employment settings. The intervention resulted in an increase in the number of communicative turns taken with coworkers without disabilities and an increase in the number of different topics discussed at these times.

Personal Areas of Expertise   School programs must play a role in helping individuals develop personal areas of expertise prior to graduation. Although movement through the traditional curriculum is important for individuals who will obtain a high school degree or move on to postsecondary education (see Chapter 5), special consideration is needed for those who will not be following a traditional educational path. Some individuals who use AAC may wish to continue their education after high school but either do not want to attend traditional postsecondary programs or have not yet developed the literacy skills needed to be successful in those environments (McNaughton & Bryen, 2007). Bryen, Slesaransky, and Baker (1995) have been active in developing and researching the impact of specialized postsecondary programs targeting employment, literacy, and assistive technology skills. The Augmentative Communication and Empowerment Supports program was developed to provide adults with significant physical and speech disabilities with training in the use of their AAC devices. These individuals had received a device through their educational or vocational programs, but most needed additional training in the operation of the device. Over a 6-year period, 17 adults with significant physical and speech disabilities participated in the intensive summer program. After a 2-week immersion program and 1 year of follow-up training and support, most participants reported that learning to use an AAC device had substantially helped them in many major life activities, including communicating with unfamiliar people or in groups, maintaining a source of income, and acquiring new skills (e.g., how to engage in advocacy activities; Bryen et al., 1995).

A follow-up program, Augmentative Communication Employment Training and Supports, focused on strategies for obtaining employment (Cohen et al., 2003). Six individuals who used AAC attended 5 days of employment-related training and then participated in 1 year of online job coaching. The coaching was meant to assist them in dealing with frequently encountered employment challenges, including identifying accessible transportation and arranging personal assistance services. Participants reported an increase in job-hunting skills, overall communication skills, and information technology skills. The number of participants who held part-time jobs increased from one to three, and four of the six participants reported increasing their monthly earned income.

Work Ethic   Employers frequently describe the importance of a strong *work ethic,* or an employee's demonstrated interest in completing an activity to a high level of quality. For adolescents with severe disabilities, having any kind of an impact on the environment—let alone completing a task to a high level of quality—is often challenging. At the same time, some adults who use AAC and who are employed have reported that they were sometimes in their first job before they got honest feedback on their performance—as children and young adults, they had known nothing but praise and so had little experience with corrective feedback (McNaughton et al., 2006).

For caregivers and educators who are trying to raise self-determined children, this is a challenging situation. It is important that young adults be provided with support and recognition for their effort, but it is also important that they receive realistic feedback on their performance. Adults who use AAC have described their frustration with inappropriately low expectations they encountered during school and the negative impact this had when they entered the work force. Sam, who provides consultation to software manufacturers on the development of speech synthesis technology, left high school because of his frustration with the "watered-down" curriculum:

> In school we were only taught half or less of what the other kids were learning, because at that time, it was believed we couldn't understand as much…(now) my boss "kicks my butt" a lot, and sometimes I hate it. Yet because of how far I am now, I wouldn't want it any other way. (McNaughton et al., 2006, p. 190)

Some parents and caregivers have spoken of the importance of providing young children with regular opportunities to complete small activities or household chores in order to build a sense of how to begin and complete a task. In his article "Heading for Work," Michael B. Williams (1998) wrote about how young children who used AAC contributed to their families: L.D., age 11, had the responsibility for dusting nonbreakable areas with a feather duster and walking the dog; Candice, age 8, was responsible for helping to sort the laundry and remembering her library book on Wednesday. The importance of early experiences in building a strong work ethic for all individuals, including those with severe disabilities, was succinctly summarized by Faith Carlson: "How can you expect to get a job if you don't start in preschool?" (1994, p. 32).

Exploring Job Interests and Matches

Part-time and summer employment helps many teenagers explore an interest in particular work activities, gives them a better idea of the time commitment associated with different jobs, and introduces them to a variety of (potential) future employers (Trainor et al., 2008). Unfortunately, many individuals with disabilities find it difficult to access these job opportunities independently, and part-time and summer employment rates for individuals with disabilities are substantially lower than those for people without disabilities (Carter, Ditchman, et al., in press).

Carter, Trainor, Ditchman, Owens, and Swedeen (in press) provided a description of a promising approach to dealing with this challenge. The researchers implemented a three-part intervention package that involved 1) *intentional student planning,* including a planning document used by the student and other stakeholders (e.g., teachers, parents, potential employers) to identify both long-term and short-term employment goals and available resources; 2) *community connectors,* or school employees to assist in identifying available resources and supports; and 3) *employer liaisons* to help create links between the schools and potential employers. The program had a dramatic impact on the summer experiences of the participants. More than 65% of the students in the employment program participated in paid or unpaid employment at some point during the summer— only 18% of the youth in the comparison group had a similar experience.

The experience of planning to participate in the workplace and getting feedback from potential employers is invaluable to the transition planning process. Scott Palm, an individual who uses AAC to communicate, described the positive impact of real-world interactions:

> My job developer came up with the idea of me giving a speech to the city council about my job. I was scared to death. I had just put the speech-giving program into my Liberator but I did not know if it would work when I needed it. . . .Then the night of the speech came. My scared feeling was replaced with a blend of emotions. I was excited but nervous. I was excited because I knew I could do it. I was nervous about how it would turn out. I invited my speech language pathologist to be there, and she was in the audience. After some technical issues with the mike, I did the speech. Something started to happen. I began to have the feeling that I was in charge of the entire room. Everybody was listening to me. It was really intoxicating. I never had a full room of people listening to me before. The speech was a huge success. (2007, p. 70)

Since giving that speech, Scott has gone on to create a successful business, Palmtree Enterprises, and has obtained contracts with two school districts to provide support services for children who use AAC (Palm, 2007).

Developing Effective Supports

In order to ensure workforce participation, many individuals with complex communication needs will require assistance with activities of daily living, technology, access to assistive technology, and ensuring a broad network of support.

Managing Personal Care Assistance   Coordinating personal care assistance requires that an individual have a good understanding of his or her care needs, an appropriate way to communicate these needs, and the ability to self-advocate when these needs are not being met (see Chapter 9). These are all skills that can and should be learned in school as part of a larger effort to support the development of self-determination skills (Wehmeyer, 2005).

Technology   Assistive technology enables many individuals with severe disabilities to demonstrate their competence in the workplace (Burgstahler, 2003). The effective use of assistive technology, however, requires more than merely the provision of a device. Randy Horton, an individual who learned to make effective use of an AAC device after 96 hours of training, described the importance of organized instruction: "People without disabilities receive 12 years of writing and language teaching during school . . . Usually the consumer is given 2 to 6 hours of teaching how to use the device. Extensive, intensive teaching during implementation is the key to success" (Horton, Horton, & Meyers, 2001, p. 49).

Developing a Broad Network of Support   Bryen, Potts, and Carey (2006) described the importance of *social capital*—in this case, the size and nature of an individual's job contact network—in obtaining a job. Although important for all individuals, social capital is especially important for individuals with disabilities, who are most likely to learn of job openings through friends and family members (McAfee & McNaughton, 1997). Inclusive educational programs play an important role in building one's social network: As the individual with a disability and his or her peers without disabilities learn about one another's skills and interests, they build social networks. After graduation, the *social network* developed while in school becomes important as an *employment network.* Bobby O'Gurek (2007) described how the combination of personal skills (a community college degree in web development, expert use of a SGD) and a strong social network developed during an inclusive educational program led to his employment as a web designer:

> A year and a half passed (after graduation) and my two friends John Shemansik and Dave Ogozalek opened a computer business in Summit Hill. They asked me if I would be interested in working for their business as a web developer. I was definitely interested in working for them.
>
> I started to work for them back in August and it is going great. This is really special to me, because S & O Computers is owned by my two best friends who I went to grade school and high school with. I was lucky to make life long and true good friends being mainstreamed in the Panther Valley School District at such at a young age.

FUTURE RESEARCH DIRECTIONS

The projected workplace of the future holds both promise and challenge for individuals with complex communication needs (Bureau of Labor Statistics, 2007). Employed individuals with more severe physical disabilities are most likely to work for the government or a disability advocacy organization (McNaughton et al., 2002). Although some AAC users have been successful in high-tech workplaces, the areas in which job growth is expected to be slow (i.e., government and advocacy organizations) have traditionally provided important employment opportunities for individuals who use AAC (McNaughton & Bryen, 2007). In addition, the high growth expected in the temporary, contract, and part-time work force may hold limited benefit for individuals who use AAC, as these jobs do not provide the employment stability and benefits packages that are critical for individuals with severe disabilities. Future research should examine ways in which appropriate transition services can ensure that individuals who use AAC acquire valued skills, needed workplace supports are available, and support is provided for the development of appropriate matches.

Skills

Research has demonstrated the positive impact of innovative approaches such as structured summer experiences (Carter, Trainor, et al., in press), e-coaching (Bryen, Cohen, & Carey, 2004), and job skill workshops (Bryen et al., 1995) on the acquisition of employment-related skills. Future research should examine ways in which high school transition programs can help individuals with severe disabilities acquire needed workplace skills, including proficiency in the use of both AAC and workplace technology, while at the same time supporting participation in the general education curriculum.

Trembath, Balandin, Togher, and Stancliffe (2009) have also provided some initial research on the participation of individuals who use AAC in volunteer activities. Volunteer activities can provide important benefits in acquiring new skills, developing a social network, and building self-esteem. Continued research is needed, however, to examine the impact of volunteer experiences on future employment activity for those individuals who choose to pursue paid employment at a later time.

Match

Only a relatively small number of employers give serious consideration to hiring an individual with severe disabilities (McFarlin et al., 1991). Although employers who do hire individuals who use AAC are more likely to do so in the future, this is a slow way to build a pool of potential employers. Future research should investigate ways in which to increase the pool of potential employers by effectively communicating the benefits of hiring individuals who use AAC and by addressing employer concerns about hiring individuals with severe disabilities.

Supports

There is increasing evidence of the viability of employment for individuals with complex communication needs. The central challenge is to ensure that needed supports are available to create an ongoing positive work experience for both the employee with complex communication needs and the employer. To further broaden the number of employment options, research is needed in three areas: 1) the use of technology to expand the range of employment activities for individuals with cognitive disabilities or severe physical disabilities; 2) techniques for providing AAC users with access to reliable, appropriate personal care assistance in the workplace; and 3) public policy changes to enable individuals with extensive medical and personal care needs to participate in part-time and contract employment.

CONCLUSION

As an adolescent, Anthony Arnold began to plan for the life that he wanted as an adult:

> As seventh grade rolled around . . . this was when I began seriously considering working at either the Prentke Romich Company or somewhere else where I could help people communicate. Throughout my middle school and high school years, I remember continuously talking about this goal and boring people with talking about what I wanted to do in the future.
>
> However, I did have one teacher who loved saying, "Anthony, stop dreaming, you will never work at the Prentke Romich Company." And . . . this year, I celebrated my fifth anniversary there, so I'm proud to say "I taught the teacher something." I did meet up with her once at a conference where I was representing the company, and I received the best apology I have ever experienced. She thanked me for teaching her what's actually possible for people with disabilities. (Isakson et al., 2006, p. 70)

Anthony's attention to needed skills, his exploration of possible vocational matches, and his ability to obtain needed vocational supports have resulted in employment success. A greater awareness of what is possible for people who use AAC—and a greater societal commitment to educating both individuals who use AAC and their potential employers—will help to ensure that more individuals who use AAC are ready to participate in and benefit from employment activities.

REFERENCES

Balandin, S., & Iacono, T. (1999). Crews, wusses, and whoppas: Core and fringe vocabularies of Australian meal-break conversations in the workplace. *Augmentative and Alternative Communication, 15,* 95–109.

Beukelman, D.R., & Mirenda, P. (2005). *Augmentative and alternative communication: Supporting children and adults with complex communication needs* (3rd ed.). Baltimore: Paul H. Brookes Publishing Co.

Bryen, D.N., Cohen, K.J., & Carey, A. (2004). Augmentative Communication Employment Training and Supports (ACETS): Some employment-related outcomes. *Journal of Rehabilitation, 70,* 10–19.

Bryen, D.N., Potts, B., & Carey, A. (2006). Job-related social networks and communication technology. *Augmentative and Alternative Communication, 22,* 1–9.

Bryen, D.N., Potts, B.B., & Carey, A.C. (2007). So you want to work? What employers say about job skills, recruitment and hiring employees who rely on AAC. *Augmentative and Alternative Communication, 23,* 126–139.

Bryen, D.N., Slesaransky, G., & Baker, D.B. (1995). Augmentative communication and Empowerment Supports: A look at outcomes. *Augmentative and Alternative Communication, 11,* 79–88.

Bureau of Labor Statistics. (2007). *Employment projections: 2006-16 summary.* Retrieved September 17, 2009, from http://www.bls.gov/news.release/ecopro.nr0.htm

Burgstahler, S. (2003). The role of technology in preparing youth with disabilities for postsecondary education and employment. *Journal of Special Education Technology, 18,* 7–20.

Carlson, F. (1994). How can you expect to get a job if you don't start in preschool? In R.V. Conti (Ed.), *Proceedings of the Second Annual Pittsburgh Employment Conference for Augmented Communicators* (pp. 32–38). Pittsburgh: Shout Press.

Carter, E.W., Ditchman, N., Sun, Y., Trainor, A.A., Swedeen, B., & Owens, L. (in press). Summer employment and community experiences of transition-age youth with severe disabilities. *Exceptional Children.*

Carter, E.W., Trainor, A.A., Ditchman, N., Swedeen, B., & Owens, L. (in press). Evaluation of a multi-component intervention package to increase summer work experiences for transition-age youth with severe disabilities. *Research and Practice for Persons with Severe Disabilities.*

Chapple, D. (2000). Empowerment. In M. Fried-Oken & H. Bersani (Eds.), *Speaking up and spelling it out: Personal essays on augmentative and alternative communication* (pp. 153–160). Baltimore: Paul H. Brookes Publishing Co.

Cohen, K., Bryen, D., & Carey, A. (2003). Augmentative Communication Employment Training and Supports (ACETS). *Augmentative and Alternative Communication, 19,* 199–206.

Creech, R. (1993). Productive employment for augmented communicators. In R.V. Conti & C. Jenkins-Odorisio (Eds.), *Proceedings of the First Annual Pittsburgh Employment Conference for Augmented Communicators* (pp. 105–108). Pittsburgh: Shout Press.

Creech, R. (2001). My experiences with personal care assistance and employment: A 20 year history. In R.V. Conti, P. Meneskie, & C. Micher (Eds.), *Proceedings of the Eighth Pittsburgh Employment Conference for Augmented Communicators* (pp. 1–3). Pittsburgh: Shout Press.

Griffin, C., & Targett, P. (2006). Job carving and customized employment. In P. Wehman (Ed.), *Life beyond the classroom: Transition strategies for young people with disabilities* (4th ed., pp. 289–308). Baltimore: Paul H. Brookes Publishing Co.

Hamm, B., & Mirenda, P. (2006). Post-school quality of life for individuals with developmental disabilities who use AAC. *Augmentative and Alternative Communication, 22,* 134–147.

Horton, R., Horton, K., & Meyers, L. (2001). Getting the literacy and language skills needed for employment: Teaching is the solution. In R.V. Conti, P. Meneskie, & C. Micher (Eds.), *Proceedings of the Eighth Pittsburgh Employment Conference for Augmented Communicators* (pp. 46–51). Pittsburgh: Shout Press.

Isakson, C.L., Burgstahler, S., & Arnold, A. (2006). AAC, employment, and independent living. *Assistive Technology, 3,* 67–79.

Levy, J.M., Jessop, D.J., Rimmerman, A., Francis, F., & Levy, P.H. (1993). Determinants of attitudes of New York State employers towards the employment of persons with severe handicaps. *Journal of Rehabilitation, 59,* 49–54.

Levy, J.M., Jessop, D.J., Rimmerman, A., & Levy, P.H. (1992). Attitudes and practices regarding the employment of persons with disabilities in Fortune 500 corporations: A national study. *Mental Retardation, 50,* 67–75.

Light, J., Stoltz, B., & McNaughton, D. (1996). Community-based employment: Experiences of adults who use AAC. *Augmentative and Alternative Communication, 12,* 215–229.

Mank, D., Cioffi, A., & Yovanoff, P. (1997). Analysis of the typicalness of supported employment jobs, natural supports, and wage and integration outcomes. *Mental Retardation, 35,* 185–197.

Mawhood, L., & Howlin, P. (1999). The outcome of a supported employment scheme for high-functioning adults with autism or Asperger syndrome. *Autism, 3,* 229–254.

McAfee, J., & McNaughton, D. (1997). Transitional outcomes: Job satisfaction of workers with disabilities—Part one: General job satisfaction. *Journal of Vocational Rehabilitation, 8,* 135–142.

McFarlin, D.B., Song, J., & Sonntag, M. (1991). Integrating the disabled into the work force: A survey of Fortune 500 company attitudes and practices. *Employee Responsibilities and Rights Journal, 4,* 107–123.

McNaughton, D. (n.d.). *Supporting transitions to the adult world for individuals who use AAC* [AAC-RERC webcast series]. Available at http://mcn.ed.psu.edu/dbm/transition/index.htm

McNaughton, D., & Bryen, D.N. (2002). Enhancing participation in employment through AAC technologies. *Assistive Technology, 14,* 58–70.

McNaughton, D., & Bryen, D. (2007). AAC technologies to enhance participation and access to meaningful societal roles for adolescents and adults with developmental disabilities who require AAC. *Augmentative and Alternative Communication, 23,* 217–229.

McNaughton, D., Light, J., & Arnold, K.B. (2002). "Getting your wheel in the door": Successful full-time employment experiences of individuals with cerebral palsy who use augmentative and alternative communication. *Augmentative and Alternative Communication, 18,* 59–76.

McNaughton, D., Light, J., & Groszyk, L. (2001). "Don't give up": Employment experiences of individuals with amyotrophic lateral sclerosis who use augmentative and alternative communication. *Augmentative and Alternative Communication, 17,* 179–195.

McNaughton, D., Light, J., & Gulla, S. (2001, August). *Autism, employment, and AAC.* Presentation at the Third Annual Pennsylvania Autism Institute, State College, PA.

McNaughton, D., Light, J., & Gulla, S. (2003). Opening up a "whole new world": Employer and co-worker perspectives on working with individuals who use augmentative and alternative communication. *Augmentative and Alternative Communication, 19,* 235–253.

McNaughton, D., Rackensperger, T., Benedek-Wood, E., Krezman, C., Williams, M.B., & Light, J. (2008). "A child needs to be given a chance to succeed": Parents of individuals who use AAC describe the benefits and challenges of learning AAC technologies. *Augmentative and Alternative Communication, 24,* 43–55.

McNaughton, D., Symons, G., Light, J., & Parsons, A. (2006). "My dream was to pay taxes": The self-employment experiences of individuals who use augmentative and alternative communication. *Journal of Vocational Rehabilitation, 25,* 181–196.

McNeill, M., McNaughton, D., & Light, J. (2008, August). *Micro-enterprise employment for individuals who use AAC.* Presentation at the International Society for Augmentative and Alternative Communication, Montreal, Canada.

Mirenda, P. (1996). Sheltered employment and augmentative communication: An oxymoron? *Augmentative and Alternative Communication, 12,* 193–197.

Odom, A., & Upthegrove, M. (1997). Moving toward employment using AAC: Case study. *Augmentative and Alternative Communication, 4,* 258–262.

O'Gurek, R. (2007). *Edwin and Esther Prentke AAC Distinguished Lecture.* Retrieved September 10, 2009, from http://www.aacinstitute.org/Resources/PrentkeLecture/2007/RobertO%27Gurek.html

Palm, S. (2007). The therapeutic value of one augmented communicator helping another augmented communicator is without parallel. In R.V. Conti, P. Meneskie, & C. Micher (Eds.), *Proceedings of the Eleventh Pittsburgh Employment Conference for Augmented Communicators* (pp. 70–74). Pittsburgh: Shout Press.

Prentice, J. (2000). With communication, anything is possible. In M. Fried-Oken & H. Bersani (Eds.), *Speaking up and spelling it out: Personal essays on augmentative and alternative communication* (pp. 207–314). Baltimore: Paul H. Brookes Publishing Co.

Rackensperger, T., Arnold, A., McNaughton, D., Baker, C., & Dorn, D. (2005, August). *Work is at home and home is at work: The benefits and challenges of Telework for individuals who use augmentative and alternative communication.* Presentation at the 10th Biennial Conference on Employment for Individuals who use Augmentative and Alternative Communication, Pittsburgh.

Rakhman, S. (2003). Catching favorable winds: Supporting the U.S. Navy and other benefits of working life. In R.V. Conti & T.J. McGrath (Eds.), *Proceedings of the Ninth Pittsburgh Employment Conference for Augmented Communicators* (pp. 33–35). Pittsburgh: Shout Press.

Rakhman, S. (2005). Catching favorable winds II: Building a civilian career at the U.S. Navy: Successful communication strategies. In S. Osgood, R.V. Conti, & Z. Sloane (Eds.), *Proceedings of the Tenth Pittsburgh Employment Conference for Augmented Communicators* (pp. 42–43). Pittsburgh: Shout Press.

Rifkin, J. (1995). *The end of work: The decline of the global labor force and the dawn of the post-market era.* New York: GP Putnam.

Staw, B.M., Sutton, R.I., & Pelled, L.H. (1994). Employee positive emotion and favorable outcomes at the workplace. *Organization Science, 5,* 51–71.

Storey, K., & Provost, O. (1996). The effect of communication skills instruction on the integration of workers with severe disabilities in supported employment settings. *Education and Training in Mental Retardation and Developmental Disabilities, 31,* 123–141.

Trainor, A.A., Carter, E.W., Owens, L.A., & Swedeen, B. (2008). Special educators' perceptions of summer employment and community participation opportunities for youth with disabilities. *Career Development for Exceptional Individuals, 31,* 144–153.

Trembath, D., Balandin, S., Togher, L., & Stancliffe, R.J. (2009). The experiences of adults with complex communication needs who volunteer. *Disability & Rehabilitation,* 1–14.

Wagner, M., Newman, L., Cameto, R., Garza, N., & Levine, P. (2005). *After high school: A First look at the postschool experiences of youth with disabilities. A report from the National Longitudinal Transition Study-2 (NLTS2).* Retrieved August 3, 2009, from http://eric.ed.gov/ERICWebPortal/contentdelivery/servlet/ERIC Servlet?accno=ED494935

Wehman, P., Brooke, V., & West, M.D. (2006). Vocational placements and careers: Toward inclusive employment. In P. Wehman (Ed.), *Life beyond the classroom: Transition strategies for young people with disabilities* (4th ed., pp. 309–353). Baltimore: Paul H. Brookes Publishing Co.

Wehmeyer, M.L. (2005). Self-determination and individuals with severe disabilities: Re-examining meanings and misinterpretations. *Research and Practice for Persons with Severe Disabilities, 30,* 113–120.

Wiesenfeld, B.M., Raghuram, S., & Garud, R. (2001). Organizational identification among virtual workers: The role of need for affiliation and perceived work-based social support. *Journal of Management, 27,* 213–229.

Williams, M.B. (1994). The monster in the closet. *Alternatively Speaking, 1*(3), 1–3.

Williams, M.B. (1998). Heading for work. *Alternatively Speaking, 4*(1), 8.

Williams, M.B., Krezman, C., & McNaughton, D. (2008). "Reach for the stars": Five principles for the next 25 years of AAC. *Augmentative and Alternative Communication, 24,* 194–206.

Wolf-Heller, K., Allgood, M.H., Davis, B., Arnold, S., Castelle, M., & Taber, T. (1996). Promoting nontask-related communication at vocational sites. *Augmentative and Alternative Communication, 12,* 169–178.

IV

Relationships and
Social Engagement

7

"Activity Brings Community into Our Lives": Recreation, Leisure, and Community Participation for Individuals Who Use AAC

John Dattilo, Elizabeth Benedek-Wood, and Lateef McLeod

> Activity brings community into our lives. Community brings us support, and thus when life seems to bring us down, we are able to rely on our own community to lift our spirits and root us on to bigger and better challenges. ("Colton," a 31-year-old man who uses augmentative and alternative communication, as quoted in Dattilo et al., 2008, p. 20)

Recreation activities, especially those that involve community participation, play an important role in the lives of all individuals. Unlike the demands of school or the workplace, *recreation* activities are designed primarily for the purpose of experiencing enjoyment (Dattilo, 2002). In addition, recreational activities have as their goal the attainment of a state of *leisure:* an experience in which an individual freely chooses an activity, enjoys the activity, and is intrinsically motivated to continue the activity (Leitner & Leitner, 2004). The experience of leisure is highly individualized—not all activities typically identified as recreation will result in an experience of leisure for an individual (Dattilo & Kleiber, 1993).

In addition to the experience of enjoyment, recreation activities can also provide opportunities to develop friendships and social networks (Bullock & Mahon, 1997; Kleiber, 1999), experience autonomy and independence (Bregha, 1985; Dattilo et al., 2008; Dattilo & Williams, 2000), develop feelings of self-competence and self-respect (Dattilo et al., 2008), and engage in self-expression (Kleiber, 1999). People who use augmentative and alternative communication (AAC), however, may experience challenges to participating in recreation activities (Dattilo, 2002; Dattilo & Light, 1993; MacDonald & Gillette, 1986). They may face barriers related to recreation opportunities (e.g., restrictive government policy, barriers imposed by traditional practices, lack of facilitator skills and knowledge, negative societal attitudes) and communication access (the individual's challenges in communicating with others). To support the development of a wide variety of recreation activities for individuals with complex communication needs, this chapter addresses the following questions: 1) What is known about the recreation experiences of individuals who use AAC? 2) What are the benefits of accessing and participating in recreation activities for these individuals? 3) What are the challenges to and recommended practices for increasing the participation of these individuals in recreation activities? and 4) How can future research improve accessibility and participation for these individuals as they participate in recreation activities?

OVERVIEW OF RECREATION, LEISURE, AND COMMUNITY PARTICIPATION

There are numerous requirements for adolescents and young adults associated with participation in structured, goal-directed experiences during school, work, and activities of daily living (Adkins

& Matson, 1980; Cheseldine & Jeffree, 1981). Typically, expectations for these activities are established by authority figures (e.g., teachers, employers) and are meant to result in achievement of some goal valued by society (e.g., learning to do a math problem, mastering a vocational skill). In contrast, *recreation* is an activity designed primarily for the purpose of experiencing enjoyment (Dattilo, 2002). Although recreation is sometimes conceptualized as simply the absence of work (Gist & Fava, 1964), important benefits to recreation activities have been identified, including the formation of a personal identity, the development of friendships, and opportunities for self-expression (Kleiber, 1999).

Increased attention to the role and importance of recreation and leisure for individuals with disabilities is a relatively recent phenomenon. Prior to the movement of the late 1960s and 1970s, most individuals with severe disabilities received minimal opportunities to participate in community recreation activities (Bullock & Mahon, 1997). Although creation of local group homes since the 1980s has enabled these individuals to live in the community, support networks for recreation have been poorly developed, leaving many people with disabilities with few opportunities to participate in community recreation activities (Dattilo, 2002). To address the lack of recreational activities, targeted programs such as the Special Olympics were developed to provide individuals with disabilities with an opportunity to participate in sporting events with other people with disabilities (Special Olympics, 2009). However, in some cases these programs did not offer a true choice because they were the only opportunity available to individuals with disabilities, and they did little to facilitate community participation and interaction with individuals without disabilities (Dattilo, 2002).

Data from the National Longitudinal Transition Study-2 (Wagner, Newman, Cameto, Garza, & Levine, 2005) provided evidence that individuals with multiple disabilities continue to experience difficulty in accessing community recreation activities (Wagner, 2005). Following high school, only 23% of individuals with multiple disabilities engage in community groups (e.g., sports teams, hobby clubs, religious groups), and this level of engagement appears to drop dramatically as students grow older (Wagner, 2005).

Descriptive research documenting the experiences of individuals who use AAC has made it clear that although some individuals who use AAC enjoy a range of recreational activities (Hamm & Mirenda, 2006), many adolescents and young adults encounter significant barriers to participation. Dattilo, Light, St. Peter, and Sheldon (1995) compared the recreation and leisure experiences of children who used AAC to those of their siblings without disabilities. They reported that the children who used AAC were less likely to be given a chance to independently select recreation activities and were more likely to require assistance to participate in these activities.

The lack of recreational activities is problematic not only in terms of the lost opportunities to experience the benefits of recreation but also in terms of difficulties dealing with a surplus of unstructured free time (Kreiner, 2005). Time without meaningful activity can lead to boredom, and boredom can lead to maladaptive behavior (Alberto & Troutman, 2003). People with disabilities need the same balance of activity, relationships, and recreation in their lives as individuals without disabilities (Kreiner, 2005).

BENEFITS OF RECREATION

Although there are significant challenges to obtaining and participating in recreation and leisure experiences, there are also clear benefits.

Experiencing Enjoyment

Recreation is meant to provide enjoyment, and as such the identification of an activity as preferred can be highly individualized. In 2008, Dattilo et al. reported results of an online focus group discussion in which eight adults who used AAC described their leisure experiences. These adults described deriving enjoyment from a wide range of activities, including enjoying the arts (e.g., attending movies, watching television or renting movies, listening to music, going to concerts/plays), shopping and eating out, engaging in adult activities (e.g., gambling), going to church or synagogue, playing games (e.g., puzzles or board games, cards, computer games), participating in physical activities and exercise (e.g., bird watching, fishing, lifting weights, gardening, walking or running, dancing, swimming), doing crafts and hobbies (e.g., baking or cooking, painting, poetry or creative writing, collecting objects), and socializing (e.g., communicating on AOL Instant Messenger, traveling, visiting friends or going to parties, social dating).

Building Friendships and Enhancing Social Interactions

Recreation activities, especially those activities involving community participation, provide opportunities for building friendships (Bullock & Mahon, 1997). Many individuals with severe disabilities do not have the same levels of participation in postsecondary education and employment activities as individuals without disabilities (Garza, 2005), and so community-based recreation activities take on an even more important role as an opportunity for creating new friendships.

Participants in the Dattilo et al. (2008) study frequently discussed the importance of recreation activities as a way to enhance their social lives and community involvement. One participant commented, "The main benefit to participating in activities is to interact with people. I want to make new friends, date, and just go out" (p. 20). These new social networks not only provide friendships but are important in terms of supporting individuals in times of challenge. Successful community living requires a rich social and interpersonal network (Halpern, 1994); recreation activities can provide important opportunities for individuals with severe disabilities to develop new relationships (Dattilo & Jekubovich-Fenton, 1995).

Increasing Autonomy and Independence

Individuals with severe disabilities typically have limited input into decisions affecting their lives (Kreiner, 2005); however, the opportunity to exercise personal choice is strongly associated with quality of life (Halpern, 1994). By definition, leisure experiences are freely chosen by the individual and therefore provide an opportunity for making decisions that may not be available in other situations (e.g., school, the workplace). The ability to make and act on independent decisions is one of the most positive outcomes associated with recreation activities for people with severe disabilities (Dattilo et al., 2008).

Improving Self-Confidence and Self-Esteem

Recreation activities can provide an opportunity to experience a sense of achievement and success, thereby increasing self-confidence and self-esteem (Hoge, Dattilo, & Williams, 1999). In the Dattilo et al. (2008) study, many of the recreation activities identified by participants resulted in the creation of tangible products (e.g., gardening, painting, creative writing) or physical changes in the individual (e.g., weight-lifting, running, swimming).

Participation in recreation activities also provides individuals who use AAC with an opportunity to educate others about their skills, interests, and abilities (Schleien & Green, 1992). Promoting positive societal views of individuals who use AAC is a valuable social contribution and may lead to enhanced self-confidence and self-esteem for the individuals who are promoting these positive views. According to Michael B. Williams, an expert in the use of AAC,

Every time you step out of your home, cruise down the street, catch the eye of a stranger, make a purchase, attend a ball game, or say hello to a child, you are making a significant change in the expectations
the world has of augmented communicators. Interacting with people as you live your life is a major contribution to society. (Williams, Krezman, & McNaughton, 2008, p. 203)

Engaging in Self-Expression

Many individuals who use AAC choose recreational activities such as painting, poetry, or creative
writing that provide opportunities for self-expression. Individuals who use AAC frequently describe the impatience of speaking individuals within communicative interactions and their own
frustration with being encouraged to truncate their communication to meet the expectations of
others (Rackensperger, Krezman, McNaughton, Williams, & D'Silva, 2005). The growing number of recognized poets (Creech, 1992; McLeod, 2008a, 2008b), painters (Hohn, 2000; Keplinger,
2009), and authors (Cardona, 2000; Joyce, 2000) who use AAC speaks to the importance of art as
an outlet for self-expression. Indeed, the creative activities of some of these individuals are so well
recognized that they might better be described as vocation rather than recreation. Often, art serves
to communicate an individual's belief in the importance of self-expression. Dan Keplinger, an internationally recognized artist who uses AAC, wrote

> In high school my teacher started to give me the tools to have art say what I wanted it to. My art speaks
> what I would be saying with words. It also says the feelings that are inside of me. Those feelings would
> make people close to me scared and worried about me. Maybe I want people to see these feelings, so they
> know everything is not happy in my world. Translating myself onto canvas became my language, some-
> thing I needed to exist. ("Q&A," 2009)

BARRIERS TO RECREATION

Many factors influence an individual's participation in recreation activities. The participation
model (Beukelman & Mirenda, 2005) serves as a guide for conducting assessments and designing
interventions to increase participation in communication activities, including recreation, for individuals who use AAC. The model divides participation barriers into two major categories: opportunity barriers and access barriers. The term *opportunity barriers* is used to describe those barriers
that prevent the individual who uses AAC from being a part of the activity—these include exclu-
sion because people do not know how to adapt the activity to support the individual who uses
AAC, negative beliefs about the value of inclusion, or physical barriers such as a lack of transportation (Beukelman & Mirenda, 2005). *Access barriers* refer to challenges that exist primarily because
of the capabilities of the individual and/or the limitations of the communication system (Beukelman & Mirenda, 2005). Individuals who use AAC systems often experience difficulty conversing
with others during recreation activities because of limitations imposed by either the AAC system
or their level of communication skills (Dattilo & Light, 1993; Dattilo & O'Keefe, 1992).

Barriers to Recreation Opportunities

"Better Things to Do"
Oh no, it's me again
strolling down in my wheelchair
you don't want to talk to me
so you plot a course to avoid me
and I understand

really, I do
'cuz you have better things to do
going to Berkeley
and you don't have time to talk to me
especially since I have to type each word on my talker . . . (McLeod, 2008a, p. 18)

Lateef McLeod is a 28-year-old man who completed a bachelor of arts degree in English from the University of California, Berkley, and a master of fine arts in creative writing from Mills College. He also uses a DynaWrite (DynaVox Mayer-Johnson) to communicate. His poem "Better Things to Do" describes his frustration with the negative attitudes he frequently encounters. Opportunity barriers are not directly under the control of the individual but rather are imposed by prospective communication partners and society. Factors of policy, practice, facilitator skill, facilitator knowledge, and, perhaps most of all, attitudes of others can serve to diminish or support participation in recreation activities (Beukelman & Mirenda, 2005).

Policy barriers include policies determined and set by decision makers (Beukelman & Mirenda, 2005). These barriers can prevent access via structural, architectural, and environmental barriers that prevent an individual from participating fully. For example, policies can determine the amount of funding allotted for transportation and technologies that have an impact on an individual's level of independence and enjoyment when participating in recreation activities. An individual who uses AAC and who participated in the Dattilo et al. study described a frequently encountered problem for individuals with severe disabilities—public transportation:

The disabled transportation where I live is a joke. If you can't take the city buses, then they have a bus system just for disabled people, like a door to door service, that's an even bigger joke. In order to go somewhere with this service you have to book a day or two beforehand and they will call you back with your pick up time but they call after closing hours. They leave a message on our machine saying my pick up time and sometimes it's 2 hours before I have to be there, and we can't call them back. I like to be spontaneous, go when I want to go. So my husband has to drive me wherever I have to go. (2008, p. 23)

Practice barriers include procedures that have become *common practice* but are not necessarily actual policies (Beukelman & Mirenda, 2005). Such practices are often mistaken as polices; therefore, they have a similar impact on participation and can influence other opportunity barriers, such as facilitator knowledge and attitudes.

Facilitator skill and knowledge barriers contribute to restricted communication and social opportunities during recreation activities for individuals who use AAC. Because recreation activities are meant to be freely chosen by the participant, this presents a unique opportunity for individuals to make decisions based on their interests and needs. However, when communication partners fail to provide necessary communication opportunities, individuals who use AAC are forced to depend on others to communicate preferences and make choices (Dattilo, 2002; Dattilo, Kleiber, & Williams, 1998; Dattilo & Williams, 2000; McDonald, 1980). As McLeod makes clear in an excerpt from his poem "Wall," this lack of conversational control can be deeply frustrating:

I yell myself hoarse like a bullfrog
but I cannot get my family and
friends to get close to me
so they really know
my dreams, thoughts, desires,
and feelings
I shiver behind this clear wall
and wait for someone to notice me
wait for a chance to speak. (2008b, p. 9)

Attitudes, especially the attitudes of peers who do not have disabilities, often have an impact on the leisure experiences of individuals with severe disabilities (Mulderij, 1997). Individuals who use AAC often describe the challenge and frustration of developing friendships with others, a challenge that is especially difficult during adolescence (Light et al., 2007). Friendships and recreation activities are often intertwined, so to experience difficulty in developing friends is to experience difficulty in gaining access to leisure experiences that are important during adolescence (Smith, 2005).

Participants in the Dattilo et al. study reported that lack of concern for people with disabilities presents a serious challenge to community participation. One individual discussed such an experience:

> I was 15 feet away from a friend's house and stuck in some snow and ice on the sidewalk. It was freezing outside, I couldn't move, nobody was stopping to help, and I thought to myself, I could actually die out [here]. (2008, p. 21)

Barriers to Recreation Access

Unlike opportunity barriers, access barriers can be reduced or eliminated by implementing an intervention with the individual or providing an appropriate communication system (Beukelman & Mirenda, 2005). Successful participation in recreation activities may require an individual to quickly access a large vocabulary and to successfully develop and maintain a shared, interactive conversation. This requirement can pose significant challenges for many individuals who use AAC. Recreation activities engaged in by adolescents and young adults often include communication exchanges that cover a wide range of topics, and topics change at a rapid pace (Smith, 2005). According to Smith, these exchanges typically occur within the context of social conversations, and, when an individual lacks the skills to participate, social isolation may follow. Communicating with others in a variety of settings and developing friendships becomes increasingly difficult during adolescence, a period when people often form and maintain social cliques (McNaughton et al., 2008). Given the important role that communication and activity skills play in increasing opportunities for participating in recreation activities and experiencing leisure, identifying access barriers is an important step in promoting the participation of individuals with severe disabilities. McLeod expressed his frustration with the challenge of using his AAC system to participate in conversations in the following excerpt from "Wall":

> I can't use my 3000 dollar
> lightwriter as a paperweight
> a tortoise tries to crawl a race
> with a bullet train
> the word-prediction capabilities
> don't shield me from the
> impatient faces that tap their toes
> their eyes always wander
> looking for the next novelty (2008b, p. 7)

Light (1989) described the contributions of four interrelated areas to an individual's communicative competence: linguistic, operational, social, and strategic competence. *Linguistic competence* refers to mastery of language required to effectively communicate and includes skills such as applying and comprehending vocabulary, grammar, and symbols (Light, 1989). The development of linguistic skills occurs throughout a person's life and becomes more complex as the person ages (Smith, 2005). Furthermore, Smith stipulated that understanding complex vocabulary, grammar, and figurative language are critical for adolescents who wish to interact with peers.

Operational competence refers to the skills needed to properly operate an AAC system (Light, 1989). When an individual's AAC system is not a good match for his or her skills and needs, that individual is unlikely to continue to use the system (Scherer, 2000). After examining the postschool outcomes of five individuals with complex communication needs, Hamm and Mirenda (2006) found that only one participant continued to use the AAC system that was provided in school. The school had recommended systems that were inappropriate and irrelevant for the other four individuals. One parent described the school-recommended system as "a toy and a joke . . . that used a lot of abstract symbols that [her daughter] couldn't relate to" (p. 139).

Social competence, or knowledge of the social rules of communication (e.g., making appropriate eye contact, balancing listening and talking), also plays a critical role in conversations that occur during participation in recreation activities (McNaughton et al., 2008; Smith, 2005). In addition, participating in conversations requires the individual to understand the topic and contribute meaningfully to the conversation. Larson and McKinley (1998) reported that conversation topics often include recreation activities, and Smith found that stories of recreation experiences often dominate social conversations. These observations illustrate the interactive relationship between leisure experiences and communication skills: A lack of knowledge and skills in one area can limit participation in the other.

Strategic competence includes adapting one's communication to assist the communication partner in understanding the message (Light, 1989). For example, individuals who use AAC reported that it can be difficult to use AAC systems to make quick interjections during conversations; therefore, these systems tend to inhibit spontaneity (Dattilo et al., 2008). One participant in Dattilo et al.'s study stated,

> I can not cut into a conversation because I am a slow thinker and I can not type fast enough to contribute to a conversation; that frustrates [me] the most. I don't know how to go back to that subject, so I just don't say anything. (2008, p. 21)

RECOMMENDED PRACTICES FOR INCREASING OPPORTUNITY AND ACCESS

Providing adaptations and supports can assist individuals in experiencing success and enjoyment in recreation activities. According to the participation model (Beukelman & Mirenda, 2005), after current participation patterns and communication needs have been described, the first step to improving the participation of individuals who use AAC is identifying barriers to participation (Beukelman & Mirenda, 2005). Once barriers are identified, it is important for professionals, family, and friends to 1) develop and adapt recreation opportunities, 2) provide supports and/or interventions to help the individual learn new recreation and communication skills, 3) educate communication partners to provide recreation choices and support communication, and 4) change societal attitudes and expectations.

Developing and Adapting Opportunities

Ongoing assessment of the individual's performance and the environment are necessary to provide appropriate adaptations and supports. In many countries, there are now legal safeguards against overt discrimination in the provision of transportation, telecommunications, and government services (Americans with Disabilities Act [ADA] of 1990, PL 101-336); however, it may still be difficult for individuals with disabilities to access and participate in activities.

One promising model for recreation participation is a model of social participation (Beukelman & Mirenda, 2005). This approach recognizes that although individuals who use AAC may not assume an *influential* (or leadership) role in every activity, there is good reason to think that they can be supported in being *active* participants in many activities (i.e., making choices, being involved, and making friends with peers). For example, Rebecca Beayni is a young woman with physical disabilities who participates in a liturgical dance group, the Spirit Movers, in Toronto, Ontario, Canada (Beayni & Beayni, 2005). Rebecca does not have independent control of her wheelchair but is helped to be a part of the dance troupe by her peers. The group has performed throughout the province of Ontario and has even performed for Pope John Paul II (Spirit Movers, 2009).

Use of social networking opportunities on the Internet may also provide a way to bypass at least some of the structural and attitudinal barriers to participation for individuals with disabilities. Bryen, Potts, and Carey (2006) surveyed 38 adults who use AAC and reported that more than 80% used e-mail to stay in touch with others. Among those individuals who used e-mail, average use was more than 2 hours a day.

Lateef McLeod is also one of many individuals who use AAC who are active participants on Internet-based social networks such as Facebook and MySpace. Many individuals who use AAC report that using the Internet has increased their social networks and their opportunities to communicate (Bryen et al., 2006). A future challenge is to support Internet participation for individuals with cognitive challenges. For example, researchers in the National Longitudinal Transition Study-2 found that individuals with intellectual disability are the least likely of any group with a disability to use the computer (Wagner, 2005).

It can also be difficult to ascertain the recreation preferences of individuals with more severe cognitive challenges; however, the use of assistive technology may be helpful in some situations. For example, to assess leisure preferences, Mirenda and Dattilo (1987) provided three children with severe disabilities (ages 10–12 years) with a switch-activated computer. The students were provided with a choice of two options from an array of five leisure activities (i.e., using a blender and drinking a milkshake, watching a slide show, watching action videos, listening to music, or feeling vibrations). All three students successfully used the switch-activated computer to consistently communicate their preferences and make choices.

Supporting the Individual

One important support for enhancing the leisure experience for individuals with severe disabilities may be identification of preferred recreational activities followed by identification of necessary supports to increase an individual's activity and communication skills. Professionals can improve and increase recreation participation by providing individuals who use AAC with opportunities to develop activity-related skills. Lack of skills and knowledge may prevent individuals from participating fully in desired activities (Bullock & Mahon, 1997). As Calculator (1996) reported, individuals with disabilities may be nominally included in activities (i.e., they may be present in the room while the activity is held), but they do not always receive the opportunity to participate.

A variety of approaches can be used to develop the activity skills of individuals who use AAC. Lilienfield and Alant (2005) implemented a peer-training program with peers of an adolescent who used AAC to determine its impact on adolescent–peer interaction patterns in three different contexts: 1) teacher-directed time, 2) small-group discussion, and 3) informal time. The intervention consisted of eight 50-minute workshops focusing on specific areas of difficulty as reported by the individual who used AAC. Target skills included communicating, listening, maintaining conversation, achieving group consensus, providing feedback and clarification, and enhancing rate of speech and negotiation. The workshops included discussion, training videos, and supported activities in which peers interacted with the adolescent. After the intervention, the individual's frequency of interactions with peers increased both in number of messages per hour and number of messages per interaction.

After teaching individuals how to effectively communicate and participate in recreation activities, it is important to provide them with an opportunity to practice the skills they have learned.

McCarthy and Light (2001) provided a theater arts program for two children who used AAC and several children without disabilities. The program occurred five times per week over a 2-week period and included activities that promoted theater arts techniques such as pantomime, unscripted role play, and scripted role play. All participants demonstrated increases in 1) level of engagement across theater activities, 2) opportunities for communication, 3) fulfillment of communication opportunities, and 4) success during communication. Success plays a critical role in skill acquisition, motivation, and participation for all individuals; the more success a person experiences, the more likely he or she will participate in that activity in the future (Eggen & Kauchak, 1994). Therefore, providing opportunities for children who use AAC to experience success is extremely important for increasing both their motivation to participate in recreation activities and their engagement during these activities.

Organized leisure education programs may play an important role in promoting leisure for individuals with disabilities. Hoge et al. (1999) examined the effects of a leisure education program on 19 adolescents and young adults with mild to moderate intellectual disability. The 18-week program focused on developing leisure appreciation, self-determination and decision-making skills, social interactions and friendships, and leisure resources. Each unit (e.g., leisure appreciation, self-determination and decision making) included group discussion and activities to teach individuals about the topic (e.g., what it means, why it is important, skills related to the topic). Some learning activities included role plays and field trips that gave individuals the opportunity to practice and apply target skills. Significant improvement in achievement of educational objectives and an increase in perception of freedom when choosing activities were identified across individuals following the program and at a 2-month follow-up.

Because communication and social interaction play a large part in many recreation activities, ensuring access to communication is critical. Adolescence provides significant challenges for using AAC systems. Individuals with complex communication needs want systems with rapid access to a wide range of vocabulary (Bryen, 2008; Williams et al., 2008), including uniquely adolescent vocabulary (i.e., slang); they also need systems that are attractive to their peers and can be used in a variety of environments (DeRuyter, McNaughton, Caves, Bryen, & Williams, 2007).

In addition to access to vocabulary and an appropriate device (i.e., linguistic and operational competence), individuals who use AAC may require specific training in the social skills and strategies needed to participate in conversations. Dattilo and O'Keefe (1992) found that some individuals who used AAC rarely initiated and maintained conversations; therefore, the researchers implemented an intervention to increase the conversational control of such individuals. The ultimate goal of the intervention was to improve leisure experiences by teaching individuals communication strategies and skills to help them initiate and share conversations as well as state their preferences and make decisions within the context of recreation activities. The specific skills targeted included responding to partner initiations and taking control of the conversation. Participants increased the percentage of turns they took in a conversation from 27% to 36% and maintained or increased their gains after the intervention was over.

Not only is the number of conversation turns important, but so is the ability of the individual who uses AAC to be a positive and valued communication partner. Light, Binger, Agate, and Ramsay (1999) discussed the significance of individuals being "other oriented"—that is, demonstrating an interest in others rather than focusing on themselves (Argyle, 1969; Spitzberg & Cupach, 1984).

Light et al. (1999) investigated the impact of teaching individuals who use AAC how to ask partner-focused questions during conversations. Questions included those that expressed an interest in the other person, such as "What did you do last weekend?" and "How are you doing?" The researchers found that all participants learned how to ask partner-focused questions and learned how to generalize the use of partner-focused questions to new communication partners as well as to new environments.

Supporting Communication Partners

Given the important role family and friends play in supporting the individual who uses AAC, it is important to provide them with supports as well. Support should be provided on how to promote participation in recreational activities, including by providing new opportunities for communication and choice within activities, as well as how to support participation within a particular activity.

Professionals, family, and friends can increase individuals' communicative interaction and participation in recreation activities by ensuring that individuals can successfully access and use their communication system and by supporting the development of a responsive environment. To increase participation, it is important to assist individuals by 1) providing access to communication, 2) teaching individuals activity-related skills, and 3) providing opportunities to practice learned skills in recreational activities.

As with leisure education for individuals with disabilities, formal training can be provided to those who interact with an individual who uses AAC. This training can increase the opportunities of individuals with disabilities to participate in recreation activities of their choice. For example, Jones et al. (1999) found that after staff were trained on how to provide active support for individuals in a community residence, individuals with disabilities demonstrated an increase in engagement during activities. The training was implemented during a 2-day workshop and focused on teaching staff how to 1) effectively plan and schedule both mandatory and nonmandatory activities (i.e., activities of the individual's choice), 2) consult with residents during planning, and 3) assist individuals when participating in these activities. In addition, the staff received a 3-day follow-up training in which the trainer assisted each staff member in applying what he or she had learned with the residents. This study demonstrates the importance of training for those who work with individuals who use AAC in order to increase 1) the number of opportunities for individuals who use AAC to participate in activities of their choice, 2) the engagement of these individuals during these activities, and 3) the quality of their participation.

People who interact with individuals who require AAC may also benefit from instruction on how best to develop and support communication. Conversation is a transactional process that occurs between individuals; communication interventions for communication partners can be beneficial for improving the quality of leisure experiences. Dattilo and Light (1993) implemented an intervention for communication partners of individuals who use AAC. Family members and friends were taught to use specific strategies when conversing, including 1) providing opportunities for the individual who uses AAC to initiate conversations, 2) providing the individual with adequate time to respond, 3) responding appropriately to all communication attempts by the individual, and 4) providing opportunities for the individual to elaborate on messages. The intervention resulted in increased participation by the individual with complex communication needs.

In addition to teaching skills to support communicative interaction, it may also be important to provide training to partners regarding the technical operation of the AAC device. In a study designed to assess the needs, priorities, and preferences of families of adolescents and young adults with complex communication needs, Angelo, Kokoska, and Jones (1996) found that mothers and fathers of adolescents and young adults reported that increasing their knowledge of the communication device was one of their top priorities.

Increasing Public Awareness

Opportunity barriers may not be eliminated simply by implementing an intervention or providing an AAC device (Beukelman & Mirenda, 2005). Many frustrations that individuals who use AAC experience during recreation result from lack of awareness, knowledge, and concern on the part of others. Therefore, it is important for individuals who use AAC, as well as their family, friends, and professionals, to play an active role in educating the public and in creating awareness of the challenges associated with having complex communication needs. Although change to accommodate the differences of an individual who uses AAC can sometimes first be seen as an imposition, it often brings many benefits. Sometimes the best way to create systems change is with the change brought about by the participation of one individual. For example, Rebecca Beayni has significant cognitive and physical challenges but has an active life volunteering 1) in schools (listening to children read), 2) at museums (guiding visitors at an interactive exhibit), and 3) as part of a traveling dance troupe (Henderson, 2007). In describing Rebecca's impact on others, her mother, Susan, wrote the following:

> Rebecca's school and later work experience is a testament to how one person can change the entire culture that exists around them. Teachers, administrators, fellow students, and co-workers always say that Rebecca's mere presence changes the very fabric of their relationships, making them more collaborative, more compassionate, and more intuitive to strategies that advantage all persons. (Beayni & Beayni, 2005, p. 1)

FUTURE RESEARCH

There is limited understanding of the recreation experience of adolescents and young adults who use AAC. Although there have been glimpses of what is possible, it is clear that for many individuals, recreation experiences are limited in both quantity and quality. Future research should help describe both the barriers to leisure experiences and innovative approaches for increasing both opportunity and access. Dattilo et al. (2008) is the only study to date that has examined the perspectives of young adults who use AAC about their leisure experiences. Because of the nature of the online focus group, only individuals with literacy skills were included in this study; therefore, further investigation of the perspectives of individuals who use AAC (including those who do not have literacy skills) may provide useful information on barriers and key supports.

In addition, more information is needed on how leisure education and appropriate transition services can serve to promote positive outcomes for individuals with complex communication needs. Although there is some documentation of successful programs supporting the development of recreation skills for school-age individuals (e.g., McCarthy & Light, 2001; Uys, Alant, & Lloyd, 2005), more work is needed on how best to prepare individuals who use AAC to ensure successful leisure experiences. Additional work is also needed to identify effective interventions to increase opportunities and support for the recreation experiences of individuals who use AAC.

CONCLUSION

Participating in recreation activities provides individuals with the opportunity to freely choose a desired activity and to experience the positive emotions of enjoyment and satisfaction associated with the leisure experience. Clearly, there are numerous challenges to participating in recreation activities in today's society, and supporting such participation among individuals who use AAC may require interventions to increase both opportunities and access. However, the benefits of recreation, both to the individual and to society, are clear. As "Colton," a 31-year-old man who uses his foot to control a tracking ball for an AAC device, made clear in the following quote, recreational activities and community participation are an integral part of a complete and satisfying adult life:

> I think my attitude towards life has a lot to do with the barriers I have overcome. Yes, I have a physical disability, but everybody has some type of barrier. I think we all have a choice to make. . . . I've chosen to live life abundantly, and because I have, I have been given solutions to barriers. It isn't all easy, but I know anything is possible. You just have to be willing to try it. . . . You only have one life to live, so you might as well live it to the fullest. (Dattilo et al., 2008, p. 23)

REFERENCES

Adkins, J., & Matson, J.L. (1980). Teaching institutionalized mentally retarded adults socially appropriate leisure skills. *Mental Retardation, 18,* 249–252.

Alberto, P.A., & Troutman, A.C. (2003). *Applied behavioral analysis for teachers* (6th ed.). Columbus, OH: Merrill/Prentice Hall.

Americans with Disabilities Act (ADA) of 1990, PL 101-336, 42 U.S.C. §§ 12101 *et seq.*

Angelo, D.H., Kokoska, S.M., & Jones, S.D. (1996). Family perspective on augmentative and alternative communication: Families of adolescents and young adults. *Augmentative and Alternative Communication, 12,* 13–20.

Argyle, M. (1969). *Social interaction.* Chicago: Aldine Atherton.

Beayni, R., & Beayni, S. (2005). *Presentation to the United Nations Ad Hoc Committee on the Rights and Dignity of Persons With Disabilities, August 3, 2005.* Retrieved May 12, 2009, from http://www.planinstitute.ca/ ?q=learnfromus/library/rebecca_beaynis_presentation_united_nations

Beukelman, D.R., & Mirenda, P. (2005). *Augmentative and alternative communication: Supporting children and adults with complex communication needs* (3rd ed.). Baltimore: Paul H. Brookes Publishing Co.

Bregha, F.J. (1985). Leisure and freedom re-examined. In T.A. Goodale & P.A. Witt (Eds.), *Recreation and leisure: Issues in an era of change* (2nd ed., pp. 35–43). State College, PA: Venture.

Bryen, D.N. (2008). Vocabulary to support socially-valued adult roles. *Augmentative and Alternative Communication, 24,* 294–301.

Bryen, D.N., Potts, B.B., & Carey, A.C. (2006). Job-related social networks and communication technology. *Augmentative and Alternative Communication, 22,* 1–9.

Bullock, C.C., & Mahon, M.J. (1997). *Introduction to recreation services for people with disabilities: A person-centered approach.* Champaign, IL: Sagamore.

Calculator, S. (1996). Introduction. In S. Calculator & C. Jorgensen (Eds.), *Including students with severe disabilities in school* (pp. xxiii–xxvii). San Diego: Singular Press.

Cardona, G.W. (2000). Spaghetti talk. In M. Fried-Oken & H.A. Bersani (Eds.), *Speaking up and spelling it out: Personal essays on augmentative and alternative communication* (pp. 237–244). Baltimore: Paul H. Brookes Publishing Co.

Cheseldine, S.E., & Jeffree, D.M. (1981). Mentally handicapped adolescents: Their use of leisure. *Journal of Mental Deficiency Research, 25,* 49–59.

Creech, R. (1992). *Reflections from a unicorn.* Greenville, NC: R.C. Publishing.

Dattilo, J. (2002). *Inclusive leisure services: The rights of people with disabilities* (2nd ed.). State College, PA: Venture.

Dattilo, J., Estrella, G., Estrella, L.J., Light, J., McNaughton, D., & Seabury, M. (2008). "I have chosen to live life abundantly": Perceptions of leisure by adults who use augmentative and alternative communication. *Augmentative and Alternative Communication, 24,* 16–28.

Dattilo, J., & Jekubovich-Fenton, N. (1995). Leisure services trends for people with mental retardation. *Parks and Recreation, 30*(5), 46–52.

Dattilo, J., & Kleiber, D.A. (1993). Psychological perspectives for therapeutic recreation research: The psychology of enjoyment. In M.J. Malkin & C.Z. Howe (Eds.), *Research in therapeutic recreation: Concepts and methods* (pp. 57–76). State College, PA: Venture.

Dattilo, J., Kleiber, D., & Williams, R. (1998). Self-determination and enjoyment enhancement: A psychologically-based service delivery model for therapeutic recreation. *Therapeutic Recreation Journal, 32,* 258–271.

Dattilo, J., & Light, J. (1993). Setting the state for leisure: Encouraging reciprocal communication for people using augmentative and alternative communication systems through facilitator instruction. *Therapeutic Recreation Journal, 27,* 156–171.

Dattilo, J., Light, J., St. Peter, S., & Sheldon, K. (1995). Parents' perspectives on leisure patterns of youth using augmentative and alternative communication systems. *Therapeutic Recreation Journal, 29,* 8–17.

Dattilo, J., & O'Keefe, B.M. (1992). Setting the state for leisure: Encouraging adults with mental retardation who use augmentative and alternative communication systems to share conversations. *Therapeutic Recreation Journal, 26,* 27–37.

Dattilo, J., & Williams, R. (2000). Leisure education. In J. Dattilo (Ed.), *Facilitation techniques in therapeutic recreation* (pp. 165–190). State College, PA: Venture.

DeRuyter, F., McNaughton, D., Caves, K., Bryen, D.N., & Williams, M.B. (2007). Enhancing AAC connections with the world. *Augmentative and Alternative Communication, 23,* 258–270.

Eggen, P., & Kauchak, D. (1994). *Educational psychology: Classroom connections* (2nd ed.). Englewood Cliffs, NJ: Macmillan.

Garza, N.M. (2005, April). Engagement in postsecondary education, work, or preparation for work. In M. Wagner, L. Newman, R. Cameto, N. Garza, & P. Levine (Eds.), *After high school: A first look at the postschool ex-*

periences of youth with disabilities. A report from the National Longitudinal Transition Study-2 (NLTS2) (pp. 3-1–3-6). Menlo Park, CA: SRI International. Retrieved May 20, 2009, from http://www.nlts2.org/reports/2005_04/nlts2_report_2005_04_ch3.pdf

Gist, N.P., & Fava, S.F. (1964). *Urban society.* New York: Crowell.

Halpern, A.S. (1994). The transition of youth with disabilities to adult life: A position statement of the Division on Career Development and Transition, the Council for Exceptional Children. *Career Development for Exceptional Individuals, 17,* 115–124.

Hamm, B., & Mirenda, P. (2006). Post school quality of life for individuals with developmental disabilities who use AAC. *Augmentative and Alternative Communication, 22,* 134–147.

Henderson, H. (2007, January 20). *Similar case, vastly different approaches.* Retrieved June 4, 2009, from http://www.rebeccabeayni.com/NewspaperArticles_SimilarCase_(Redo).html

Hoge, G., Dattilo, J., & Williams, R. (1999). Effects of leisure education on perceived freedom in leisure of adolescents with mental retardation. *Therapeutic Recreation Journal, 33,* 320–332.

Hohn, R. (2000). Making people laugh and cry. In M. Fried-Oken & H.A. Bersani (Eds.), *Speaking up and spelling it out: Personal essays on augmentative and alternative communication* (pp. 215–220). Baltimore: Paul H. Brookes Publishing Co.

Jones, E., Perry, J., Lowe, K., Felce, D., Toogood, S., Dunstand, F., et al. (1999). Opportunity and the promotion of activity among adults with severe intellectual disability living in community residences: The impact of training staff in active supports. *Journal of Intellectual Disability Research, 43,* 164–178.

Joyce, M. (2000). A fish story. In M. Fried-Oken & H.A. Bersani (Eds.), *Speaking up and spelling it out: Personal essays on augmentative and alternative communication* (pp. 87–96). Baltimore: Paul H. Brookes Publishing Co.

Keplinger, D. (2009). *Dan Keplinger, artist.* Retrieved June 3, 2009, from http://www.kinggimp.com/index_static.html

Kleiber, D.A. (1999). *Leisure experience and human development: A dialectical interpretation.* New York: Basic Books.

Kreiner, J.L. (2005). *Development of a vocabulary-free leisure interest assessment instrument for individuals with severe developmental disabilities and communication difficulties.* Unpublished doctoral dissertation, Kent State University, Kent, OH.

Larson, V.L., & McKinley, N.L. (1998). Characteristics of adolescents' conversations: A longitudinal study. *Clinical Linguistics & Phonetics, 12,* 183–203.

Leitner, M.J., & Leitner, S.F. (2004). *Leisure enhancement* (3rd ed.). Binghamton, NY: Haworth Press.

Light, J. (1989). Toward a definition of communicative competence for individuals using augmentative and alternative communication systems. *Augmentative and Alternative Communication, 5,* 137–144.

Light, J., Binger, C., Agate, T.L., & Ramsay, K.N. (1999). Teaching partner-focused questions to individuals who use augmentative and alternative communication to enhance their communicative competence. *Journal of Speech, Language, and Hearing Research, 42,* 241–255.

Light, J., McNaughton, D., Krezman, C., Williams, M., Gulens, M., Galskoy, A., et al. (2007). The AAC Mentor Project: Web-based instruction in sociorelational skills and collaborative problem solving for adults who use augmentative and alternative communication. *Augmentative and Alternative Communication, 23,* 56–75.

Lilienfield, M., & Alant, E. (2005). The social interaction of an adolescent who uses AAC: The evaluation of a peer-training program. *Augmentative and Alternative Communication, 21,* 278–294.

MacDonald, J., & Gillette, Y. (1986). Communicating with persons with severe handicaps: Roles of parents and professionals. *Journal of The Association for Persons with Severe Handicaps, 11,* 276–285.

McCarthy, J., & Light, J. (2001). Instructional effectiveness of an integrated theater arts program for children using augmentative and alternative communication and their nondisabled peers: Preliminary study. *Augmentative and Alternative Communication, 17,* 88–98.

McDonald, E.T. (1980). Early identification and treatment of children at risk for speech development. In R.L. Schiefelbusch (Ed.), *Nonspeech language and communication: Analysis and intervention* (pp. 49–80). Baltimore: University Park Press.

McLeod, L.H. (2008a). Better things to do. In *A declaration of a body of love* (pp. 18–19). San Mateo, CA: Café Press.

McLeod, L.H. (2008b). Wall. In *A declaration of a body of love* (pp. 7–9). San Mateo, CA: Café Press.

McNaughton, D., Rackensperger, T., Benedek-Wood, E., Krezman, C., Williams, M.B., & Light, J. (2008). "A child needs to be given a chance to succeed": Parents of individuals who use AAC describe the benefits and challenges of learning AAC technologies. *Augmentative and Alternative Communication, 24,* 43–55.

Mirenda, P., & Dattilo, J. (1987). Instructional techniques in alternative communication for students with severe intellectual handicaps. *Augmentative and Alternative Communication, 3,* 143–152.

Mulderij, K.J. (1997). Peer relations and friendship in physically disabled children. *Child: Care, Health and Development, 23,* 379–389.

Rackensperger, T., Krezman, C., McNaughton, D., Williams, M., & D'Silva, K. (2005). "When I first got it, I wanted to throw it off a cliff": The challenges and benefits of learning AAC technologies as described by adults who use AAC. *Augmentative and Alternative Communication, 21,* 165–186.

Scherer, M.J. (2000). *Living in the state of stuck: How assistive technology impacts the lives of people with disabilities* (3rd ed.). Cambridge, MA: Brookline Books.

Schleien, S.J., & Green, F.P. (1992). Three approaches for integrating persons with disabilities into community recreation. *Journal of Parks and Recreation Administration, 10,* 51–66.

Smith, M. (2005). The dual challenges of aided communication and adolescence. *Augmentative and Alternative Communication, 21,* 67–79.

Special Olympics. (2009). *What we do.* Retrieved June 4, 2009, from http://www.specialolympics.org/What _We_Do.aspx

Spirit Movers. (2009). *Spirit Movers.* Retrieved May 12, 2009, from http://www.larchedaybreak.com/spirit-movers.aspx

Spitzberg, B., & Cupach, W. (1984). *Interpersonal communication competence.* Beverly Hills: Sage.

Uys, C.J.E., Alant, E., & Lloyd, L.L. (2005). A play package for children with severe disabilities: A validation. *Augmentative and Alternative Communication, 17,* 133–154.

Wagner, M. (2005, April). The leisure activities, social involvement, and citizenship of youth with disabilities after high school. In M. Wagner, L. Newman, R. Cameto, N. Garza, & P. Levine (Eds.), *After high school: A first look at the postschool experiences of youth with disabilities. A report from the National Longitudinal Transition Study-2 (NLTS2)* (pp. 7-1–7-26). Menlo Park, CA: SRI International. Retrieved May 20, 2009, from http://www.nlts2.org/reports/2005_04/nlts2_report_2005_04_ch7.pdf

Wagner, M., Newman, L., Cameto, R., Garza, N., & Levine, P. (Eds.). (2005, April). *After high school: A first look at the postschool experiences of youth with disabilities. A report from the National Longitudinal Transition Study-2 (NLTS2).* Menlo Park, CA: SRI International. Retrieved May 20, 2009, from http://www.nlts2.org/reports/2005_04/nlts2_report_2005_04_complete.pdf

Williams, M.B., Krezman, C., & McNaughton, D. (2008). "Reach for the stars": Five principles for the next 25 years of AAC. *Augmentative and Alternative Communication, 24,* 194–206.

8

The Language of Love

Sexuality and People Who Use AAC

Dave Hingsburger

> Communication leads to community, that is, to understanding, intimacy and mutual valuing. (Rollo May)

Perhaps more than any other area of human existence and experience, sexuality is laden with anxiety and fear (Crooks & Baur, 2007). Questions are uncomfortable to ask, answers are difficult to hear. Add to the already high discomfort of sexuality the issue of disability, and predictably there are problems (Hingsburger & Tough, 2002). The willingness of surgeons to cut into the body of women such as Carrie Buck (the first woman with a disability sterilized in the United States under eugenics laws) demonstrates how far society is willing to go to curb the sexual behavior of those with disabilities (Lombardo, 2008). Ironically, although one may proclaim disgust at historical approaches to managing the sexuality of those with disabilities, many agencies continue to have policies that limit opportunities for relationships, limit sexual behavior, and limit access to information (Griffiths, Richards, Federoff, & Watson, 2002). They may not use a surgeon's knife, but the effect is chillingly similar.

For those who use augmentative and alternative communication (AAC), the topic of relationships and sexuality brings up important issues about power and control, about prejudice and preconceptions, about decisions and attitudes (Collier, McGhie-Richmond, Odette, & Pyne, 2006). Picture three people ready to tell their stories. Each has a unique experience as a person who uses AAC, and each brings a topic to the table. Each was referred to a sexuality clinic providing service to people with intellectual disabilities wherein I worked as both a therapist and a consultant. We begin, at the beginning, with people and their experiences.

WENDY

Frustrating is the only word to describe my feelings at that moment. I was faced with doing an interview with a woman who had an AAC system about the possibility that she had been abused by her taxi driver. The first time I met her, she arrived with a staff person but without her communication board. The staff person was shocked that I wanted to actually try and understand her, that I was not just going to look at Wendy but then talk to the staff member to get information. The staff person expressed disbelief that I thought it was even worth trying to interact with Wendy. I was told that "she has a communication board but doesn't use it." I've heard this before and I know that it most often means "she has a communication board but the staff don't bother to use it." An appointment was made for the following day for her to come in, with board, for a chat with me.

When Wendy arrived, I asked the staff person to leave. The staff person protested, saying that I would need her help to understand Wendy. Because her "help" had resulted in Wendy having to make another appointment to come in, I continued with my demand for time alone with Wendy. I pulled out the communication board and set it up. The first word that Wendy pointed to was THANK YOU. I then tried to talk to Wendy about what had happened. Even though this was not a police investigation, Wendy's family wanted to know if their child had been victimized by the taxi driver. He had been convicted of molesting two others with disabilities, and they had suspected something was wrong when Wendy would act up before getting in the cab, something out of character for her.

The communication board was broken into categories of words. The only body words she had were EYE, HAND, MOUTH, and EARS. That was it. She had emotion words, four of them. She had a symbol for TAXI. There were hundreds of other words but none for private parts of her body, none for *touch,* and the word *private* did not exist on her board. I knew that I could ask her yes and no questions, but I was told that, when anxious, she would always answer those types of questions in the affirmative.

After it was all over I met with Wendy's parents and suggested that there needed to be language on the board that was more reflective of both her age (she was 24 at the time) and her needs; that she really should have words about the sexual body parts, and that beyond that I thought the words should be introduced as part of a sex education/abuse reduction class. The words should be learned in the context of their meaning, not just appear suddenly one morning.

Both parents took it "under advisement" but in the end decided that they were going to ensure that she was more "protected" and therefore less "vulnerable." I tried to explain that the more they tried to protect Wendy by limiting her knowledge and vocabulary, the more vulnerable she would really be. I tried to explain that she had a right to language and a right to know about her body.

They informed me that these ideas were "nonsense" and that if I knew their daughter better I would see that her disability would never allow her to be an adult and that she would forever need the protection of others. They were opposed to additional vocabulary, and they would not agree to additional instruction for Wendy............

JONATHON

It was all there in the teacher's notes. Jonathon was a boy in his early teens who was beginning to show a real interest in girls. When he struggled to ask questions regarding sexuality and girls, the questions were seen as inappropriate and even somewhat deviant. The following is a direct comment from a note by the school psychologist: "Jonathon is a pleasant looking boy of 14 who seems to have an obsessive interest in female anatomy." *Hmmm,* I thought to myself, *what 14-year-old boy doesn't?* I had been called in, I thought, to help deal with Jonathon's questions and help him deal with being a teenager in a world that has confusing rules and shifting boundaries. Ultimately, when Jonathon was described to me by a disapproving teacher and an uncomfortable psychologist as "almost pathological," I reminded them that his behavior—the one that resulted in the referral to me—was *staring.* Yes, he stared at women's breasts and butts. For teenage boys, that's pretty typical behavior.

In a tone she usually reserved for only students, the teacher said to me, "You don't understand, Jonathon has a *cognitive* disability along with all of his physical problems." I told her that I did understand that he had cerebral palsy and a mild intellectual disability but that he was still a teenage boy.

As Jonathon used Blissymbolics as his primary communication mode, I brought a few of the booklets I had worked on several years before, booklets that introduced the facts, concepts, and language of sexuality to Blissymbol users. The teacher glanced at one, closed the book, and called a halt to the meeting.

We spoke on the phone the next day and she told me that she needed to compose herself because the idea that I would "sully the innocence" (she actually said *sully*) of one of the children in her classroom was upsetting to her. I pointed out that Jonathon was a teen, a pubescent teen at that, and that he was not a child. His staring at the breasts of women told me that he wasn't an "innocent." He needed education, I said, to ensure that he understood that his interests were normal and his questions valid. Without education, his interests would maybe lead to impulses that could lead to serious trouble for him.

The "team" decided that it would be best simply to use a behavioral approach, to punish staring and reinforce (I'm not kidding) "appropriate looking." Jonathon was expelled from school a few months later for grabbing a teen mentor's breasts. ············

JASON

Jason came to our office for one-to-one education on relationships and sexuality. He took well to the new vocabulary and was respectful in the questions he asked. He wanted to know more about relationships than he did about sexuality. He wanted to be loved and to love someone else. That was his main desire. He was a wonderful guy.

The care home that had referred him for the education classes was, at first, pleased at his progress and his interest in attending. However, he was pulled out of the classes for attempting to ask a woman at his day program out on a date. His agency had a no sex policy, and agency staff were quite surprised that Jason had acted on his desire for a relationship by asking someone out. ············

These scenarios, all based on real individuals, highlight the main problem faced by people with disabilities in regard to relationships and sexuality. That problem? They are under the control of others. Although this is true for all people with intellectual disabilities, for those who use AAC the problems are multiplied. Not only are care providers in control of much of their lives, including their sexuality, they are also often in control of their language. The availability of a symbol for *penis* is fine, but if a care provider decides not to allow that symbol on the board, it may as well not exist.

THE MYTH OF PROTECTION

The fact that people with disabilities are vulnerable to abuse is a surprise to no one. The research is conclusive that having a disability makes it more likely that a person will be a victim of sexual abuse (Powers et al., 2002; Powers, McNeff, Curry, Saxton, & Elliott, 2004). The response to this fact leads many to decide that "protection" is the best way to go (Hingsburger, 1995). Protection is a valuable concept, but the concern is that many believe this really means "protection by others" rather than "protection by self." Their version of protection invariably looks like restriction and punishment. Ensuring that an individual is constantly monitored, constantly in view, constantly accompanied is impossible. And even if possible, it would lead to a life of very limited quality. People with disabilities, then, often end up with fewer rights, less freedom, and more restrictions than those serving jail terms for crimes.

But beyond the inequity of "punishing" those with a disability in the name of protection, the approach also does not work. Given that most victimization is done by those in care-providing roles—and that it is those in care-providing roles who are doing the supervision—the problem becomes evident (Hingsburger, 2006). Protection by self is a far more appropriate and productive approach. Ensuring that people with disabilities have an understanding of the nature of abuse and the language to report it may seem radical, but it is the only way that makes sense.

Given that abuse is conceived of as a crime of power, anything that equalizes power will contribute to a successful strategy to prevent victimization (Crossmaker, 1986). Teaching a few basic concepts and a few words can have a dramatic effect on individuals' ability to repel abuse and protect themselves. How? Abusers, cowards at the best of time, are intimidated by those who can effectively report. By increasing the odds that abusers will be caught, one can decrease the odds that abuse will occur—one important aspect of real protection (Crossmaker, 1989).

LANGUAGE EQUALS POWER

Sex education is linguistic education. It gives a person the language to communicate about his or her body, and thereby it gives power (Patterson, 1991). One can only imagine the pain that Wendy felt first as a result of being victimized and then from being denied the ability to tell her story, to seek justice, to protect herself.

There are many ways of being victimized, many ways of being disrespected, many ways of being denied power. I remember attending a self-advocate meeting about individual rights. A woman with a disability sat next to her boyfriend and expressed her frustration with the barriers to learning about sex and in particular about pregnancy and disease. She and her boyfriend did not want a baby, and they did not want to get sick, but no one would answer their questions, and no one would give them information. She wanted to know "who decided" that they would have this information withheld from them (Hollo, 2003).

Years ago there were few curricula about sexuality for those with disabilities. This is no longer true; now a variety of curricula address a wide variety of needs and abilities (American Association on Intellectual and Developmental Disabilities, 2009). So in fact this young woman was right. If people with a disability of any sort—and particularly those who use AAC—cannot communicate about sexuality and about their bodies, then a decision has been made to withhold both vocabulary and information (Burke, Bedard, & Ludwig, 1998).

So what words do people need in their working vocabularies? The words that protect against abuse are also the words that are needed for establishing consent to participate in sexual activity (Lyden, 2007). Some words are labels for body parts; for example, *vulva, vagina, anus, breast, nipple, stomach, thigh, penis, testicles, erection, pubic hair, mouth*. (Of course there should be words for all body parts; the words listed here are specific to the subject of sexuality.)

Other words are related to concepts (e.g., *private, consent* [want], *non-consent* [not want], *okay, not okay*), actions (e.g., *ejaculate, intercourse, insert, threaten, force, touch*), and feelings (e.g., *happy, pleasure, scared, angry*). Research by Diane Bryen (2008) firmly established that few of these words are typically provided in the preprogrammed vocabulary of AAC devices. In follow-up work, Bryen and colleagues developed comprehensive vocabulary lists to enable individuals who use AAC to gain access to needed concepts and terms (Institute on Disabilities at Temple University, 2009).

It becomes obvious that it is impossible to add the language of sexuality to someone's communication system without doing sex education. Each word comes with a multitude of questions, each word leads to a discussion, each word answers one question but asks another. A number of years ago when the Blissymbolics Communication Institute decided to create words regarding sexuality, they realized that to simply create the symbols and then toss them onto communication boards would be a travesty of the trust that the symbol users had in them. Instead, they asked me and Susan Ludwig, a public health nurse, to create a series of books that introduced the language of sexuality in the context of the information that is necessary for the understanding and the use of these words (Ludwig & Hingsburger, 1993).

For those who use communication systems that are publicly visible, such as on a communication board, there is sometimes a concern that the presence of "adult" language can lead some communication partners to initiate inappropriate interactions. The fact that explicit language is there "for the pointing at" may encourage those with abusive intentions to persuade individuals who use AAC to participate in unwanted interactions and to discuss topics that were formerly inaccessible.

For this reason many have devised ways to keep private language private. One fellow had a symbol for PRIVATE BOOK, and when he pointed there the support staff would get an attachable board out from the back of his wheelchair. Another woman had one part of her communication board velcroed shut. An attached note said that she was the only person to decide if it was to be opened.

But what is noteworthy in both of those situations is that suddenly the individual communicator is the one in the decision-making position. As this person now has adult things to say, he or she is given the adult responsibility of deciding when and where to use that language.

ATTITUDES BASED ON PREJUDICE

As discussed earlier, a failure to provide sex education is the result of a decision, not a lack of resources. Although many people with disability remain woefully uneducated about sexuality, this is because of a lack of will on the part of care providers. When faced with providing or not providing information about sexuality and relationships, someone decided to withhold information. What is the source of this decision? Disability brings with it a lot of assumptions, a lot of preconceptions. Disability, which is simply a different way of being in the world, is often seen as an impediment to growth, development, and adulthood (Owen, Griffiths, & Endicott, 2009). This has huge ramifications when it comes to sexuality. The mere idea of sexuality is an outrage to those who see people with disabilities as perpetual children, as existing in a "presexual" state of needing not information but protection, not education but supervision (Earle, 2001; Pendler & Hingsburger, 1991). For individuals who hold this view, sex education promotes sexuality rather than prevents abuse. The introduction of sexual terminology or sexual facts is believed to "put ideas into innocent heads" (Swango-Wilson, 2008).

This view of someone with a disability as a perpetual child is difficult for someone who is an AAC user to combat (Lever, 2003). Others with more typical communication are not restricted by circumstance as to how they may access language and terminology. They can more easily self-advocate, as their vocabulary comes from a variety of sources. What guardians desire to withhold, television can easily grant. What parents try to control, friends can supply. What staff hope to conceal, media will inevitably reveal. Thus, with a myriad of sources for learning words combined with a tongue that works—parents, guardians, and staff can be clearly told where to get off.

For AAC users, there is the horrifying possibility of learning words that would lead to a reexamination of possibilities but never, ever, being able to use them. Forced to live within the limits set upon one's language by others can only be seen as an abuse of power of the highest order (Glennen, 1997). Sarah Lever, in individual who uses AAC, wrote the following:

> Sometimes even when we want to speak out, we don't have the right words to do so. Most communication aids don't come with vocabulary necessary to end the silence about crime and abuse. Many of us don't have easy access to the right vocabulary in our communication devices. Not having adequate vocabulary raises the risk of people who rely on AAC being victimized because we are identified as unable to tell anyone when crime or abuse occurs. It allows those who would commit crimes against us to continue undeterred. We need adequate vocabulary to talk about crime and abuse, and we need to know how to use that vocabulary. (2003, p. 4)

Being forced to use only words approved by one's mother, vetted by one's team, and scrubbed clean by the most conservative of one's staff is to be robbed of the most basic freedom—communication—by those who "know best." This goes beyond sexuality to question the basic rights of all with disabilities.

Oddly, the other main sexual myth that has led to harsh attitudes and harsher practices is the idea that, rather than being sexually innocent, people with disabilities are sexually uninhibited and dangerous (Bogdan, Biklen, Shapiro, & Spelkoman, 1990). The irony is that, as happened with Jonathon, one's actions and restrictions can be the genesis for extremely inappropriate behavior. This then can be a self-perpetuating mistake, in that restrictions lead to inappropriateness, and inappropriateness leads to further restriction (Griffiths, Quinsey, & Hingsburger, 1989). There is no research supporting the hypothesis that those with disabilities are less inhibited sexually than others (Rowe, Savage, Ragg, & Wigle, 1987).

Ironically, though, sexual disinhibition is often a feature of practice and parenting. A young man attending a conference with his mother stopped by a booth where I was working. She noted, loudly, that he needed changing and began to take his pants off right there in front of me, others working the booth, and people looking over materials for sale. I suggested that she do this in private. She said, "He doesn't know the difference," to which I responded, "How can he when he's never been given the dignity of privacy?" Although she was angered by my comment, we spoke later and she stated that she had never thought about the issue of changing him publicly before; even though he was clearly a man, she thought about him as a child. She began wondering if she had acclimatized him to inappropriateness from living with and possibly learning poor boundaries. I suggested that she add the words *public* and *private* to his communication board and that she begin teaching these concepts to her son. She caught me at the end of the conference and told me, teary eyed, that she did not have to teach him the concepts, that he knew them. And as soon as the symbols were put on his communication board, he pointed at PRIVATE over and over again as if he were scolding her for years of exposing him to the public.

CONFRONTING PREJUDICE

Perpetual children. Holy innocents. God's babies. People with disabilities in general have to fight against these kind of stereotypes, but those with intellectual disabilities live with them daily (Wood, 2004). Although the fight for the right to education or language is a difficult one, the fight for the right to relationships is even more difficult. Oddly, many agencies, although they provide sex education, still have policies that forbid any form of romantic attachment (May & Simpson, 2003). In many cases, the more "disabled" an individual is seen as being, the stronger the stance against sexuality (Tepper, 2000).

Although it may cause anger to refer to this as prejudice, it simply is. To come to a belief that a whole group of people lack the ability to love, the need for sex, the longing to be special to someone else, is as ignorant as any prejudice can be. Research into attitudes toward sexuality and disabilities shows clearly that there are many who simply believe that masturbation should be the limit ("as long as it's not on my shift") for people with disabilities (Cuskelly & Bryde, 2004), and to date only a few have dared to even raise the topic (Earle, 2001).

Here's the real problem, though. It is frequently those individuals with negative attitudes who are also those who hold the power. A gay person with a homophobic neighbor may be bothered by the attitude, but this attitude does not have any direct power over the gay person's living of life. This is not true for people with disabilities. The simple fact is that anti-sexuality feelings regarding disability run deep and pose serious challenges to those who want to begin relationships. Those who have managed to traverse the dangerous ground of agency disapproval have tended to be those who are quite able, very verbal, and good at self-advocacy. These individuals are cutting new ground within agencies, but for those who use AAC, sometimes the opportunities that are gained by a few are not accessible to the rest of those who receive agency services.

In spite of the challenges, however, the work of attitude change falls on the shoulders of those with disabilities. It always has. In Canada, the language for referring to disability has changed as a direct result of the self-advocacy movement (People First of Canada, 2006). In the United States, the acceptance of segregated housing for people with disabilities ended and institutions closed as a direct result of the self-advocacy movement (Castles, 1996). There is power in groups, and there is power in one. Neither should be discounted.

These changes in language, in housing options, and in other areas of disability advocacy confirm my belief that the only thing that leads to attitude change is confrontation. And it has to be confrontation between the right people. Let me give an example. Years ago, when working at a sexuality clinic, I was often asked by people with disabilities to speak to their parents about their interest in a relationship. I saw this as my job, and I did it. Not once did I change an attitude or garner permission. I finally realized that I was going to a parent and saying "Your child is competent to be in a relationship," but by speaking for that individual I was communicating nonverbally "Your child isn't capable of speaking for herself."

We changed our policy such that we would support someone in speaking to their family, but we would no longer do the talking. Our first experience was with a man with whom I held several practice sessions. When we went to speak to his mother, whose face was set to refuse, he so beautifully communicated his desire to be in a relationship and his desire for her to be happy with him that we could hear her heart melting.

A fundamental tenet for those of us serving people with disabilities should be "Never do work for your clients that belongs to them." These are not our families, and these should not be our discussions. It is our job to ensure that individuals have enough skill to speak for themselves, no matter how they speak. They need vocabulary *and* they need backbone. In other words, they need to be adults.

ATTITUDES BASED ON FEARS

Sometimes it isn't prejudice, it's fear. Given the reasons to fear sexual relationships, it's amazing that sexual contact is ever made at all. Consider the "Big Three" concerns that parents bring forward: exploitation, disease, and unwanted pregnancy. Should parents be concerned about these issues? Of course, they are huge concerns.

How does one know that someone has the knowledge and the skill to navigate the dangers of sexuality? This question was asked by YAI in New York City (YAI Network, 2009). They had established themselves as an agency that served adults, and that meant that the opportunity for adult relationships would be possible for those who could give informed consent to sexual encounters. Now that they had acknowledged the importance of informed consent, they needed to figure out a way to assess individuals' ability to provide informed consent and a way to teach individuals the skills necessary to do so.

After years of work, YAI created a means of assessing the ability of an individual with a disability to provide consent. The YAI consent assessment (YAI Sexuality Rights and Advocacy Committee, 1995) is broken into five areas of understanding (discussed in the next section) and uses practical, real-world questions to assess if an individual has the information and skills needed to make healthy decisions. The test is used in Canada, and it is noteworthy that it was accepted in a court case as a reasonable measure of consent in someone with a disability (S. Tough, personal communication, March 24, 2005).

Too often the discussion over a person's ability or perceived lack of ability to provide consent comes down to opinion. My opinion versus yours. An agency opinion versus a guardian's opinion. The YAI consent test takes the discussion out of the realm of opinion and into the arena of fact (Blasingame, 2005). The test clearly identifies gaps in knowledge that can lead to poor decisions and serious mistakes. If an individual fails the test, the intent is for him or her to receive training in the area of concern and then take the test again.

The consent test is a huge friend to all with disabilities, but especially for those who use AAC. People who may not have been provided with opportunities to demonstrate their competence can prove themselves to be as knowledgeable as anyone else. One woman who used a speech output device to speak said that after 1 hour of testing she proved to everyone around her that she "wasn't a little girl any longer." The grin on her face said it all. Suddenly everyone had to look at her differently. It wasn't just about sex, as it turned out; it was about the cutesy way that staff spoke to her, the "goo goo" tones in the voice. This test enabled this woman to demonstrate her knowledge and helped support her entry into new forms of relationships in every part of her life.

There are those who would restrict because of their fear that an individual lacks needed knowledge and skills. The consent test allows these people to reassess their understanding of who an individual with a disability truly is—and to begin to ask better questions about how to provide the services needed to support relationships and a richer quality of life.

ASSESSING CONSENT (AND CONFRONTING FEAR)

A growing awareness of the rights of individuals with disabilities has led to increased interest in ways of assessing an individual's ability to provide informed consent (Ames & Samowitz, 1995; Lyden, 2007). To address the fears of caregivers that an individual does not understand the implications of a particular activity or know how to protect himself or herself from unwanted consequences (Lyden, 2007), the YAI test (YAI Sexuality Rights and Advocacy Committee, 1995) measures knowledge in five main areas.

1. The individual "has an awareness of the nature of the sexual act under consideration and of having a choice to engage in or abstain from the type of sexual contact under consideration" (p. 1). The "acts under consideration" can include hugging, touching of private parts, and intercourse. There is no need for an individual to have extensive language about the inner workings of the body—knowledge about fallopian tubes, vas deferens, and the like is not necessary. The individual only needs to be able to define sexual activity and then be able to indicate the ability to say no to unwanted touch and unwanted sexual activity. The ability to say no is revisited a number of times in this test, as the test was structured to ensure that individuals have the clear understanding that they are the ultimate decision makers when it comes to sexuality and sexual acts.

2. "The person has an understanding of how to prevent an unwanted pregnancy and diseases which are sexually transmitted" (p. 3). This area requires a little more technical knowledge and language that reflects that knowledge. People are required to be able to identify at least one method of birth control, one sexually transmitted disease, and one method of protection from sexually transmitted disease. What is clear is that in order to establish informed consent, individuals need to be aware of the possible consequences of sexual activity. Moreover, it is important that individuals know that there are ways of being sexual and being safe at the same time.

Having the ability to discuss the prevention of unwanted pregnancies and sexually transmitted diseases also increases the likelihood that the individual will be able to describe, in situations of abuse, exactly what has happened. The behavior of a partner (e.g., the use or lack of use of a condom) may have both medical and legal ramifications, and it is important for the individual to be able to accurately describe any events that took place.

3. "The person has an understanding of the need for restriction of sexual behavior as to time, place, or behavior" (p. 4). Here the concepts of *public* and *private* are emphasized. It is of utmost importance that an individual understand the various layers of privacy. There are private places, private spaces, private parts, private thoughts, private topics of conversation. It is important that an individual learn to match behavior with place.

These concepts can be very hard for a person with significant disabilities to learn, as often, in receiving care, typical boundaries are violated. It is hard for people to speak of the *bathroom* and *bedroom* as private spaces when they are assisted by others, sometimes even strangers, in meeting very private needs. First, it is important for care providers to maximize privacy by ensuring that the individual is not exposed to public view, doors are closed, and voices lowered. Second, it is important to adapt any curriculum to the needs of those with greater disabilities. None of the existing curricula address the concepts of *public* and *private* from the point of view of those with more significant needs. Therefore, it is important to define *private* in a new and more sophisticated way. For an individual who needs assistance with toileting, the bathroom is "private plus one to help" and the bedroom is "private plus one to help." They are still very different rooms than the front room and the kitchen. Furthermore, sitting on a toilet is vastly different from sitting on a couch, and masturbating is very different from drawing. But these differences can be difficult to understand for those who live constantly in the presence of others. So "private plus one to help" is a concept that can more readily be learned.

4. *"The person has an understanding that certain sexual activities are against the law and could result in or have dire consequences"* (p. 6). The questions in this area address the individual's understanding that sexual behavior is a consensual private act between adults. If it is not consensual, if it is not private, or if it is not between adults capable of providing informed consent, then it is illegal and can have drastic consequences.

This information is best presented in an empowering rather than threatening way. These laws exist to protect as much as to prosecute. Ensuring that people know that they are the only ones who can give permission for sexual activity is followed by the corollary that they cannot touch others sexually without permission. Teaching about personal power and personal control is an important part of teaching the language of sexuality.

5. *"The person understands risk in a potentially harmful sexual situation and is capable of making a reasonable plan for removal from the situation"* (p. 7). Part of the reason sex education is so important is that it gives an opportunity, in the benign setting of a class, to talk about what can happen in the explosive setting of a relationship. Learning how to assert oneself in a relationship is of vital importance in maintaining healthy, nonabusive relationships. These questions address individuals' ability to recognize risk and take appropriate actions to remove themselves from a potentially harmful situation.

Thinking about conflicts that may arise and knowing how to deal with high-risk situations is particularly important for those with mobility or communication disabilities. Strategies for escape or for reporting are of vital importance (Center for Research on Women with Disabilities, 1999). Research indicates that the more significant the disability, the more likely the abuse (Sobsey, 1994). Having training in how to escape, possessing language to report abuse, and having the opportunity to practice the use of these skills can give a sense of personal power and safety where there was none before.

ASSESSMENT AND INSTRUCTION FOR INFORMED CONSENT

Using an established consent test such as the YAI as a basis for identifying and developing a curriculum simply makes sense. It allows an instructor to focus on what is truly important in the area of sexuality and to address an individual's current capacity and his or her information and skill needs. It also demonstrates that much of what is traditionally covered in sexual education is really not necessary for someone to be capable of giving consent. Information on how to correctly identify the location of a fallopian tube or describe the journey of sperm from ejaculation to fertilization is nowhere to be found. Ironically, people without disabilities often expect those with disabilities to know more than they know and to be able to name body parts that most have forgotten exist.

In addition, the language needed in order to be able to show consent, report abuse, or discuss sexual issues with a doctor frequently overlaps. Making sure that people have access to this kind of language is of great importance to their personal dignity and safety in a variety of situations. A woman who is deaf once explained to me how a lack of language had affected her safety, her self-esteem, and her relationship with her family:

> My parents refused me any opportunity to take sex education and would not discuss the issue with me. Even though my parents are hearing, they learned sign, and when I tried to ask them about sex or about the changes in my body, they would just shut down and say that I shouldn't talk about those kinds of dirty things.
>
> When I was in high school I was molested by one of the teachers. I tried to tell my mother, and when I pointed to my vagina, because I didn't have the dignity of the word, she just stopped me. Then I tried to tell my doctor, and it took a while for him to understand because he thought I was being inappropriate. What was really distressing, though, was that the police brought an interpreter, but how could she interpret language I didn't have? I think my credibility was lowered because I couldn't effectively tell my story. I felt shamed sitting with a male police officer pointing at my groin and grimacing. It was humiliating. Nothing happened to the teacher. I am still so angry at my family. I haven't forgiven them. I haven't seen them for years. (Anonymous, personal communication, June 28, 2009)

The use of an assessment tool such as the YAI is a catalyst for an important discussion of how individuals perceive themselves and how societal views of individuals may need to change. The mere ability to discuss sexual activity and protection from diseases or unwanted pregnancy automatically raises the perception of an individual from unable to informed. It is impossible to have a discussion with someone who is able to talk confidently about responsibility without beginning to see him or her as responsible.

TEACHING IN THE REAL WORLD

Classroom style teaching may not always be the most effective way of providing instruction to those with intellectual disabilities. Using strategies in real-world situations and everyday occurrences may be more effective.

Boundaries

Although assessment materials such as the YAI can help determine what should be taught to an individual with a disability, careful thought will need to be given to how new information is taught. As mentioned earlier, because of the public nature of the lives of those with significant disabilities, key concepts such as *public* and *private* can be very difficult to learn.

One of the best ways of making these abstract concepts more concrete is to place the symbol for *private* underneath the picture of a closed door and the symbol for *public* underneath the picture of an open door. Then use this symbol throughout the life space of the individual. Place the PUBLIC symbol on the door to the front room and the PRIVATE symbol on the door to the bedroom. Place the PUBLIC symbol on the drawers that hold public clothing and the PRIVATE symbol on the drawers that hold private clothing. Use the language of privacy throughout the training. If the individual wants to leave the bedroom in his or her underclothing, say, "Hold on, are you wearing public clothes or private clothes? Is the front room a public room or a private room? What do you need to do?" Getting the person to think about matching clothing, behavior, and topics of conversation to appropriate places is a good first step in establishing this concept.

For individuals who are dressed by others and therefore do not have the opportunity to learn by error and get better by practice, it is important that those providing assistance also provide language, context, and concepts. For example, "Okay, now you have your private clothes on, but it's important for you to change into public clothes because we're going into a public room. What would you like to wear?" Conversations that describe what is happening are called *parallel talk*— these conversations allow an individual to learn about the decision-making process. This is a wonderful opportunity to learn the reasons for the rules and to begin to make decisions and assert power over an area in which passivity may have been rewarded in the past.

Moreover, care providers can easily demonstrate the flexible nature of public and private. If an individual comes into his or her office (a public room) and wants to talk about something private, he or she can simply say, "Right now the door is open, so this is a public room. What can we do to make it private?" Once it is identified that the door needs to be closed, the person can simply place the PRIVATE symbol on the inside of the door, comment on it, and then begin the discussion.

It is important for staff to rigorously follow public and private rules. Doors are made to be closed, and when staff are providing service to someone in private areas, doors should be closed and eyes should be averted so that the person has the maximum amount of privacy possible. As another example, staff should be careful not to wear clothing that confuses. Men who wear pants with underwear that shows or women who wear blouses that allow view of bras or bra straps simply confuse the issue. Many agencies do not wish to impose dress codes; however, dress codes can help to establish a professional atmosphere as well as clear boundaries for residents or clients.

Privacy is a learned skill. It is learned through respectful treatment and clear boundaries. People with disabilities have a right to learn about privacy and a right to experience privacy. The right to privacy is a basic human right—it is not a privilege granted by munificent agencies.

Consent

"No means no" is a popular slogan regarding sexual relationships and personal power. In the real world, "no" does not always mean "no." In fact, look at two common scenarios:

Abel lives in a group home with two other residents. An outing has been planned to the mall. A staff person approaches Abel and says, "Abel, do you want to go to the mall?" Abel indicates no. The other two residents are in the van and waiting. There are not enough staff to support one person at home and two at the mall. What is going to happen? Most likely, the staff person is going to grab a coat and say "Abel, do you want to get your coat on now?" Abel indicates no. What happens now? Probably the coat will be put on Abel and he will be taken to the van for the outing.

A staff member notices that Candy has not done the dishes, and it's almost time for lights out. Calling to her, the staff person says, "Candy, do you want to do your dishes now?" Candy shakes her head no. What's going to happen? The staff person will probably up the volume and the means of the request: "It's your night to do dishes, everyone has to contribute, that's the rule. Now, do you want to do dishes?" Candy shakes her head no. What happens now? Probably the staff person will come and "assist" Candy into the kitchen and get her to do the dishes.

In both of these situations, Abel and Candy learn that "no means force." This is a dangerous lesson to teach to those in care. Later on, in a sexual situation, if Candy says no to Abel, he may simply choose to do what he has learned to do a thousand times over—force her. Candy, of course, will not be surprised, because in her life "no" has seldom meant "no"—it has almost always meant "force."

One needs to ask the following question: "How do I expect someone to say no to a penis when we've never given them the opportunity to say no to peas?" Those of us who work with individuals with disabilities need to do two things. First, we need to ensure that they have the opportunity to say no and practice saying no to people in positions of power. The simple fact is that people with disabilities are rarely abused by strangers—most often the abuse comes from care providers (Sobsey, 1994). So there needs to be a lot of practice regarding assertion. Vita Community Living Services, an organization that serves people with disabilities in the city of Toronto, Canada, has a Bill of Rights written by self-advocates within the agency. One of the rights is the following: The right to learn about personal power and a chance to use it every day. Second, we need to ensure that all care providers come to understand the difference between a demand and a choice. The confusion between these two things is what leads to lesson after lesson wherein "no means force" is repeated over and over again.

Learning to Say No

Many people with AAC are limited in their communication of the word *no.* Most communication boards simply have the word or symbol NO that can be pointed to in some manner. For those with speech, there tend to be two types of no. The softer no of a "no thank you" and the harsher assertive *no!* that demonstrates that the person means business. It is important that these two types of no exist for AAC communicators, too. Having a *no!* that is exclusively used to deal with unwanted touch or undesired interactions is hugely important. It immediately demonstrates to an abuser that the individual can discriminate what is going on and can respond to it. The belief that "they don't understand, so they can't report" is shattered the first time an emphatic *no!* is said in response to unwanted touch or unwanted sexual play.

Once the two words are created, it is important to use them. Set up situations in which the individual needs to say no. Start out with those that need simply the soft no. Here are some examples used by staff to provide opportunities for an individual to practice the use of the soft no:

Larry: So what vegetable would you like for supper tonight?

Hank: Carrots.

Larry: Okay, peas it is.

Hank: No. Said carrots.

And another:

Ann: What color blouse would you like to wear?

Dee: Green.

Ann: Here you are. [Hands a blue one.]

Dee: No. Said green.

Caregivers should not be surprised if, at first, the individual simply acquiesces to the switch. It takes a lot of practice to speak up and be assertive when for most of one's life compliance and complacency have been rewarded. These little opportunities may seem trite or even silly, but they are radical to many who live within systems and who have learned that the "right answer" is "what staff want" (Heal & Sigelman, 1995). In fact, many staff complain that it is hard to know what people with disabilities are thinking or what they want because they always seem to tell them what they think they want to hear. With a shift in perspective, one gets a glimpse into someone's past interactions with those in power, if the individual with a disability is afraid to even say "carrots" when the staff so clearly like peas. Once an individual has learned to say the softer no, it is time to practice the louder *no!* Again, doing some role plays that involve someone using a more forceful no can be very useful, however it will be important that everyone understand the nature and goal of the role-play activity. It is important that the role play proceed only if all participants demonstrate an ongoing understanding of the fictional aspect of the activity.

Choices Versus Demands

Even when ensuring increased choices for people with disabilities, to be successful in life everyone has to develop demand tolerance for appropriate requests. This means that when the boss says to do something, people do it—like it or not. When it's time for rent to be paid, people pay it—like it or not.

Of course the world should be full of choices for people with disabilities, but by the same token it should not be free of demands. To eliminate demands is to infantilize people with disabilities into noncontributing, nonproducing people. So before speaking, caregivers need to ask themselves "Is a 'no' possible here?" If it's not, it's not, so don't offer a choice. In the earlier example, Abel is asked if he wants to go on the outing. Everyone else is going, no staff will be at the home to provide support, so clearly he is going to go, too. We could get into a philosophical argument about group homes, group living, and so forth, but right now, let's simply be practical. The staff could offer a choice about something for which there is a choice: "Do you want to wear a coat or a sweater?" But for things for which there is no choice because of health or safety concerns (e.g., a person cannot be left unattended at home), instead of saying "Do you want to go on the outing?" it is best to say "It's time to get in the van to go to the mall" and proceed from there.

OPPORTUNITIES

Once the hurdle of education and language is crossed, another major roadblock to relationships is having access to opportunities to meet and socialize with potential partners. In this regard, one needs to look at the partner pool and initiating action.

Partner Pool

Many people with disabilities suffer from internalized *disphobia,* which is a fear and loathing of one's own disability that evidences itself in fear and loathing of others with disabilities (Hingsburger, 2005; Hingsburger & Tough, 2002). These individuals do not wish to ever be in the company of others with disabilities, would never consider someone with a disability as a potential partner, and want to relate "up and out" of disability. These individuals may say "I would never date someone *like that,*" with the "like that" meaning "with a disability."

Disphobia reduces the potential partner pool significantly in much the same way as not having the opportunity to meet people without disabilities limits the partner pool of those with disabilities. It is important that people with disabilities have a wide social circle, one that includes a variety of people with a variety of interests. Who knows where love will bloom? But if it blooms in a garden in which the individual would never step foot, a lifetime of loneliness is ensured.

Part of the philosophy of integration and inclusion is to eschew any activities in which people with disabilities get together (Chappell, 1997). In practice, this philosophy can teach people with disabilities to be prejudiced against disability, to fear association with others with disabilities, and to *disidentify* with the disability community. It is important to challenge these antiquated ways of thinking and develop a more pro-disabled outlook. People with disabilities are simply part of the mosaic of the world and therefore should be reasonably represented in the mosaic of social opportunities.

The saying "You can't love others until you love yourself" is quite true here. People who are *self-accepting* are almost always also people who are successful at a variety of relationships. People with disabilities are beginning to speak of the concepts of *disability pride* and *disability community* (Disability Pride Parade, n.d.). These are relatively new concepts, but they are beginning to address the issue of internalized disphobia in powerful ways.

It is also important that those who support people with disabilities be careful not to use negative language regarding disability and not to make judgments about people with disabilities and their choice of being with or not being with others with disabilities. It is simply no one's business whom one befriends or whom one loves.

Initiating Action

People relate to other people in a variety of ways, but one of the most obvious is through common interests. Oddly, staff often report that individuals with disabilities ask them to find them a boyfriend or girlfriend. This is probably because of a lifetime of having things *done for* them rather than *doing for oneself.* But it is important that people with disabilities realize that this is their quest and their quest alone. They may need assistance getting to places, having alone time, or even communicating if both people use boards or other devices, but they must be the ones making decisions and initiating action.

It is impossible to set general rules for these situations, with the exception of one major rule: Let the individual lead in deciding how and when to approach someone for conversation or contact. Ask the individual to give guidance as to what kind of care provider assistance he or she needs. As long as the request is not illegal (such as procuring a prostitute), the individual needs to be assisted with little argument. Remember that hurt is part of the relationship game and that it is not appropriate for a care provider to protect an individual from the bumps and bruises that come from social interactions. Every boy who has ever walked the thousand-mile journey across a gym floor to ask a girl to dance and then had to walk the million-mile journey back after being rejected knows that risks come from every encounter. These are part of the learning journey.

MAGIC DOES HAPPEN

The topics of relationships and sexuality are vast and can seem overwhelming. From another perspective, it is as simple as two people enjoying time together and letting the relationship grow.

Anne is a woman with cerebral palsy who lives with her husband in Toronto, Canada. She is an active artist, author, and advocate for disability rights (see http://www.artistanneabbott.com), and she uses an alphabet board (and a computer for the Internet) to communicate. Her story describes the importance of trying new ways to develop friendships and how some friendships may develop into intimate relationships:

> At twenty-nine I was resigned that I would die an old maid, a virgin, forever without a mate. If that is how things were going to be, then so be it, I thought. I had tried my best.
>
> And then, one day, something happened that changed my life. A friend of mine talked me into purchasing a computer and a modem. My friend also showed me how to access a computer bulletin board system (BBS) and communicate with people. From then on, I spent up to three hours a day in on-line "chat rooms" with total strangers talking about just about anything and everything. One day I logged onto a BBS and began chatting with a fellow named Rob. He seemed sweet and funny, and I liked him, as he liked me, almost instantly. We chatted for hours and soon found out that we had many things in common. Even so, I didn't feel comfortable enough at first to tell him that I had cerebral palsy. I was afraid of how he might react. I couldn't face another rejection! However, because he kept asking me if he could meet me and because he told me he thought he was falling in love with me, I felt like I had to break my silence.

Amazingly, Rob didn't care about my disability. He still thought I was a wonderful person, he said, and wanted to meet me. All my family and friends thought I was insane to go meet someone I had only chatted with for a month over a BBS, but I didn't care. I knew Rob would be just as he had seemed in the chat rooms of the BBS. I was right, of course. When we met that day, it was as if we had known each other all of our lives. We started dating after that, and soon fell in love. Neither of us could have been happier. It was as if we had been made especially for each other. (Abbott, 1998, pp. 3–4)

For there to be more stories like Anne's, people with complex communication needs must have opportunities to meet and interact with a wide variety of communication partners, must have access to an augmentative communication system with vocabulary to support adult conversations, and must have the skills and experience to support the development of adult relationships.

Equally important, they must live in a world that recognizes the right and ability of individuals with complex communication needs to participate in intimate relationships and that works to combat the discrimination and prejudice that these individuals often face. By educating *all* individuals of the importance of these basic principles, hopefully more individuals will enjoy experiences like Anne's.

CONCLUSION

In sign language, the sign for LOVE is placing two crossed arms over one's heart. It is a wonderful sign to make, because doing so gives a sense of being hugged and being held. The need for closeness and the desire to be with another is part of the human condition. As human beings, we need love. We need touch. We need affection. But there is more. We need respect. We need education. We need opportunity.

Do what's right.

REFERENCES

Abbott, A. (1998). Sex and the woman with a disability. *Communicating Together, 15*(1). Retrieved September 13, 2009, from http://www.accpc.ca/Speak_Up/Sex_&_Woman_w_Disabilities.pdf

American Association on Intellectual and Developmental Disabilities. (2009). *Sexuality and intellectual disability.* Retrieved September 13, 2009, from http://www.aamr.org/content_198.cfm

Ames, T.R., & Samowitz, P. (1995). Inclusionary standard for determining sexual consent for individuals with developmental disabilities. *Mental Retardation, 33,* 264–268.

Blasingame, G.D. (2005). *Developmental disabled persons with sexual behaviour problems: Treatment, management and supervision.* Oklahoma City, OK: Wood & Barnes.

Bogdan, R., Biklen, D., Shapiro, A., & Spelkoman. D. (1990). The disabled: Media's monster. In M. Nagler (Ed.), *Perspectives on disability* (pp. 138–142). Palo Alto, CA: Health Markets Research.

Bryen, D.N. (2008). Vocabulary to support socially-valued adult roles. *Augmentative and Alternative Communication, 24,* 294–301.

Burke, L., Bedard, C., & Ludwig, S. (1998). Dealing with sexual abuse of adults with a developmental disability who also have impaired communication: Supportive procedures for detection, disclosure and follow-up. *Canadian Journal of Human Sexuality, 7,* 79–92.

Castles, E.E. (1996). *We're people first: The social and emotional lives of individuals with mental retardation.* Westport, CT: Praeger.

Center for Research on Women with Disabilities. (1999). *National Study of Women with Physical Disabilities: Major findings.* Retrieved October 12, 2009, from http://www.bcm.edu/crowd/national_study/MAJORFIN.htm

Chappell, A.L. (1997). From normalization to where? In L. Barton & M. Oliver (Eds.), *Disability studies: Past, present and future* (pp. 45–62). Leeds, England: Disability Press.

Collier, B., McGhie-Richmond, D., Odette, F., & Pyne, J. (2006). Reducing the risk of sexual abuse for people who use augmentative and alternative communication. *Augmentative and Alternative Communication, 22,* 62–75.

Crooks, R., & Baur, K. (2007). *Our sexuality* (10th ed.). Belmont, CA: Wadsworth.

Crossmaker, M. (1986). *Empowerment: A systems approach to preventing assaults against people with mental retardation and or developmental disabilities.* Columbus, OH: National Assault Prevention Center.

Crossmaker, M. (1989). *Increasing safety for people receiving mental health services.* Columbus, OH: National Assault Prevention Center.

Cuskelly, M., & Bryde, R. (2004). Attitudes towards the sexuality of adults with an intellectual disability: Parents, support staff, and a community sample. *Journal of Intellectual and Developmental Disability, 29,* 255–264.

Disability Pride Parade. (n.d.). *Our mission.* Retrieved October 29, 2009, from http://www.disabilityprideparade.com/whypride.php

Earle, S. (2001). Disability, facilitated sex and the role of the nurse. *Journal of Advanced Nursing, 36,* 433–440.

Glennen, S.L. (1997). Introduction to alternative and augmentative communication. In S.L. Glennen & D.C. DeCoste, *Handbook of alternative and augmentative communication* (pp. 3–20). San Diego: Singular.

Griffiths, D.M., Quinsey, V.L., & Hingsburger, D. (1989). *Changing inappropriate sexual behavior: A community-based approach for persons with developmental disabilities.* Baltimore: Paul H. Brookes Publishing Co.

Griffiths, D., Richards, D., Federoff, P., & Watson, S.L. (2002). *Ethical dilemmas: Sexuality and developmental disability.* Kingston, NY: NADD Press.

Heal, L.W., & Sigelman, C.K. (1995). Response biases in interviews of individuals with limited mental ability. *Journal of Intellectual Disability Research, 39,* 331–340.

Hingsburger, D. (1995). *Just say no! Understanding and reducing the sexual victimization of people with disabilities.* Eastman, Quebec, Canada: Diverse City Press.

Hingsburger, D. (2005). *The R word: Helping people with intellectual disabilities deal with bullying and teasing.* Eastman, Quebec, Canada: Diverse City Press.

Hingsburger, D. (2006). *Black ink: Practical advice and clear guidelines for dealing with reports of sexual abuse from people with intellectual disabilities.* Angus, Ontario, Canada: Diverse City Press.

Hingsburger, D., & Tough, S. (2002). Healthy sexuality: Attitudes, systems and policies. *Research and Practice for Persons with Severe Disabilities, 27,* 8–17.

Hollo, W. (2003). *The rights stuff: Self advocates determining their own rights.* Angus, Ontario, Canada: Diverse City Press.

Institute on Disabilities at Temple University. (2009). *Vocabulary set: Sexuality, intimacy and healthy sex.* Retrieved September 13, 2009, from http://disabilities.temple.edu/aacvocabulary/SEXUALITY.shtml

Lever, S. (2003). Speaking out: Access to vocabulary. *Alternatively Speaking, 6*(3), 4–5.

Lombardo, P.A. (2008). *Three generations, no imbeciles: Eugenics, the Supreme Court, and* Buck v. Bell. Baltimore: Hopkins Fulfillment Service.

Ludwig, S., & Hingsburger, D. (1993). *Being sexual.* East York, Ontario, Canada: Sex Information and Education Council of Canada.

Lyden, M. (2007). Assessment of sexual consent capacity. *Sexuality and Disability, 25,* 3–20.

May, D., & Simpson, M.K. (2003). The parent trap: Marriage, parenthood and adulthood for people with intellectual disabilities. *Critical Social Policy, 23,* 25–43.

Owen, F., Griffiths, D., & Endicott, O. (2009). *Challenges to the human rights of people with intellectual disabilities.* Baltimore: Jessica Kingsley.

Patterson, P.M. (1991). *Doubly silenced: Sexuality, sexual abuse and people with developmental disabilities.* Madison: Wisconsin Council on Developmental Disabilities.

Pendler, B., & Hingsburger, D. (1991). Sexuality: Dealing with parents. *Sexuality and Disability, 9,* 123–130.

People First of Canada. (2006). *About us.* Retrieved from October 9, 2009, from http://www.peoplefirstofcanada.ca/about_us_en.php

Powers, L.E., Curry, M.A., Oschwald, M., Maley, S., Saxton, M., & Eckels, K. (2002). Barriers and strategies in addressing abuse: A survey of disabled women's experiences. *Journal of Rehabilitation, 68,* 4–13.

Powers, L.E., McNeff, E., Curry, M., Saxton, M., & Elliott, D. (2004). *Preliminary findings on the abuse experiences of men with disabilities.* Portland: Oregon Health & Science University Center on Self-Determination.

Rowe, W.S., Savage, S., Ragg, M., & Wigle, K. (1987). *Sexuality and the developmentally handicapped: A guidebook for health care professionals.* Queenston, ON: Edwin Mellen Press.

Sobsey, D. (1994). *Violence and abuse in the lives of people with disabilities: The end of silent acceptance?* Baltimore: Paul H. Brookes Publishing Co.

Swango-Wilson, A. (2008). Caregiver perceptions and implications for sex education for individuals with intellectual and developmental disabilities. *Sexuality and Disability, 26,* 167–174.

Tepper, M.S. (2000). Sexuality and disability: The missing discourse of pleasure. *Sexuality and Disability, 18,* 283–290.

Wood, M. (2004). Sexuality and relationships: Education for people with Down syndrome. *Down Syndrome News and Update, 4*(2), 42–51.

YAI Network. (2009). *History.* Retrieved October 12, 2009, from http://www.yai.org/about/History.html

YAI Sexuality Rights and Advocacy Committee. (1995). *Consent tool.* New York: YAI.

V

Living in Society

9

Preparing Youth Who Use AAC to Communicate with Their Personal Assistants

Barbara Collier and Hazel Self

> A good personal assistant or attendant can be my arms and legs for certain daily activi-
> ties. That frees me up to get on with my work and my life without having to worry about
> how I'll get to the bathroom or have a cup of coffee. When an assistant is good, life is so
> much easier. When an assistant is bad, it can be devastating. (A. Abbott, personal com-
> munication, June 20, 2006)

Personal assistance services (PAS) are a critical component of the daily experiences of many people with complex communication needs. PAS are provided by people who are often referred to as personal assistants, attendants, or support workers. Their role is to assist with tasks that an individual would do independently if he or she did not have a disability (Litvak, Zukas, & Heumann, 1987). Individuals with disabilities may require assistance with a wide variety of activities, including meal preparation, eating and drinking, personal hygiene, and housekeeping. These supports may be needed in a variety of locations, including home, workplace, academic, medical, and social settings. As noted in the quote by Anne Abbott, a woman who uses augmentative and alternative communication (AAC) and a consumer of PAS, receiving appropriate PAS represents a key component in making societal inclusion and personal freedom a reality for individuals with disabilities (Matsuda, Clark, Schopp, Hagglund, & Mokelke, 2005).

In the past, individuals with complex communication needs had few choices about where and how to receive needed supports for activities of daily living, and they were often given no choice but to live in government care facilities or nursing homes (Lakin & Stancliffe, 2007). As recently as 1977, more than 85% of Americans with significant developmental and intellectual disabilities lived in state institutions or nursing homes (see Figure 9.1). Individuals who needed a high level of assistance were often "warehoused" in large government institutions, typically at a great distance from family members and their home communities. Also, because the workers in these settings dealt with dozens of individuals in a day, care was not individualized, and individuals who could not communicate or advocate for themselves often received inadequate care. Rick Creech, an individual with severe physical disabilities, described his memories of the bathing routine in the institution in which he lived as a child: "They had 60 minutes to bathe twenty children, an assembly line of babies....today, I start to panic if water is poured over my face" (1992, p. 41).

There have since been three major trends in changes in living arrangements for adults with disabilities. These have been guided by the principles of self-determination, community inclusion, and the independent living movement (Lozano, 1993; Stancliffe & Lakin, 2007): 1) the decreasing use of large institutions and the increasing use of community living, 2) the decreasing size of community settings, and 3) the increasing numbers of people living in homes that they themselves

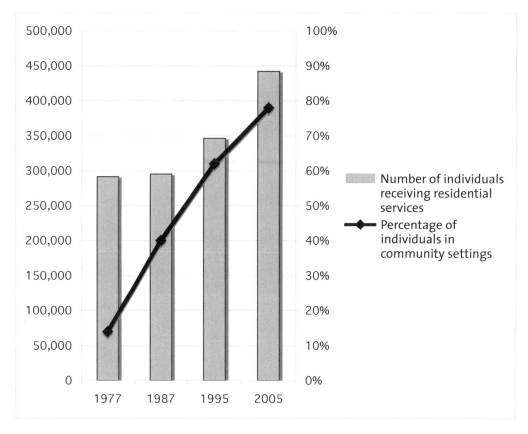

Figure 9.1.   People with intellectual and/or developmental disabilities receiving residential services in community settings in the United States in 1977, 1987, 1995, and 2005. (From Lakin & Stancliffe, 2007; adapted by permission.)

own or rent (Lakin & Stancliffe, 2007). For example, in 2005 in the United States, although a greater number of individuals received support for their living arrangements, 22% lived in institutional settings (e.g., state institutions or nursing homes), and 68% lived in community settings (e.g., group homes and supported independent living; Lakin & Stancliffe, 2007). In addition, new models of consumer-managed services are emerging whereby consumers or families receive funds to directly purchase and control their PAS, which in turn provides consumers with more control and choices for where and how they want to live. These new living arrangements provide new potential benefits (and challenges) for individuals with complex communication needs, especially with respect to access to PAS.

     There are many different models of PAS delivery, and the provision of services can vary widely in terms of the location of service delivery, the types of services provided, the background experiences and training level of the PAS provider, and the funding support. In this chapter we describe both traditional and new models of PAS, as well as ways to ensure that both the PAS provider and the individual who uses AAC have the skills needed to ensure appropriate service provision.

PERSONAL ASSISTANCE SERVICES PROVISION MODELS

People with disabilities who receive PAS represent many different living arrangements. Although large national surveys provide information on the experiences of individuals with a wide variety of disabilities (Lakin & Stancliffe, 2007), there is only limited information on the experiences of individuals with complex communication needs, typically a group with a greater-than-average level of service need. A survey of 26 adults who use AAC by Collier, McGhie-Richmond, Odette, and Pyne (2006) identified four major approaches to living arrangements and PAS provision: 1) Eight individuals received *informal supports* from family members, which were often augmented with family-directed agency services; 2) eight received services in an *agency-operated group home,* in which paid staff provided services to individuals with disabilities; 3) nine people lived independently in their communities and received *agency-delivered services*—for example, in the Ontario Supportive Housing model, PAS are provided in a community apartment complex in which a specific number of apartment units are occupied by people needing PAS; and 4) one person used *consumer-managed services,* living in an apartment of her own choosing and receiving government funding to hire and manage her own services. Each of these four approaches is commonly experienced in the disability community (Felce & Perry, 2007; Stancliffe & Lakin, 2007).

Informal Supports

Living at home with family members has traditionally been the most common living arrangement for individuals with disabilities (Lakin & Stancliffe, 2007) and continues to be common for individuals who use AAC (Hamm & Mirenda, 2006; Lund & Light, 2006). People with disabilities who live at home with their parents often report great satisfaction with the quality of daily personal services and care they get from family members (Benjamin, Matthias, Franke, Stoddard, & Kraus, 1998; Lund & Light, 2006). Family members are typically very familiar with the care needs and communication systems of the individual with complex communication needs. In addition, family members can play a key role in advocating for the person who uses AAC, in obtaining needed services, and in helping the individual participate in community activities. Many adults who use AAC who live with their families augment their caregiving supports with agency-based PAS.

Although this arrangement suits many people who use AAC, some report that living with family members restricts their ability to make decisions and to pursue their own personal lifestyle. In 2006, Augmentative Communication Community Partnerships Canada (ACCPC) hosted a peer support group discussion among nine adults who use AAC. One woman communicated about her experience living with her family:

> When I was young my mother knew everything I wanted. She could read my mind. But as I got older, I had my own opinions and it was hard to tell my mother that I wanted her to do things differently and to butt out of my private life. (personal communication)

Other members of the group commented on the challenges of communicating with loved ones in areas relating to self-determination and privacy and of being assertive in difficult situations. One man explained, "My sister reads all my mail. I have no privacy. I'm afraid I will hurt her feelings if I tell her to stop."

Some individuals reported difficulties in finding ways to communicate independently and privately during community social and health services without family members speaking on their behalf.

Another concern with relying upon family members for service provision is that there is sometimes significant stress associated with providing care for a family member with a disability, and the physical care for an individual becomes increasingly challenging for parents as they themselves grow older (Emerson, Robertson, & Wood, 2004). Individuals with complex communication needs may also worry about overburdening their parents and may feel uncomfortable about requesting changes or additional supports (Creech, 1992).

Agency-Operated Group Home Settings with Internal Supports

Small communal-style living environments represent a change from the institutional settings of the past and represent an increasing trend both in North America and internationally (Stancliffe & Lakin, 2007). In this setting, typically five to seven individuals with disabilities live in a family-style home in their community. Many people who use AAC and who have complex PAS needs find that this living arrangement meets their needs in that they are provided with a small number of round-the-clock staff and a mixture of full-time and part-time staff. In addition to PAS, residents in these settings may also receive support in participating in leisure activities and in accessing community events and services, thus reducing the risk for social isolation that is frequently a concern for people with complex communication needs. The communal home environment can also be a good setting for residents who require support in self-directing their PAS and handling their finances. One consumer commented, "I love where I live. Everyone is like my family. The staff is great" (anonymous, personal communication, March 12, 2006).

The training expectations for staff can vary widely. In Ontario, Canada, the typical training requirement for staff is a community college course for personal support workers. This course trains students to provide personal care to seniors and people with disabilities. Topics covered include assistance with mobility, personal care, safety, household management, and meal preparation. There is no training in communication or in working with people who have communication needs. Staff training specific to the needs of individual residents is typically provided through on-the-job training from consumers, families, and other staff and through workshops on specific topics.

Most group home organizations assist their residents in scheduling and communicating at medical, seating, communication, and therapy-related services. In the absence of any clear protocols to provide communication assistance, the quality of such assistance is dependent on either the ability of the consumer to direct the staff person or the staff person's own innate skills to assist with communication.

As with any service delivery model, there may be downsides to the communal or group home model. Many of these organizations emerged as a result of deinstitutionalization, and some may still be rooted in a philosophy of taking care of residents who had traditionally received minimal services while living in state institutions (Felce & Perry, 2007). Staff and managers who are unable to effectively communicate with individuals with complex communication needs may have limited expectations for the involvement of these individuals in making decisions about service delivery. Although some consumers who use AAC may not want or expect to play a strong role in directing their own care, others may be frustrated by their lack of self-determination and autonomy. One man who uses AAC commented on the difficulty of obtaining recognition for his opinions: "My parents love me but they make decisions about my life and communicate with staff and managers behind my back. The staff will phone them about everything and they don't ask me. I'm so frustrated" (anonymous, personal communication, March 12, 2006).

Finally, one problematic approach adopted by some residential service providers in large urban areas is the grouping of consumers by the type of support they require. Although this may provide consumers who use AAC with staff who have more training and resources to support them, it may also restrict their socialization with other residents. This is particularly true for consumers who rely on partners to co-construct their messages and who cannot independently communicate with others.

Independent Living with Agency-Provided Services

One community-based PAS model is the use of agency-provided services within an individual's home. For example, in Ontario, Canada, individuals may choose to live in an apartment complex in which a small percentage of the total number of apartments are occupied by people sharing either onsite or visiting agency PAS services. Services are prebooked and are shared among consumers in the building. To be eligible for community-based agency-provided PAS, people must demonstrate that they can 1) live independently (or with minimal supports) in the community, 2) have their service needs met with a limited number of service hours, and 3) direct all aspects of their assistant services (Centre for Independent Living, 2009).

As one consumer explained,

It's not enough to tell him (my attendant) to lift me from my bed to my wheelchair. I need to tell him how I want to be lifted and positioned. Getting services done in the way I want is all about communicating the details involved in that activity. (A. Shelbourne, personal communication, November 13, 2007)

One frequently identified concern with the combination of agency-provided services and independent living is that the pressure staff feel to provide services quickly does not allow for sufficient time for communication during service routines. One female consumer noted,

Staff will just go through the motions. If I need anything different done, I don't get a chance to communicate about it—the assistant might ask a few questions that I can answer "yes" and "no" to, but she rarely lets me use my communication board to tell her what I want. She says she doesn't have time to let me use my board and she needs to go to the next person on her list. (A. Abbott, personal communication, June 20, 2006)

In some situations, the provision of PAS is restricted to the building in which the consumer lives. This means that consumers who require PAS or communication assistance in the community must rely on other sources of support for these services. Aaron Shelbourne uses partner-assisted scanning to access his communication display, and he described the inequity of this situation:

If I was deaf, I could get help from a sign language interpreter to help me communicate with people. People who cannot speak have no services like this. I need someone to help me communicate. The person would understand how I communicate with my eyes and tell people what I am communicating. If I had someone like that, I could communicate with lots of people and get better services. (personal communication, October 9, 2007)

Agencies who provide PAS typically hire staff who have completed certified training programs in personal support services. However, consumers who direct their PAS emphasize over and above this formal training the importance of attitude and a willingness to learn and to be directed by the consumer. Consumers typically take responsibility for training their attendants and managers in how they communicate and frequently report that they often encounter challenging situations with staff and managers. One male consumer commented on staff training as follows: "I try to train my assistants in communication but lots of times, they don't let me communicate or don't follow my instructions. When I complain, managers do nothing" (Anonymous, personal communication, March 12, 2006).

Despite the limitations of this model, agency-provided PAS can work well for some people who use AAC. One male consumer who communicates using an alphabet board commented on his services:

I like the independence it gives me and I love living in my own place. I have some very excellent assistants and I don't need assistance when I'm in the community. I don't want the hassle of all the bookkeeping and reporting that is associated with consumer-managed services. (T. Diamanti, personal communication, October 9, 2007)

Independent Living with Consumer-Managed Services

There is growing evidence that consumer satisfaction increases when consumers have more choice and control over their support services (Benjamin, Matthias, & Franke, 2000, Kendrick, Jones,

Bezanson, & Petty, 2006). In this respect, consumer-managed services afford the highest level of control. In traditional systems, resources are generally tied to service organizations, and people have few choices in terms of where they live or what their support services will look like. Individualized funding and consumer-managed services ensure that people and their networks have control over their own resources (Lord & Hutchinson, 2007). In a typical consumer-managed model, the government provides funds directly to the consumer to hire and manage his or her own assistants. Not only does this model allow for maximum consumer control, but there is evidence that it is also the most financially efficient model (Roeher Institute, 1997).

As with any publicly funded service, there are restrictions on accessing these funds. Although 70% of U.S. states provide consumer-managed programs (Paraprofessional Health Care Institute, 2003), individuals in these states typically must pass a challenging "test" to obtain access to funds. To be eligible for this service in Canada, consumers must demonstrate that they can independently hire and manage all aspects of their PAS as well as maintain bookkeeping services and be accountable to the government funding source in financial matters.

Evidence of the challenge of obtaining these funds can be seen in the fact that despite widespread interest in increased consumer control within service models, a survey found that only 1 of 26 adults in Ontario who use AAC used consumer-managed services (Collier, McGhie-Richmond, et al., 2006). This individual described the benefits of high levels of consumer control:

> I have less service time using direct funding, but I have never been happier. I can choose who works with me, and that has a major impact on the quality of my life. Before when I used agency-directed services, I had to take whomever they sent to assist me. Some assistants were good, others were not, and I used to dread thinking about who would walk in the door to get me up every morning. Being in control of who works with me means I get a good assistant, and a good assistant is a good communicator. Good support services can minimize the challenges of daily life for people with disabilities. (A. Abbott, personal communication, March 6, 2007)

A review of the steps needed to obtain consumer-managed services, however, provides insight into the procedural barriers that restrict access to these services. In Ontario, the process to obtain consumer-managed services involves a written application and face-to-face interview. One consumer who used partner-assisted eye gaze to communicate via a wordboard reported that he was not allowed to bring an experienced communication assistant to aid in the interview process. He was disqualified on the basis that the interviewer could not understand how he communicated. Another consumer who used AAC was disqualified because she lacked the knowledge and skills required to independently manage her PAS. She reported that she had obtained no preparatory training or experience while she was growing up and so lacked the knowledge, vocabulary, and communication skills to direct and manage her PAS.

Clearly, there is a need to educate administrators about accommodating the needs of consumers who use AAC in terms of qualifying for and using consumer-managed PAS. Consumers who use AAC and who want to access these types of services may also require support in obtaining the information, tools, and skills to hire and manage their PAS.

RECOMMENDATIONS FOR IMPROVING THE QUALITY OF PERSONAL ASSISTANCE SERVICES

Although PAS provides essential services and many benefits for people with disabilities, individuals who use AAC have described three common challenges that occur in a large number of PAS contexts (ACCPC, 2005; Chappel & Moats, 2001; Creech, 2001; Hohn, 2001; Pecunas, 2001; Prentice, 2001; Williams, 2000). First, there is a need to promote positive *communication;* consumers frequently make comments such as "They (staff) need to know how to 'read' our boards" ("talk more to us," "stop talking for us," "help us communicate with other residents who use AAC," and "know our body language"). Second, there must be ways to improve *staff attitude;* consumers communicate that personal assistants should "show an interest in us," "be sensitive," and "be kind." Third, there should be strategies to promote *consumer empowerment;* consumers "want to make our decisions about things that are important to us" and "want people outside of the home to help us when we have problems with the staff and management."

In working to address these concerns, it becomes clear that these concerns are in many ways intertwined. For example, lack of access to appropriate vocabulary makes it difficult for individuals with complex communication needs to act in a self-determined manner. Negative staff attitudes and low expectations for communication by caregivers may lead to reduced opportunities and failed attempts at communication.

In this section, therefore, we offer recommendations for enhancing the quality of life of individuals who use AAC and receive PAS and for how to address communication, staff attitude, and consumer empowerment in a variety of contexts. We first discuss the issue of communication broadly, because it is central to many of the issues discussed here. We then provide examples of how individuals with complex communication needs can be supported in specific communication contexts associated with PAS, including developing service routines, giving feedback and handling conflict, ensuring personal safety, and communicating in the community.

Communication

"The three things you need in order to have a good relationship with your workers are communication, communication, communication" (Feucht, 2001, p. 30). Although not all consumers who use AAC experience challenges communicating with personal assistants and using PAS, many report that they frequently experience communication barriers with their assistants and service managers that have an impact on the quality of their lives (Balandin, 2001; Collier, 2000a). Successful communication requires skills on both sides. The skills and strategies required for successful augmented interactions are not intuitive and need to be taught. Positive communication partner skills include 1) knowing how the person who uses AAC communicates, 2) asking questions in ways that the person who uses AAC can understand and answer, 3) recognizing and providing opportunities for the person to initiate and respond, 4) giving the person sufficient time to construct messages, and 5) using strategies to confirm and/or repair communication breakdowns (Blackstone, 1999).

Preparing PAS providers to communicate with individuals with complex communication needs may pose additional challenges. For example, some studies have indicated that group home staff are more likely to communicate with one another than with the individuals they were hired to assist (Jones et al., 1999). In addition, consumers in group homes frequently describe staff as being overly directive as well as unresponsive to initiations by consumers (Balandin, 2001). In the Unites States and Canada most group home workers receive little formal training before beginning their work with consumers. Therefore, the consumer and his or her family members may have to assume the role of instructor in educating personal assistants and managers about how the individual communicates and what he or she wants them to do to support communication.

As a first step, Collier and Diamanti (2007) suggested that individuals who use AAC complete a *personal communication passport* (Millar, 1997) to explain how they communicate and what they want their communication partner to do when communicating with them (see a sample personal communication passport at http://www.accpc.ca/pdfs/Passport.pdf).

Consumers need this information if they are to train others in how to communicate with them. The topics can also be used as part of a performance appraisal process that consumers can complete with their assistants and managers as a means of giving feedback on communication skills.

The broad range of skills and activities listed in Table 9.1 speaks to the need for ongoing and organized instruction for personal assistants. At the same time, however, the PAS industry is characterized by high turnover and limited staff training.

Table 9.1.   Communication training for personal assistants

Context	Sample training topics
Direct face-to-face communication	Acquiring knowledge and skill relating to
	How the consumer communicates using his or her formal AAC systems (e.g., communication display, signs, speech-generating device)
	What the consumer wants his or her communication partner to do when communicating (e.g., where to sit or stand, whether to say words aloud when selected, whether to guess at meaning)
	Interpreting and responding to unaided communication (e.g., body language, vocalization, speech, gestures, facial expression) when formal AAC systems are not accessible during services
	Verifying and clarifying techniques during services
	Asking questions in ways the consumer can answer with and without formal AAC systems
	Providing opportunities for communication during time-sensitive routines
	Ensuring consumer choice and autonomy during services
	Setting up, charging, cleaning, and maintaining the consumer's AAC systems
Telephone communication	Answering the telephone on behalf of the consumer (e.g., script that is authorized by consumer)
	Delivering a message via a telephone call on behalf of the consumer (e.g., introduction script)
	Assisting the consumer to communicate directly over the phone
	Managing telephone messages
Written communication	Setting up the computer for consumer use
	Assisting with reading documents
	Assisting with signatures, correspondence, record keeping, and so forth
Communication assistance with another person	Conveying messages accurately and effectively between the consumer and another person
	Encouraging direct communication between the consumer and another person
	Demonstrating authorship of consumer message to another person
	Safeguarding the privacy of the consumer around communication matters
	Supporting communication between two or more people who speak and who use AAC

In summarizing the training approaches used by the eight participants in her focus group, Collier (2007) reported that some participants made personal videotapes to train their staff. Others used a two-step training process. The first step consisted of using a generic training videotape such as *Communicating Matters: A Training Guide for Personal Attendants Working with Consumers Who Have Enhanced Communication Needs* (Collier, 2000a). Then, in the second step, they provided individualized information describing techniques for setting up and maintaining their AAC system as well as interacting in common communication contexts (e.g., asking questions during routines when the consumer may not have access to his or her AAC device or display, facilitating communication with the public, supporting the consumer in using a communication display to communicate over the phone, ensuring privacy for a consumer who uses AAC; Collier & Diamanti, 2007).

It can be difficult to change the behavior of staff who are used to providing care in a particular way (Purcell, McConkey, & Morris, 2000), and individuals with complex communication needs report mixed results from providing training for PAS workers. Sometimes one key piece of information can have a dramatic impact. One female consumer who lived in a communal setting noted that an attendant who had worked with her for 6 years did not know that she lifted her leg to indicate that she wanted to use her communication display—the attendant had interpreted her signal as meaning that the individual wanted to be left alone. Simply informing the attendant of the intent of the consumer's signal made a major difference to the quality of the woman's interaction with that assistant. Other outcomes are not as straightforward or satisfactory. After a 10-week training program for attendants that included group attendant sessions and individual coaching with the consumers, one female consumer noted, "The good attendants are better, the poor attendants are the same" (anonymous, personal communication, May 6, 2006).

In many cases in which communication with their assistants is cited as a barrier, consumers report that managers should play a more active role in supporting the consumers to ensure effective communication with staff. Ensuring that attendants communicate effectively with consumers who use AAC is ultimately the responsibility of the manager of an attendant service agency. Collier and Diamanti (2007) recommended that consumers train managers in addition to frontline staff and, if necessary, engage family members or AAC clinicians to advocate for thorough staff training.

Developing Service Plans

My parents encouraged me to communicate with lots of people and to direct my services from a young age. For example, instead of just taking off my coat, they expected me to ask someone to do that and to tell that person how I wanted it done. (T. Diamanti, in Collier, 2007)

Many individuals with disabilities, whether or not they use AAC, develop service plans with their attendant agencies. A service plan outlines how the consumer wants a specific service to be provided. Service instructions may become part of a formal contract between the consumer and the service agency. Unlike consumers who can augment their written service plans by talking through the details with their attendants (e.g., adding details to instructions for individual attendants, giving feedback), consumers who use AAC may need to prepare messages to direct their services or to create detailed written documentation to describe their service provision.

Collier and Haans (2000) described a multistep process used with six adults for identifying needed vocabulary during service routines. First, participants identified the communication contexts that were significant for them. Second, prior to the training program, the participants were observed communicating within their identified contexts. For example, a male consumer who identified assistance with drinking as a targeted context was observed asking a person who was unfamiliar with his needs to give him a drink. After the helper provided assistance, the consumer's shirt was wet. Third, consumers were asked what the ideal service provision would have included. When asked what the helper could have done to avoid wetting his shirt, the consumer in the previous example indicated that the helper could have used a towel. Although the consumer knew what he needed, he had assumed that his helper also knew this; this incident was found to be typical of many in which the consumer expressed anger and dissatisfaction with his services rather than constructively communicating about what could be done to improve the situation.

Fourth, consumers were supported in developing detailed service plans for services that were predicable and routine (e.g., transfers into and out of a wheelchair, positioning in a chair, using the washroom, assistance with drinking and eating). Each service plan provided step-by-step instructions as to how the consumer wanted the service to be performed.

Participants worked on their service plans with a facilitator who guided them through the process by asking questions, confirming details, and supporting the consumers in documenting the instructions in ways that would be easily followed by new attendants. Service plans were documented in binders and/or programmed into speech-generating devices (SGDs). Some consumers used photographs to show how they wanted things done (e.g., how they wanted to be positioned in their wheelchair) or used simple message devices such as talking photo albums. These communication supports were then placed in locations (e.g., the bathroom for reminders on bathroom routines) where they could be conveniently activated by the consumer or by the attendant. See Box 9.1 for a sample service routine for nail care.

> **BOX 9.1.   Sample service routine for nail care**
>
> **When cutting or cleaning my nails, it is important to know that:**
>
> My hand may clench. This is due to my spasticity. It does not help to ask me to relax or open my hand. I cannot control it.
>
> **The best thing to do is:**
>
> - Gently pry open each finger.
> - Hold each finger firmly when you cut or clean the nail.
> - Cut my nails short.
> - File any jagged nails because I might scratch myself.
>
> From Collier, B., Janzen, P., & Blackstien-Adler, S. (2006). *Communicate 4: Supporting youth and adults with physical disabilities in communicating about their services and participating in their communities.* Pittsburgh: DynaVox Systems; reprinted by permission.

Fifth, once consumers had developed their services plans, they were encouraged to practice using them in role-playing situations. This gave them the opportunity to test out their service plans and to refine their documents so that unfamiliar attendants would have the necessary information. Participants were encouraged to use their new tools and skills in real-life situations and to report back to the group.

For some consumers, the documented service plan alone made a significant change in how their services were provided. One male consumer noted,

> I spent a year writing up my service plans for different situations. I put them in a binder. I have instructions on how I want people to talk to me; how I can communicate with them; what I want done every morning; how to assist me when I am eating; how to lift me out of my wheelchair, etc. This is one of the best things I have ever done. It made a major difference when I went to camp where people didn't know me. I wish I had done it when I was younger. (anonymous, personal communication, May 15, 2006)

Consumers may need vocabulary to communicate about skin care, medications, physical assistance, sexuality, human rights, violation of rights, and so forth. A number of context-based vocabulary lists may be relevant to communicating with personal assistances (e.g., ACCPC, 2004, 2006; Balandin & Iacono, 1998; Balandin & Iacono, 1999; Beukelman & Yorkston, 1982; Collier, 2000b; Collier, 2003; Elder & Goossens, 1996; Fried-Oken & Stuart, 1992; Myers, Gibbons, Fried-Oken, & Bersani, 1996; Stuart, Beukelman, & King, 1997). Based on their experience working with adults, Collier, Janzen, and Blackstein-Adler (2006) developed a series of 250 communication pages containing more than 9,000 vocabulary items for use in dynamic SGDs to assist individuals in communicating in 26 PAS communication contexts. More information, including information on a home study guide to support youth in learning how to communicate with attendants, is available online (http://www.dynavoxtech.com/products/software/communicate4.aspx).

Giving Feedback and Handling Conflict

> It's good to begin young and encourage children who use AAC to tell you how well you or another person treated them. For example, ask a young child to give you feedback. Did I do a good job, an OK job, or a bad job? If bad, what was wrong? This gives children a sense of control and responsibility to tell us when things are not right. (Collier, 2007)

People who speak and who use attendant services frequently describe the importance of giving positive and constructive feedback to the staff who work with them (Prentice, 2001). However, informal observations of individuals who use AAC interacting with PAS workers provides evidence that few if any consumers give any feedback to their assistants (Collier, 1998). This may be because of the effort and time involved in communicating what some may consider an unnecessary comment, or it may be that this reflects a consumer's feeling of being disempowered in these situations. As one consumer commented, "It doesn't matter what I think or say" (Anonymous, personal communication, May 18, 2006).

Giving feedback on how a service is performed reinforces the roles and expectations within the relationship, instills a sense of control in the consumer, and provides an opportunity for the PAS worker to improve his or her services (Collier, 2008). Learning strategies for giving feedback and handling conflicts not only supports consumers in evaluating and directing attendant services but empowers them to report and disclose any abusive and criminal offenses that they may experience (Collier, 1998).

Individuals who use AAC may need instruction and support to learn to communicate feedback. As noted by Jon Feucht, some individuals who use AAC will develop a personal communication style based on trial and error:

> I had a lot of problems when I first started working with attendants. The biggest problem was communication. I just didn't know how to get my point across without getting mad. Over time, I tried different techniques of getting my point across. I kept the ideas that worked and abandoned those that failed. (2001, p. 30)

Although each individual will clearly need to develop a personal style that works for him or her, there are significant costs associated with "failures" in interpersonal communication, such as personal anger and frustration as well as staff turnover. Giving constructive feedback, which involves clearly and politely instructing a person in how a service could be improved, may serve to prevent unwanted consequences.

Collier (2007) reported that some consumers are concerned about "sounding harsh" when giving feedback, especially when using their SGDs and when communicating with loved ones. The group brainstormed about catchphrases that could be used with feedback messages, including, "Don't take this the wrong way, but..." and "I'm sure you don't mean it, but..." Consumers reported that both preprogrammed phrases such as "That's great!" and "Thanks" as well as body language and vocalization (for quick items such as validation of satisfaction or to alert the assistant that something is wrong) may be needed to provide feedback on how services are provided.

A common concern of individuals who use AAC is the appropriate handling of interpersonal conflicts and recurring problems (Light et al., 2007). McCarthy, Light, and McNaughton (2007) used web-based instruction to teach the DOIT! problem-solving strategy (Light et al., 2007, adapted from Wehmeyer & Lawrence, 1995) to five adolescents. The acronym DOIT! stands for *D*escribe the problem, *O*utline potential ways to solve the problem, *I*dentify the outcome that best meets the situation, *T*ake action, and *!*celebrate success. These individuals practiced using the strategy with a variety of problem scenarios, including scenarios related to personal care and providing feedback, and many demonstrated increased skills during the training program.

Collier (2007) developed a modified version of the problem-solving strategy that also incorporated the use of "I-messages" so that consumers could be assisted in clearly communicating their feelings in difficult situations. Collier taught the strategy to six adults in a series of 10 group and individual sessions. The participants engaged in problem-solving activities using scenarios based on real-life situations, including the provision of PAS. Participation in the scenarios resulted in the identification of new vocabulary needed by consumers, including words and phrases to describe the problem (e.g., "I have a problem with this," "I need to talk to you about something," "When you do that, I feel . . ."), state the significance of the problem (e.g., "This is important to me," "This is not the first time this has happened"), communicate what needs to happen (e.g., "I need you to . . ." "Could you . . ." "Would you be willing to . . ."), negotiate a solution (e.g., "What do you need to happen?" "What do you think?"), monitor an agreement (e.g., "Let's try it for a week," "Let's see how it goes"), and state what will happen if the problem persists (e.g., "I'll speak with the manager," "I'll lodge a formal complaint").

One male consumer used the strategies to lodge a complaint about the inaccessibility of an exit route during a power outage in a mall. He reported, "I used the vocabulary to help me explain my rights and to negotiate what I wanted the management to do. It helped to give me confidence, and they took me seriously" (J. Jessop, personal communication, August 2, 2006).

Ensuring Personal Safety

If youth who use AAC are to be prepared for adulthood, they require information, the means to communicate, and skills relating to their rights and safety. People with disabilities and complex communication needs are 2 to 6 times more likely than people without disabilities to experience physical, mental, and sexual abuse as a result of their inability to effectively communicate (Sobsey, 1994b). Based on a survey of 40 adults who use AAC, Bryen, Carey, and Frantz (2003) reported that 45% of the individuals had experienced crime or abuse, and that 97% of those who had experienced crime or abuse knew the perpetrators. Further, of those individuals who had experience crime or abuse, 71% reported being victimized multiple times, and only 28% had reported their experiences to the police. ACCPC (2004) explored the abuse experiences of 26 people who use AAC and found that the majority had experienced a range of abuses, including violations of rights, discrimination, and criminal offenses, and that most of these offenses had occurred within the caregiving or PAS context. In addition, participants in the project had no way to communicate about these experiences; lacked the information to make informed decisions about how to take appropriate action; and could not access health, social, and justice services within their communities (Collier, McGhie-Richmond, et al., 2006). The lived experiences of many of these individuals—a lack of independent mobility, reliance on support services, limited resources, financial dependence on others, and social isolation—have all been identified as significant risk factors for abuse (Farrar, 1996; Powers et al., 2002).

Sobsey (1994a) suggested that for adults with disabilities, living safely in the community requires acquiring skills and knowledge in a number of areas, including assertive communication and social skills, self-defense and personal protection, personal rights and safety, communication and choice making, developing and maintaining adult interpersonal relationships, and money management. In 2004–2006, ACCPC provided educational sessions on ways to reduce the risk of victimization for 18 adults with complex communication needs. Participants had very diverse safety issues depending on their level of independence, access to environmental controls and communication, mobility, and life experiences. It was noted that 1) the majority of the consumers had never had any formal safety awareness training; 2) few had access to basic safety tools, such as vocabulary to communicate in an emergency, call bells, and environmental controls for opening and closing doors; and 3) only a small number could ensure the privacy of their belongings and personal information. In general, the participants wanted to know about their rights, about how to handle interpersonal conflicts with personal assistants, as well as about how to secure their belongings and safeguard their privacy (ACCPC, 2006).

Table 9.2 provides a list of the safety issues addressed in guided peer support groups with individuals who used AAC. These include individual rights and responsibilities, personal assertiveness, healthy relationships, safety tools and strategies, and the complaints process (ACCPC, 2006). In addition, consumers developed personalized emergency plans for use in the community that would inform another person about what they wanted done in an emergency. One participant commented on the value of peer support:

Table 9.2.   Safety issues for consumers who use augmentative and alternative communication

Safety area	Sample topics
Rights and re- sponsibilities	Human rights, service rights, and accessibility rights
	Recognizing abuse, discrimination, and rights violations
Assertiveness	Handling difficult situations and people
	Negotiation and conflict resolution
	Feedback and monitoring
	Handling recurring offenses
Relationships	Healthy and unhealthy relationships
	Personal boundaries
	Sexuality and sexual rights
Personal safety	Strategies and tools for home and community (e.g., emergency and evacuation plans; securing personal space, belongings, and information; monitoring the safety practices of caregivers; money management and tracking)
Complaints and appeals	What to do when not satisfied with the services provided
	Following a complaint process
	Appealing a decision
	Where to get help
Reporting abuse	What to do if abused or being abused
	Where to get help
	Legal options for dealing with abuse
	What happens when abuse is reported to the police
	What happens when an abuse case goes to court
	How abusers can be punished after a criminal trial

From Collier, B. (Producer/Director). (2007). *Pointing it out: Safety for people who use augmentative communication* [DVD and booklet]. Toronto: Augmentative Communication Community Partnerships Canada; adapted by permission.

> I learned about how other people handle similar situations to mine. For example, I never liked the fact that my assistants would just walk into my apartment and when we discussed this in the group, I was surprised and pleased that this was unacceptable (to the other people in the group). People in the group suggested that I put a note on my door and tell staff to knock before entering. I was nervous about doing this but the group gave me the support I needed to do it and everything turned out really well. It was a simple thing but I feel much more respected. (ACCPC, 2006)

Individuals with complex communication needs also frequently experience difficulty reporting abuse, so participants in the group developed a list of people from whom they could choose a communication assistant, if needed, for reporting an incident to the authorities. This strategy helps to avoid a situation in which the offender may be asked to assist the consumer in communicating with the manager or police.

Many consumers who participated in the ACCPC training reported special concerns about reporting staff behavior and said they were intimidated when it came to complaining about a staff person's behavior (ACCPC, 2007). As Anne Abbott explained,

> If you are being abused by a person that you rely on for your care, you might be afraid to complain. The person might hear about it and take it out on you. Or you might be afraid that you will lose your services if you complain. (Personal communication, July 12, 2007)

In order to learn the skills needed to effectively report inappropriate behavior, the consumers in the ACCPC educational sessions discussed various scenarios and developed possible courses of action. In addition, each PAS agency shared its complaint process, and this information was used as participants discussed a number of case scenarios.

Communicating in the Community

Individuals with severe disabilities require active support from caregivers in order to successfully participate in meaningful communication activities (Gardner & Carran, 2005); however, some personal assistants do not provide services in the community. Those assistants who do accompany the consumer at his or her request to community appointments may need to provide communication assistance for the consumer and his or her service provider. Consumers who rely on an attendant to support them in these situations often report challenges relating to the quality of the assistance they receive. For example, many adults who use AAC report that the person to whom they want to communicate (e.g., a doctor, a lawyer) may direct all communication to the assistant and ignore the consumer (Blackstone & Collier, 2008). In these situations, the attendant often takes on the role of speaking for the consumer, and, in doing so, may compromise the consumer's autonomy and privacy.

One innovative response to this challenge, the Communication Assistant Project (Collier, McGhie-Richmond, & Self, in press), identified four key support areas that must be addressed when training someone to assist in the communication between a consumer and a third party: 1) protocols for ensuring the consumer's authorship for all aspects of his or her communication, 2) techniques for conveying consumer messages effectively and efficiently in one-to-one or group settings, 3) strategies for encouraging third parties to engage in direct communication with a consumer, and 4) strategies for increasing participation of the person using AAC in an interaction. To this end, ACCPC developed a code of ethics that addresses confidentiality and safeguards necessary for ensuring the integrity of the consumer's intended meaning and the authenticity of his or her communications. In addition to training attendants to assist with communication, consumers learned how to direct, evaluate, and give feedback to their attendants in matters relating to the quality of the communication assistance.

Findings from this project indicated that many adults who use AAC can significantly increase the quality of their communication in their communities when using trained communication assistants. Participants reported increased self-esteem and autonomy and felt that they received improved health, social, and legal community services. They also reported that more people learned how to communicate directly with them after observing how the assistants interacted with them (ACCPC, 2008; Collier, 2008). One consumer reported,

> My speech can be difficult to understand, and I type messages out on my device when I am not understood. When I was in [the] hospital, I used a communication assistant to help me communicate with the doctors and nurses. It made a big difference to the quality of my care. I felt I was listened to and respected. That's not always the case when people don't understand what I am saying. (L. McQuillan, personal communication, December 4, 2007)

As human rights legislation moves forward to ensure that all people with disabilities have equitable access to their communities in which they live, it will become increasingly important to support people who use AAC in obtaining and directing their communication access supports (Blackstone & Collier, 2008).

CONCLUSION

Many individuals who make use of PAS describe frustration with the gap between what the PAS systems allow them to do and their actual needs and potential (Beatty, Richmond, Tepper, & Dejong, 1998; Matsuda et al., 2005). As PAS systems move toward being more responsive to the people they serve, consumers who use AAC must be supported in clearly articulating their PAS needs. Future research is needed to define the types of supports required by consumers to effectively communicate with and use PAS at all levels.

BOX 9.2.   Recommendations from consumers who use personal assistance services for preparing youth for adulthood

- Encourage young children to communicate about what they want done and how they want it done.

- Expect and ask for feedback on how services are provided.

- Encourage a sense of control by asking permission before providing any services.

- Foster self-esteem and confidence.

- Foster autonomy, choice making, and decision making at all times.

- Encourage and accept youth's right to communicate "no."

- Acknowledge and discuss any uneasiness that youth may have about people.

- Teach safety skills, and allow youth to take reasonable risks.

- Provide ways that youth can communicate about topics relating to directing services, rights, respect, safety, and abuse.

- Provide opportunities to discuss and learn about sexuality and abuse.

- Encourage a sense of personal privacy.

- Discuss appropriate boundaries and touch with strangers, acquaintances, friends, and so forth.

- Role-play imagined scenarios in which youth can determine what actions they would take.

From Augmentative Communication Community Partnerships Canada. (2004). *Speak Up project.* Retrieved November 18, 2008, from http://www.accpc.ca/Speak_Up/index.htm; adapted by permission.

In addition, service providers need to find better ways to prepare individuals with complex communication needs to be ready to effectively direct PAS providers. Box 9.2 provides a list of skills recommended in this regard; however, at this time service providers have only a limited understanding of how to effectively support the development of these skills. The field needs evidence-based interventions that can support individuals who use AAC in learning the communication and self-determination skills needed to pursue personal lifestyle decisions, and it needs to advocate for systemic change that addresses and accommodates the needs of consumers who use AAC. If where and how one lives is fundamental to quality of life, it makes sense that children and youth who use AAC should be provided with the tools, skills, and supports to prepare them to use PAS, many of which are linked to residence options. As noted by Lozano,

> The issue for people with intellectual and developmental disabilities should not be whether they have the skills to live on their own, but rather, how the system created to serve them can provide the necessary supports to enable them to do so. (1993, p. 261)

REFERENCES

Augmentative Communication Community Partnerships Canada. (2004). *Speak Up project.* Retrieved November 18, 2008, from http://www.accpc.ca/Speak_Up/index.htm

Augmentative Communication Community Partnerships Canada. (2005). *Resources: Attendant services.* Retrieved November 18, 2008, from http://www.accpc.ca/Resources_Attendant_Services.htm

Augmentative Communication Community Partnerships Canada. (2006). *Reducing the risk of abuse.* Retrieved November 18, 2008, from http://www.accpc.ca/rtr-resources.htm

Augmentative Communication Community Partnerships Canada. (2007). *Access to justice.* Retrieved January 20, 2009, from http://www.accpc.ca/equaljustice.htm

Augmentative Communication Community Partnerships Canada. (2008). *Communication assistants: A model for communication access.* Retrieved January 20, 2009, from http://www.accpc.ca/ca-abouttheproject.htm

Balandin, S. (2001). The pedal hits the metal: Conversations between employees who use AAC and their attendants during meal breaks. In R.V. Conti & C. Jenkins-Odorisio (Eds.), *Proceedings of the Pittsburgh Employment Conference for Augmented Communicators* (pp. 62–67). Pittsburgh: Shout Press.

Balandin, S., & Iacono, T. (1998). A few well chosen words. *Augmentative and Alternative Communication, 14,* 147–161.

Balandin, S., & Iacono, T. (1999). Crews, wusses and whoppas: Core and fringe vocabularies of meal-break conversations in the workplace. *Augmentative and Alternative Communication, 15,* 95–109.

Beatty, P.W., Richmond, G.W., Tepper, S., & DeJong, G. (1998). Personal assistance for people with physical disabilities: Consumer-direction and satisfaction with services. *Archives of Physical Medicine and Rehabilitation, 79,* 674–677.

Benjamin, A., Matthias, R., Franke, I., Stoddard, S., & Kraus, I. (1998). *Comparing client-centered and agency models for supportive services at home.* Los Angeles: University of California at Los Angeles.

Benjamin, A.E., Matthias, R., & Franke, T.M. (2000). Comparing consumer-directed and agency models for providing supportive services at home. *Health Services Research, 35,* 351–356.

Beukelman, D.R., & Yorkston, K. (1982). Communication interaction of adult communication augmentation system use. *Topics in Language Disorders, 2*(2), 39–54.

Blackstone, S. (1999, April). Communication partners. *Augmentative Communication News, 12*(1/2), 1–2.

Blackstone, S., & Collier, B. (2008, September). Communication assistance: Human supports for communication access. *Augmentative Communication News, 20*(3), 7–12.

Bryen, D.N., Carey, A., & Frantz, B. (2003). Ending the silence: Adults who use augmentative communication and their experiences as victims of crimes. *Augmentative and Alternative Communication, 19,* 125–134.

Centre for Independent Living. (2009). *Attendant services overview.* Retrieved February 9, 2009, from www.cilt.ca/overview.aspx

Chappel, D., & Moats, M. (2001). Changing jobs, keeping personal care attendants. In R.V. Conti & C. Jenkins-Odorisio (Eds.), *Proceedings of the Pittsburgh Employment Conference for Augmented Communicators* (pp. 4–6). Pittsburgh: Shout Press.

Collier, B. (1998, August). *Enhancing communication between personal attendants and AAC users.* Presentation at the 10th Biennial Conference of the International Society for Augmentative and Alternative Communication, Dublin, Ireland.

Collier, B. (2000a). *Communicating matters: A training guide for personal attendants working with consumers who have enhanced communication needs.* Toronto: Augmentative Communication Community Partnerships Canada.

Collier, B.M. (2000b). *See what we say: Situational vocabulary for adults who use augmentative and alternative communication.* Baltimore: Paul H. Brookes Publishing Co.

Collier, B. (2003). *Communicating about sexuality* [Computer software]. Solano Beach, CA: Mayer-Johnson.

Collier, B. (Producer/Director). (2007). *Pointing it out: Safety for people who use augmentative communication* [DVD and booklet]. Toronto: Augmentative Communication Community Partnerships Canada.

Collier, B. (2008, August). *Communication assistants for adults who use AAC.* Presentation at the 14th Annual Conference of the International Society for Augmentative and Alternative Communication, Montreal, Canada.

Collier, B., & Diamanti, T. (2007, March). *What we know for sure: Fostering self-advocacy in youth who use AAC.* Keynote address at the annual conference of the United States Society for Augmentative and Alternative Communication, Los Angeles, CA.

Collier, B., & Haans, N. (2000, August). *Developing assertiveness skills in AAC users.* Presentation at the Ninth Biennial Conference of the International Society for Augmentative and Alternative Communication, Washington, DC.

Collier, B., Janzen, P., & Blackstien-Adler, S. (2006). *Communicate 4: Supporting youth and adults with physical disabilities in communicating about their services and participating in their communities.* Pittsburgh: DynaVox Systems.

Collier, B., McGhie-Richmond, D., Odette, F., & Pyne, P. (2006). Reducing the risk of sexual abuse for people who use AAC. *Augmentative and Alternative Communication, 22,* 62–75.

Collier, B., McGhie-Richmond, D., & Self, H. (in press). Exploring communication assistants as an option for increasing communication access to communities for people who use augmentative communication. *Augmentative and Alternative Communication.*

Creech, R. (1992). *Reflections from a unicorn.* Greenville, NC: R.C. Publishing.

Creech, R. (2001). My experiences with personal care assistance and employment: A 20 year history. In R.V. Conti & C. Jenkins-Odorisio (Eds.), *Proceedings of the Pittsburgh Employment Conference for Augmented Communicators* (pp. 1–3). Pittsburgh: Shout Press.

Elder, P., & Goossens', C. (1996). *Communication overlays for engineering training environments* (Books 1–4). Solana Beach, CA: Mayer-Johnson.

Emerson, E., Robertson, J., & Wood, J. (2004). Levels of psychological distress experienced by family carers of children and adolescents with intellectual disabilities in an urban conurbation. *Journal of Applied Research in Intellectual Disabilities, 17,* 77–84.

Farrar, P. (1996). *End the silence: Preventing the sexual assault of women with communication disorders.* Calgary, Alberta, Canada: The University of Calgary, Technical Resource Center.

Felce, D., & Perry, J. (2007). Living with support in the community: Factors associated with quality of life outcomes. In S.L. Odom, R.H. Horner, M.E. Snell, & J. Blacher (Eds.), *Handbook of developmental disabilities* (pp. 410–428). New York: Guilford Press.

Feucht, J. (2001). Authentic voices of America. In R.V. Conti & C. Jenkins-Odorisio (Eds.), *Proceedings of the Pittsburgh Employment Conference for Augmented Communicators* (pp. 30–42). Pittsburgh: Shout Press.

Fried-Oken, M., & Stuart, S. (1992). A few selected words about word selection: Vocabulary issues in AAC. In D. J. Gardner-Bonneau (Ed.), *The Second ISAAC Research Symposium in Augmentative and Alternative Communication* (pp. 68-78). Philadelphia: ISAAC.

Gardner, J.F., & Carran, D.T. (2005). Attainment of personal outcomes by people with developmental disabilities. *Mental Retardation, 43,* 157–174.

Hamm, B., & Mirenda, P. (2006). Post-school quality of life for individuals with developmental disabilities who use AAC. *Augmentative and Alternative Communication, 22,* 134–147.

Hohn, I. (2001). How to hire a personal care assistant for the job. In R.V. Conti & C. Jenkins-Odorisio (Eds.), *Proceedings of the Pittsburgh Employment Conference for Augmented Communicators* (pp. 43–45). Pittsburgh: Shout Press.

Jones, E., Perry, J., Lowe, K., Felce, D., Toogood, S., Dunstan, F., et al. (1999). Opportunity and the promotion of activity among adults with severe intellectual disability living in community residences: The impact of training staff in active support. *Journal of Intellectual Disability Research, 43,* 164–178.

Kendrick, M., Jones, D., Bezanson, L., & Petty, R. (2006). *Key components of system change: Unlocking the code of effective systems change.* Retrieved from the Independent Living Research Utilization Community Living Partnership web site: http://www.socialrolevalorization.com/resource/MK_Articles/keyComponentsOf SystemsChange.pdf

Lakin, K.C., & Stancliffe, R.J. (2007). Residential supports for persons with intellectual and developmental disabilities. *Mental Retardation and Developmental Disablties Research Reviews, 13,* 151–159.

Light, J., McNaughton, D., Krezman, C., Williams, M., Gulens, M., Galskoy, A., et al. (2007). The AAC Mentor Project: Web-based instruction in sociorelational skills and collaborative problem solving for adults who use augmentative and alternative communication. *Augmentative and Alternative Communication, 23,* 56–75.

Litvak, S., Zukas, H., & Heumann, J. (1987). *Attending to America: Personal assistance for independent living.* Oakland, CA: World Institute on Disability.

Lord, J., & Hutchinson, P. (2007). *Pathways to inclusion: Building a new story for people and communities.* Concord, Ontario, Canada: Captus Press.

Lozano, B. (1993). Independent living: Relation among training, skills, and success. *American Journal on Mental Retardation, 98,* 249–262.

Lund, S.K., & Light, J. (2006). Long-term outcomes for individuals who use augmentative and alternative communication: Part I—What is a "good" outcome? *Augmentative and Alternative Communication, 22,* 284–299.

Matsuda, S., Clark, M., Schopp, L., Hagglund, J., & Mokelke, E. (2005). Barriers and satisfaction associated with personal assistance services: Results of consumer and personal assistant focus groups. *OTJR: Occupation, Participation and Health, 25*(2), 66–74.

McCarthy, J., Light, J., & McNaughton, D. (2007). The effects of Internet-based instruction on the social problem solving of young adults who use augmentative and alternative communication. *Augmentative and Alternative Communication, 23,* 100–112.

Millar, S. (1997, September). *Personal communication passports.* Presentation at the SENSE Conference, Westpark Centre, University of Dundee, Scotland.

Myers, C., Gibbons, C., Fried-Oken, M., & Bersani, H. (1996). Self advocacy core vocabulary for augmented speakers with intellectual disabilities. *Proceedings of the 7th Biennial Conference of ISAAC* (pp. 543–544). Vancouver, British Columbia, Canada: ISAAC.

Paraprofessional Health Care Institute. (2003). *Direct-care health workers: The unnecessary crisis in long term care.* Retrieved October 24, 2003, from http://assets.aarp.org/rgcenter/il/dd117_workers.pdf

Pecunas, P. (2001). Attendant care class. In R.V. Conti & T.J. McGrath (Eds.), *Proceedings of the 8th Annual Pittsburg Employment Conference for Augmented Communicators* (pp. 19–22). Pittsburgh: Shout Press.

Powers, L., Curry, M.A., Oschwald, M., Maley, S., Saxton, M., & Eckels, K. (2002). Barriers and strategies in addressing abuse: A survey of disabled women's experiences. *Journal of Rehabilitation, 68,* 4–13.

Prentice, J. (2001). The personal assistant: A working augmentative communicator's perspective. In R.V. Conti & C. Jenkins-Odorisio (Eds.), *Proceedings of the Pittsburgh Employment Conference for Augmented Communicators* (pp. 23–29). Pittsburgh: Shout Press.

Purcell, M., McConkey, R., & Morris, I. (2000). Staff communication with people with intellectual disabilities: The impact of a work-based training programme. *International Journal of Language & Communication Disorders, 35,* 147–158.

Roeher Institute. (1997). *Self-managed attendant services in Ontario: Final evaluation report.* Toronto: Author.

Sobsey, D. (1994a). Crime prevention and personal safety. In M. Agran, N.E. Marchand-Martella, & R.C. Martella (Eds.), *Promoting health and safety: Skills for independent living* (pp. 193–213). Baltimore: Paul H. Brookes Publishing Co.

Sobsey, D. (1994b). *Violence and abuse in the lives of people with disabilities: The end of silent acceptance?* Baltimore: Paul H. Brookes Publishing Co.

Stancliffe, R.J., & Lakin, K.C. (2007). Independent living. In S.L. Odom, R.H. Horner, M.E. Snell, & J. Blacher (Eds.), *Handbook of developmental disabilities* (pp. 410–428). New York: Guilford Press.

Stuart, S., Beukelman, D.R., & King, J. (1997). Vocabulary use during extended conversations by two cohorts of older adults. *Augmentative and Alternative Communication, 13,* 40–47.

Wehmeyer, M., & Lawrence, M. (1995). Whose future is it anyway? Promoting student involvement in transition planning. *Career Development for Exceptional Individuals, 18,* 69–83.

Williams, M.B. (2000). Just an independent guy who leads a busy life. In M. Fried-Oken & H.A. Bersani (Eds.), *Speaking up and spelling it out* (pp. 231–238). Baltimore: Paul H. Brookes Publishing Co.

10

Medical and Health Transitions for Young Adults Who Use AAC

Susan Balandin and Annalu Waller

> I had to go back to the ICU [Intensive Care Unit]. This time I said to the head doctor "Do you know much about cerebral palsy?" He said "Not much". I said "You will have to learn more about it" and my mum was there telling the doctor what I was saying. (Balandin, Dew, Llewellyn, & Kendig, 2003)

People with lifelong disability (e.g., intellectual disability, cerebral palsy) are living longer in part as a direct result of improved medical care in Western countries and many others around the world. Many individuals with intellectual disability, excluding those with Down syndrome, now experience a life expectancy similar to that of people without disability, although they are likely to experience the concomitant disabilities that are common in later life (e.g., problems with vision, hearing, and mobility; World Health Organization, 2000).

Individuals with complex communication needs who use augmentative and alternative communication (AAC) are often part of the group of people with cerebral palsy who are among those with more severe physical or cognitive disability. The life expectancy of children and adults with mild cerebral palsy is likely to be similar to that of their peers without disabilities. The life expectancy of those with the most severe disability (i.e., those who are immobile and fed by others or by gastrostomy) has also improved, with mortality rates falling by about 3.4% annually. However, for people affected by all but the most mild form of cerebral palsy, the picture is not so clear. In other words, gains in survival time are only marginally significant, approaching 1% (Strauss, Brooks, Rosenbloom, & Shavelle, 2008).

Nevertheless, there have been changes in mortality rates, and these can be expected to continue in the future (Strauss et al., 2008). Another significant shift with important implications for medical services is the movement from reliance on government institutions to community living arrangements for people with severe disabilities. Individuals with lifelong disability, including those with complex communication needs, are now likely to live in the community, selecting from either supported or independent living arrangements (see Chapter 9) and accessing generic community health care services.

Consequently, more than ever before, young adults with complex communication needs are making the transition from pediatric to adult community-based medical and health services. However, this transition may be far from smooth, despite a multitude of programs that focus on supporting young people with disabilities in making this service move (Binks, Barden, Burke, & Young, 2007; Scal & Ireland, 2005). These individuals face many challenges. As children, they typically enjoyed three important supports: 1) parents or caregivers helped manage and organize their care; 2) a children's rehabilitation or treatment center or medical facilities usually provided "one-

---

Pseudonyms are used with all quotations to protect the identities of those quoted. All quotations are from our research studies, which received ethical approval from the relevant university human research and ethics committees.

stop" coordinated services; and 3) in many countries, there were government guarantees of pediatric rehabilitation services (Young, 2007).

The health care system for adults is dramatically different: 1) Individuals or their guardians are responsible for managing health care, including identifying and advocating for needed services; 2) individuals may need to interact with and coordinate information among multiple medical professionals, including general practitioners, medical specialists (e.g., dentists, vision specialists), and rehabilitation specialists (e.g., speech-language pathologists, seating specialists); and 3) there are typically fewer guarantees of services, especially rehabilitation services (e.g., supports for AAC technology and services). Although it is clear that individuals must move from pediatric to adult health services, it is also clear that careful planning and preparation is needed to ensure a successful transition.

OVERVIEW OF THE CHAPTER

The aim of this chapter is to discuss barriers to and solutions for making a successful transition from pediatric to adult medical and health services for young adults who use AAC. In this chapter, there is a focus on young adults with cerebral palsy. The reasons for this are twofold. First, because of their wide range of health needs, young adults with cerebral palsy access physician and health services approximately twice as frequently as young adults without disability (Young et al., 2007). Second, we would argue that the experiences of this group of young adults, some of whom have intellectual disability, encapsulate those of others with lifelong disability, including young people with intellectual disability (Hudson, 2003). We suggest that, more than any other group, young people with cerebral palsy who use AAC are torn between wanting to live independently yet being reliant on others for physical help with many activities, including communication (Cooper, Balandin, & Trembath, 2009). This poses special challenges with respect to accessing needed medical services.

No research focuses specifically on health service transitions for young people who use AAC. Therefore, we extrapolate from the available literature how the use of AAC may impede or facilitate these transitions. This chapter includes an overview of the issues associated with the transition from pediatric to adult health care drawn from the literature from Australia, Europe, and North America. Using our knowledge of older adults' health care experiences, we discuss how the use of AAC might affect young adults attempting to make a successful transition to adult health care. Potential barriers to and solutions for successful transitions are explored, and the impact of AAC on the unmet health needs of the group is discussed in light of AAC practice and service delivery. Using pseudonyms, illustrative quotes from people who use AAC are incorporated throughout the text.

ACCESS TO ADULT HEALTH SERVICES

Although young people with lifelong disability will require ongoing access to knowledgeable health services across the life span (American Academy of Pediatrics, American Academy of Family Physicians, & American College of Physicians–American Society of Internal Medicine, 2002), such services may not be readily available or easily accessible. Children and adolescents with lifelong disability usually access specialized services, including health services, using an interdisciplinary team approach. Adults, in contrast, are more likely to access a complicated mix of independent health service providers, including general practitioners and medical specialists who provide services to the general community, as well as rehabilitation professionals (such as speech-language pathologists and occupational therapists) who focus on disability-related issues (Young et al., 2007). In many cases, it is the responsibility of the adult to coordinate scheduling, information, and services among these different professionals.

This presents problems for all stakeholders not only at the time of transition but also in the ensuing years. Young people and their families may feel that they have been cut adrift from services that they have known for many years, sometimes since birth.

General Practitioners

Like all people, individuals with severe disabilities require the services of a general practitioner for everyday health concerns as well as the health screening and health promotion activities that are appropriate for all adults (Binks et al., 2007; Lam, Fitzgerald, & Sawyer, 2005; Reiss & Gibson, 2002; Scal & Ireland, 2005). However, there is good reason to think that there is underutilization of general practitioner services by adults with disabilities (Andrews, Henderson, & Hall, 2001).

Limited use of general practitioner services is of special concern when we consider the difficulty that adults who use AAC may experience obtaining regular preventive services, such as mammography screening for breast cancer, as they grow older. A qualitative study of the mammography screening experiences of 87 women with disabilities (including 19 women with cerebral palsy) indicated that women with cerebral palsy who use a wheelchair or who have difficulty standing unaided may not be offered this type of screening (Poulos, Balandin, & Llewellyn, 2006; Poulos, Llewellyn, & Balandin, 2006). Mary's quote illustrates the difficulties that older adults experience in obtaining regular screening services:

> I did ask [my GP] about mammograms and she said it would be impossible because I can't stand up to the machine, if you stand up you have to be able to keep still and I can't [because of my spasms]. (Balandin et al., 2003)

Mary's general practitioner had told her that she would perform an annual manual check of Mary's breasts. However, Mary was concerned that this would not be sufficient: "I'm not very sure because my grandmother has had breast cancer, I'm just a bit concerned but I know I can't have a mammogram" (Balandin et al., 2003).

Clearly, individuals with cerebral palsy need access to the same preventive services as individuals without cerebral palsy. For example, women who are unable to stand to undergo mammography screening should be offered an alternative type of screening (e.g., ultrasound; Poulos, Balandin, et al., 2006). The cost of limited access to preventive services is clear—Strauss, Cable, and Shavelle (1999) reported that women with cerebral palsy are 3 times more likely to die from breast cancer than their peers without disabilities.

Medical Specialists

It is often difficult for individuals with severe disabilities to find specialists who are able to address specific health concerns such as vision and dental care (Burtner & Dicks, 1994). Individuals with cerebral palsy frequently have significant vision issues (Pellegrino, 1995). Individuals with disabilities also have significant dental problems frequently, in part because they have not received regular services throughout their lives, and these problems are compounded with age (Owens, Kerker, Zigler, & Horwitz, 2006).

The challenge is twofold—few medical specialists know how to provide services to people with disabilities, and many government programs only provide funding for children's services. Public advocacy is needed both to improve the limited training on working with individuals with disabilities provided to medical specialists and to ensure funding for adult services (Balandin & Morgan, 1997, 2001).

Disability-Related Services

For many individuals with moderate to profound physical disabilities, therapeutic interventions such as AAC interventions from speech-language pathologists and support with seating and mobility from occupational and physical therapists are available from infancy until the time they leave school. These therapeutic interventions, which help individuals maximize their abilities, are valued by both people with disabilities and their families. However, these services tend to dissipate when individuals with disabilities leave school. This is just the time when the need to maintain abilities is paramount: Changing social and employment situations result in new demands and in both emotional and physical stress. Therapists have shared stories of meeting young people some years after the people have left school and being devastated by the deterioration in their physical abilities because of a lack of ongoing physiotherapy. One physiotherapist even questioned whether the years of work with an individual were pointless if ongoing support was not available. Further research into the impact of reduced or nonexistent therapy on young adults is needed.

In the area of AAC, individuals may need access to communication systems that are a better fit with new work or living arrangements and may need to implement changes to their access system to reflect new skills or to take advantage of newly developed technologies. Although cerebral palsy is nonprogressive, there are ongoing challenges in terms of secondary problems such as arthritis and changes in muscle tone (Bottos, Feliciangeli, Sciuto, Gericke, & Vianello, 2001). Evidence has demonstrated that timely access to assessment for communication technology, physical support, therapeutic interventions, wheelchairs and seating, ongoing stabilizing orthotic prescriptions, and, at times, surgery helps maintain levels of personal, employment, and social independence (Williams, Krezman, & McNaughton, 2008). There is good reason to think that, at least in some countries, there are significant barriers to AAC services for adults. For example, it has been estimated that in the United States, only 2%–3% of individuals who would benefit from AAC have appropriate access to AAC technology and services (Assistive Technology Law Center, 2006).

Coordinating Medical Services

Adults who use AAC and their families have described the difficulties they experience when accessing medical and health services (Balandin, Hemsley, Sigafoos, & Green, 2007; Hemsley, Balandin, & Togher, 2004, 2007; Hemsley et al., 2001; Robillard, 1994; Williams, 1993). Indeed, it is a sad indictment of the inadequacy of support services, including health services, that in countries such as Australia, many parents still voice the hope that their adult sons or daughters with disabilities will die before they themselves do because these parents fear for the future when they will no longer be there to provide support and help navigate the various systems, including the health care system (Berg, 2009; Hemsley, 2008; Hines, 2009).

Health care teams worry about young adults dealing with services that are fragmented and that do not provide the same level of involvement and follow-up as interdisciplinary teams. Parents or team managers coordinate services and information for children. Once individuals with disabilities become adults, these responsibilities shift to them. Transitions may be further complicated by the desire of young adults who use AAC to make independent decisions while being reliant on others for support in many of their activities of daily living. The creation of a health transition plan, discussed in detail later in this chapter, is meant to assist in the process of making a smooth transition from pediatric to adult services. However, to date there is little information on what issues these plans should focus on or whether using them improves the health care experience for all stakeholders (Scal & Ireland, 2005). Furthermore, plans for health differ from plans for education in that, to our knowledge, there is no policy that all young people, regardless of level of ability, have a health transition plan.

COMMUNICATION AND HEALTH

Communication difficulties may also account for part of the reason that young adults with cerebral palsy report that they experience poorer health than their typically developing peers (Bjornson, Belza, Kartin, Logsdon, & McLaughlin, 2008). Successful communication is a two-way process in which each participant contributes and supports the contributions of his or her partner (Light, Roberts, Dimarco, & Greiner, 1998; McNaughton & Light, 1989). In this section we focus on important skills for individuals with complex communication needs; in the following section ("Educating Health Care Professionals") we focus on how health care professionals can better support positive interactions.

For individuals who use AAC, successful participation in conversations with a medical professional requires that they be able, whether alone or with support, to 1) introduce themselves and their communication system, 2) make use of appropriate vocabulary and language to communicate their concerns and needs, and 3) make use of appropriate communication strategies to ensure that their needs and concerns are addressed. Additional issues related to communication include the development of self-determination and self-advocacy skills as well as communication skills to manage daily care issues.

Introducing a Communication System

As individuals with disabilities transition to adult medical services, they will frequently encounter medical professionals who have limited experience working with individuals with complex communication needs (Balandin, 2004; Balandin et al., 2007; Buzio, Morgan, & Blount, 2002; Hemsley, Balandin, & Togher, 2004; Hemsley et al., 2007; Murphy, Molnar, & Lankasky, 1995). Both partners need to take responsibility for a successful interaction; however, individuals who use AAC need to be prepared to introduce themselves and their communication system. The importance of effective introductions was made clear in Balandin et al.'s (2003) study of the experiences of 15 individuals who use AAC interacting with their health professionals. One participant, Mark, described the positive impact of his introduction strategy, saying,

> You usually have to break the ice, there's always an icebreaking, because they don't know anything about you and you don't know anything about them . . . If you lay down your history, if you tell them up front that you have cerebral palsy, perhaps they look at you a bit weirdly to start off with, unable to comprehend. I just tell them "I'm perfectly capable of understanding what you are saying and I want to know exactly what is in store for me."

Many adults have told us that they take a friend, family member, or support worker with them when accessing health services. This person may mediate the communication of the individual who uses AAC or take primary responsibility for giving and gathering information. The distinction between these two roles is important and should be clearly identified at the beginning of any conversation—many individuals with complex communication needs have noted that they do not like to bring a speaking partner, as they risk the health professional communicating with the natural speaker rather than with them. Health professionals, including nurses (Hemsley et al., 2001), have noted that it is a great help when a natural speaker is present because the health professionals then feel that they know what is happening, and the communication is easier. Such comments, well meant by professionals who are eager to provide optimum care, support the premise that if a natural speaker is present the person who uses AAC may be ignored. Even when the person with disabilities is able to speak and answers questions, medical staff may continue to address questions to the natural speaker unless he or she overtly defers to the person with disabilities. Thus, we suggest that young people who use AAC be encouraged to prepare for any health consultation and, if they take a natural speaker with them, set clear guidelines about how they wish the appointment to progress.

Access to Appropriate Vocabulary

In order to participate in detailed discussions of medical needs, individuals with complex communication needs must have access to appropriate vocabulary. Many individuals who use AAC complain that when they were young adults, others restricted their vocabulary, and they were unable to communicate easily on topics important to teens and young adults (Williams et al., 2008). For individuals who make use of symbol representations, Bryen (2008) has identified important vocabulary for a variety of adult concerns, including issues related to health, sexuality, and abuse. It is critical that individuals with complex communication needs who act as their own advocates have access to appropriate vocabulary and that this vocabulary undergo social validation and be updated regularly to ensure that it is, in fact, useful.

The importance of access to appropriate vocabulary is apparent in the following vignette, documented as part of a larger study by Balandin et al. (2003):

············ Margaret, a woman with severe cerebral palsy living in a group home, was worried, as she was experiencing prolonged pain in her stomach but had no means of communicating this to her carers or her doctor because of the limited messages on her speech-generating device. With detailed, specific questioning this concern was pinpointed and a message was added at her request so she could talk about this problem. ············

Strategies to Improve Communication with Medical Professionals

The typical medical interview between a person without a disability and a general practitioner is approximately 20 minutes in length (Mann et al., 2001). Marvel, Epstein, Flowers, and Beckman (1999) reported that the typical patient has an average of 23 seconds to communicate his or her concern before being interrupted by the doctor. Although both patient and physician satisfaction seem to be related to factors other than simply the length of the interaction, clearly it may be challenging for individuals with complex communication needs to communicate concerns and obtain needed information without the use of specific strategies. Both patient and physician satisfaction with a medical interview can be improved through the use of strategies to quickly and efficiently communicate needs and concerns and provide opportunities for the patient to obtain desired information (Talen, Grampp, Tucker, & Schultz, 2008).

Talen et al. (2008) held focus groups with 41 medical professionals and identified the following patient characteristics that, from a doctor's perspective, lead to more successful medical exchanges: 1) knowledge of their own health, diagnosis, and current medications; 2) communication skills in presenting clear, organized descriptions of symptoms; and 3) personal attitudes of ownership, trust, and honesty about their medical condition (see Table 10.1). In order to ensure that physicians obtain a complete picture of the medical status of an individual with complex communication needs, that individual may wish to consider preparing "medical narratives" that provide detailed information on medical history and concerns that may not be recorded in medical notes. This is especially helpful in averting repeated occurrences of situations. For example, a woman with cerebral palsy discovered that some medical equipment, such as automatic blood pressure machines, is affected by the involuntary movements associated with her disability. She therefore tells a reusable narrative about a situation in which a nurse became very concerned because a device was providing a reading of high blood pressure. The woman questioned the result, and the nurse eventually found an old-fashioned, but more accurate, blood pressure gauge (after a long hunt through the health center). Telling such a narrative not only provides useful information but allows the individual who uses AAC to take control of the conversation and demonstrate his or her ability to relate a narrative within context—a clear demonstration of communicate competence (Waller, 2006). Although medical narratives are sometimes included in communication passports (Fitton, 1994), there is a danger that these may not be with the person when needed. Research is investigating the use of interactive multimedia to support access to medical narratives (Prior, Cummins, Waller, Kroll, & Balandin, 2009).

In investigating the narratives of older parents providing support to a son or daughter with cerebral palsy who uses AAC, Hemsley, Balandin, and Togher (2004, 2007, 2008b) noted that health professionals rarely talk to the person who uses AAC, often do not read information that is provided by the family, and treat the person who uses AAC differently from other patients on the hospital ward. Using these data and additional data gathered from focus groups with health professionals and adults who use AAC (Hemsley et al., 2008a, 2008b, 2008c), Hemsley developed a kit to support people who use AAC and their families when in the hospital. This kit is being tested for efficacy.

Besides being prepared, another useful strategy is to estimate the amount of time the appointment will take and to inform medical professionals if one or a range of issues will need to be discussed. Despite the best efforts of the individual who uses AAC to prepare for a meeting, conversations may go in unexpected directions, and communication will take longer. In describing his interactions with his general practitioner, who is not a native English speaker, Colin noted the need to keep repeating what he is saying (using his device) until the general practitioner understands: "It is a bit hard for him [GP] to understand it. It could be the voice" (Balandin, 2004; Balandin et al., 2003). Many adults who use AAC and who manage their own health care have told us that they always try to book a long appointment, as they may need extra time to communicate.

Self-Determination and Self-Advocacy

When individuals with complex communication needs consistently self-advocate for their medical needs it not only is in their own and their parents' best interest but also is considered a valued skill from a physician's perspective (Talen et al., 2008). Self-advocating involves not only having access to appropriate vocabulary and to an effective and efficient method of communicating but also having a belief that individuals have a right to a *voice* in their medical care.

Issues of self-determination and self-advocacy are discussed in detail in Chapter 2; research, especially in the area of pain management, has made clear the importance of self-advocacy skills for individuals with cerebral palsy (Andersson & Mattsson, 2001). Young adults with cerebral palsy are likely to experience significant levels of pain, yet like their older peers with cerebral palsy, they often do not access health services for support in coping with this pain (Andersson & Mattsson, 2001).

Bjornson et al. (2008) suggested that pediatric physiotherapy, including stretching and bracing, might account to some extent for such increased levels of pain. In consumer forums, older adults with cerebral palsy, including those who use AAC, have recounted early horror stories of therapies (including wearing braces at night) and the pain they experienced as a result. The fact that this pain was associated with past medical interventions, and the fact that past concerns with pain were ignored as the pain was viewed as being a necessary by-product of these interventions, can lead to reduced self-advocacy behaviors with medical professionals on issues related to pain.

The following anecdote reflects both the importance of self-advocacy skills and how medical practitioners often underestimate the level of reported pain in people with communication disorders. The second author, who has cerebral palsy and dysarthria, was told that ongoing hip pain was due to arthritis as a result of early aging. Surgery performed at Waller's insistence revealed a dysplastic hip that had been dislocating—only then did the surgeon concede the level of pain that Waller had been experiencing.

Learning to self-advocate within the time-pressured constraints of a medical appointment can be challenging. Adults who use AAC have told us that often they do not have enough time to discuss their health concerns with relevant health care providers, they feel that providers are impatient with their communication, and they feel that providers do not take enough time to provide information. This is a major problem for young people who are starting to take responsibility for their own health care and who may not have the literacy or motor skills to be able to search alternative sources of information (e.g., printed health promotion materials, the Internet) for themselves (Blackstone, 1996; Iacono, Balandin, & Cupples, 2001; Iacono, Cupples, Balandin, & Cassidy, 2001).

There is a delicate balance here. Liptak (2008) stressed the importance of encouraging young people to be involved in their own health care decision making. For this to happen, young people must be well informed about their health needs and their expectations for services, and they must be prepared to advocate for their needs. At the same time, individuals with complex communication needs must also be prepared to act, as much as possible, in ways consistent with physicians' expectations for a good physician–patient exchange (see Table 10.1). Acquiring some of these skills may be challenging for individuals with complex communication needs; however, all of these skills enable these individuals to perform as informed self-advocates. Just as it is important for physicians to work to meet patient expectations, patients should be aware of their doctors' expectations for a successful visit.

Developing self-determination and self-advocacy skills can be challenging. Unlike their same-age peers, young people with lifelong disability who use AAC may rely on support staff and their parents and family members not only for support with activities of daily living but also for social interaction (Cooper et al., 2009; Merchen, 1990). Nevertheless, research indicates that 76 young people ages 20–30 years with motor disorders such as cerebral palsy or spina bifida did not differ from their same-age peers in their views of their subjective age (Galambos, Darrah, & Magill-Evans, 2007). These 76 young people reported that they felt the same age as or slightly older than their chronological age, despite noting that they were treated by their parents as if they were younger than their chronological age. Galambos et al. reported that, contrary to their expectations, the young people with the most severe level of disability felt the oldest and most mature. The authors suggested that this might be because this group had more contact with older people and (because of the many physical challenges they faced) were experienced in problem solving and in dealing with the reactions of others to their disability.

Here then is a group of people who are often treated as if they are younger than their chronological age but who feel themselves to be their chronological age or older. It is no small wonder that people who use AAC consistently express frustration about being treated as if they are children or as if they are unable to understand what health care providers say (Balandin et al., 2003). Discussing what would improve his interactions with his dentist and general practitioners, Malcolm told us that he wanted to be treated like other adults:

Malcolm: Just treat me like anybody else.

Interviewer: Hmm. So you feel they don't do that? What makes you feel they don't do that?

Malcolm: Sometimes they talk down to me and it is one of my pet hates. (Balandin et al., 2003)

Managing health care systems and services is problematic for adults who have complex communication needs (Buzio et al., 2002; Robillard, 1994; Willner & Dunning, 1993). Consequently, there is an urgent need to ensure that young adults who use AAC develop the knowledge and skill to man-

Table 10.1. Patient behaviors that support successful communication, as identified by physicians

Knowledge	
Health history and family health history	Knows personal medical history, including chronic disease history and allergies
	Knows family medical history
Diagnosis	Knows diagnosis and what it means
Medications	Knows own medications (prescription and over-the-counter) and what they are for
	Knows changes in medications
Other	Knows why they made the appointment and what to expect from doctor
	Knows doctor's name
	Knows medical terms

Skills	
Preparation and organization	Brings a list of prioritized concerns
	Brings a list of current medication, test results
	Writes questions down
History of present illness: descriptive and sequential	Provides focused, precise description of problem
	Reports relevant details on how he or she feels
	Provides accurate view of severity, pain
	Knows what has been tried
Questions and comments	Asks for information, wants to know more
	Asks questions to confirm treatment plan
Other	Arrives on time
	Brings family member, caseworker to help

Attitudes	
Patient ownership of health	Takes ownership of health
	Accepts responsibility for taking medications
	Accepts diagnosis and treatment
Doctor–patient relationship	Knows there is a time limit
	Knows that there will be other follow-up visits
	Demonstrates mutual acceptance, respect
Trust, tolerance, and honesty	Shares information with other doctors
	Is honest about symptoms
Other	Shares positive health experiences
	Is optimistic

age their own health care and service decisions to the best of their ability. Young adults who use AAC may encounter barriers to optimum health care provision and must be prepared to self-advocate.

Management of Daily Care

Successful communication is important not only during focused medical discussions but also during day-to-day activities, such as mealtimes, that can affect an individual's health. Many people with complex communication needs are at risk for *dysphagia,* or difficulty eating, drinking, and swallowing (Balandin, Hemsley, Sheppard, & Hanley, 2009; Sheppard, 1991, 2002).

A study indicated that adults who use AAC vary in terms of their perceived success managing safe eating and drinking regimes (Balandin et al., 2009). Some noted that even if they have written plans, support staff and families may not read or follow them. Others noted that family members become impatient and are not always supportive.

These adults varied in the amount of control they wished to take. Some were critical of their speech pathologist and chose which advice they would follow and which they would ignore. Several passively accepted whatever management strategies were implemented. They did not always like these but reported that it was too difficult for them to implement any change. However, almost all of the 42 participants in this study agreed that dysphagia management should be implemented using a collaborative approach in which the person with dysphagia was central (Balandin et al., 2009). Thus, health care providers must be aware that a person who uses AAC and who does not complain may not be content with the service but may not know how to complain or may be too anxious to do so.

EDUCATING HEALTH CARE PROFESSIONALS

It is clear that many health care professionals lack skill in communicating with people who use AAC, despite the gradual increase in the number of study programs in which undergraduate health care providers (i.e., medical students) receive lectures from people with disabilities—including those who use AAC (e.g., Lennox & Diggens, 1999; Tracy & Iacono, 2008). Many adults who use AAC have told us that health professionals require more education (Balandin, 2004; Balandin et al., 2003, 2007). One of 15 participants in a qualitative study of the health experiences of adults with cerebral palsy (Balandin, 2004; Balandin et al., 2003), Caroline, summarized what others have said:

> I think they [health professionals] need to know about the different aspects of different kinds of cerebral palsy and disability because there's some that have got eyesight problems, intellectual problems and physically that they need to . . . understand that the brain can be damaged in three or four different ways. I believe that at [university] they are beginning to tell doctors more about cerebral palsy because my niece is doing a disability course and I think she got a little bit on cerebral palsy but a little bit could be made a bit longer. . . . It needs to happen for the older doctors and the older nurses (too) and I suppose a course [that's] not just cerebral palsy but about cerebral palsy because they never know when they're going to have them in the hospital.

James noted that many doctors recognize this gap in training themselves:

> I find that the young doctors have a far better understanding of what is cerebral palsy and how it affects you than the older doctors, they really do not have the same understanding and it's interesting that a lot of the doctors talk to me about that on the side. (Balandin et al., 2003)

The barriers faced in hospitals by those who use AAC are well documented (see, e.g., Adubato, 2004; Balandin et al., 2007; Barr, 1997; Buzio et al., 2002; Clements, Focht-New, & Faulkner, 2004; Costello, 2000; Hemsley, Balandin, & Togher, 2004; Hemsley et al., 2007, 2008b; Iacono & Davis, 2003; Juleff & Fox, 2003; Lam et al., 2005; Lo Surdo, 1996; Regnard, Mathews, Gibson, & Clarke, 2003; Robey, Gwiazda, & Morse, 2001; Robillard, 1994; Tuffrey-Wijne, Bernal, Jones, Butler, & Hollins, 2006; Young et al., 2007). It would be redundant to discuss these issues here; nevertheless, it is important to note that all people (young or old), their families, and their health care providers agree that having a functional communication system is a necessity for good health care, safety, and well-being when in the hospital. Newell noted the following:

If you have got a disability, then don't get sick. If you get sick, then don't go to a hospital. If you have to go to a hospital, then make sure that you have as much control over your care regime as possible. (1999, p. 15)

Without a functional communication system, it is impossible to exert control over what is occurring, a fact recognized not only by people with disabilities and their families but also by health professionals (e.g., nurses; Hemsley et al., 2001).

Reports on the value of education about AAC for health service providers at the undergraduate level are promising (Balandin & Armstrong, 2001, 2002; Lennox & Diggens, 1999; Tracy & Iacono, 2008). For example, 128 medical students participated in a 3-hour communication training program that involved a variety of activities, including interacting with people with a range of physical and sensory disabilities. After the program, students' attitudes toward disability as measured on the Interaction with Disabled Persons Scale (Gething, 1994) had improved significantly. Furthermore, students noted that they gained not only new insight into their own inadequacy in terms of communicating but also strategies for facilitating better communicative interactions. Similarly, 164 speech pathology students were enthusiastic in their evaluations of the involvement of people who use AAC as lecturers and noted that lectures from people who use AAC were a more powerful learning tool than hearing about communication from academic staff (Balandin et al., 2001).

Of special interest are the educational programs in which individuals with complex communication needs play a significant role in providing instruction. Recounting his experiences with health care providers (Balandin, 2004; Balandin et al., 2003), James noted the benefit of such instruction, saying,

If you have a collaborative approach to training staff then I think you'll have a far better medical service and people are going to get better a lot quicker . . . they [health professionals] need to understand that cerebral palsy's not a brain disorder. It's one function of the brain that doesn't work properly. We are intelligent, even the ones without speech are intelligent, it's just that they can't express it.

People who use AAC and the AAC community must have a role in advocating that such courses form a part of the training of *all* health professionals, including nurses, therapists, dentists, and pharmacologists. Training medical professionals to become better at listening to speaking patients is now a key area of research (Talen et al., 2008; Zandbelt, Smets, Oort, Godfried, & de Haes, 2004). Similar attention must be given to developing doctors' skills in working with individuals who use AAC. However, we would stress that such education programs require careful evaluation in terms of not only the acquisition of knowledge but also the transition of knowledge to practice. We hope that such training will have a positive impact on health transitions and health care and will make health management easier for young people with AAC who are taking on an adult role. However, further research is needed to evaluate the efficacy of training and to identify which training strategies are most effective.

TRANSITION PLANNING

There is evidence that young adults who experience a poorly managed transition to adult health services may give up on the health system and become resistant or hostile to using health services (Liptak, 2008; Whitehouse & Paone, 1998). Adolescence and young adulthood is a time of risk taking; consequently, many young adults do not go for routine health services but rather rely on emergency services if needed (Tuffrey & Pearce, 2003). Furthermore, Tuffrey and Pearce noted that young people with neurological impairments might not have the social skills needed to seek out the health services they require. We may surmise that for some young people who use AAC, communication difficulties may be a further disincentive to accessing health services. However, Tuffrey and Pearce noted that it is important that young adults make the transition to adult health services not only to optimize their health throughout adulthood but also to reinforce to themselves and their families that life as an adult is a realistic expectation. As we have noted, there is limited information about how young adults who use AAC view their transition to adulthood. In addition, there is no information on how they feel about the fact that they are likely to require ongoing health intervention and support at a higher rate than their peers without disabilities (Bjornson et al., 2008; Young et al., 2007).

There is a wide variety of reasons why young adults may experience difficulty transitioning to adult services. Clearly, there is a lack of medical professionals prepared to work with individuals who use AAC, and many individuals who use AAC have not been provided with instruction in the skills needed for successful interactions with medical professionals (see Table 10.1). Some adults who use AAC have complained to us about the health services they received as children and the false promises that some of these services held out, particularly in the areas of speech and mobility. They have also discussed how they have rejected advice from health professionals as an affirmation of their right to choose which advice they will follow and which they will reject. Despite these challenges, there is agreement that it is imperative that young people with chronic health conditions 1) have appropriate transition planning to support them in this process (Binks et al., 2007; Liptak, 2008; Nieuwenhuijsen et al., 2008; Reiss & Gibson, 2002), 2) have opportunities to learn about their health and health screening needs, and 3) learn from an early age to advocate for the services they need.

Transition Plans

Liptak (2008) argued that an appropriate transition plan is likely to optimize the health and well-being of young adults with cerebral palsy, as it helps facilitate their access to appropriate adult services. Yet despite agreement that health transition plans should be coordinated (Nieuwenhuijsen et al., 2008), be flexible, foster independence (Binks et al., 2007; Reiss & Gibson, 2002), and be well resourced (Binks et al., 2007), little is known about how best to prepare young adults who use AAC to transition into the adult health care system.

Families of someone with a lifelong disability need to plan for a future when parents either will be too frail to provide support or will have died. Research into the roles of adult siblings has indicated that both siblings with and without disabilities have considered what support will be required and how this could be managed (Dew, Balandin, & Llewellyn, 2007). Both types of siblings have noted that the support will be different from that provided by parents, and all siblings want to ensure that the person with disabilities maintains as much independence as possible. Discussing the transitions of older people with intellectual disability, Bigby (1997a, 1997b, 2000) noted that supports are usually available, even though clear planning may not have occurred. When it comes to health transitions, it is not known what plans are in place for young people who use AAC if parents are not available to provide support.

Dew and colleagues (2007) noted that people with disabilities, their siblings or family members, and service providers would benefit from collaborative planning to ensure that any transitions in care are managed smoothly to avoid crises in management and feelings of burden. Clearly, if young people who are transitioning into adult health services have to do this at a time when parents are no longer able to provide support, they will need a sibling, friend, or other person who can help them, if needed. At the same time, it is important that young people who use AAC are supported and encouraged to take as decisive a role in their health as possible, as this is part of the responsibility that goes with becoming an adult (Binks et al., 2007; Liptak, 2008).

A health transition plan can help in the shift from pediatric to adult services. These plans must address the specific needs of the individual who uses AAC as well as acknowledge the individual's desire and need to have greater control over his or her health services. It has been suggested that from the age of 14 years, all young people with special health care needs have a health plan that is created collaboratively among themselves, their families, and their health care providers (American Academy of Pediatrics, American Academy of Family Physicians, & American College of Physicians–American Society of Internal Medicine, 2002). Yet despite some agreement on the attributions of health transition plans, there is little evidence that such plans are being developed (Binks et al., 2007).

According to the American Academy of Pediatrics, American Academy of Family Physicians, and American College of Physicians–American Society of Internal Medicine, health care transition plans should reflect the following guidelines:

1. An identified health provider who oversees the process including future health care planning.
2. Identification of the core skills that health professionals need to manage health care transitions and provide appropriate transition services and ensure that these are part of health care training.
3. Prepare and maintain an up to date medical summary that is both portable and accessible. This will provide a common knowledge base between different health professionals.
4. In collaboration with the young person and his/her family, create a written transition plan by age 14. The plan should address what services will be required, who will provide them and if necessary how they will be financed. The plan should be reviewed and updated annually or at times of transition of care.
5. The same guidelines should be applied to all young people but additional supports and resources will be needed for those with disability or specialised care needs.
6. If required affordable continuous health insurance must be available. (2002, p. 1305)

Tuffrey and Pearce (2003) from the United Kingdom suggested the following as essential elements of a health transition plan:

1. *Timing:* Careful planning is required to ensure that transitions take place when a person's health is stable rather than at a time of health crisis. The young person's level of maturity and his or her educational and social context should also be considered. Tuffrey and Pearce suggested that having a target transfer age might be useful for all stakeholders and that questionnaires might be useful for ascertaining how much the young person understands about his or her health and how much responsibility he or she is prepared to take.

2. *Multidisciplinary teamwork:* All health professionals, the family, and the young person should be involved in discussions about health care transitions and planning.

3. *Evaluation:* The transition process and the new health services should be evaluated, including through user feedback.

One key step in the development of a health transition plan is the documentation of current status and services. Nieuwenhuijsen et al. (2008) noted that often parents are well informed as to their child's current medical status and the services the child receives but do not pass this information on to their sons or daughters. Clearly, if young people are to manage their own health, they need to know their own medical history and how to access the appropriate health care provider. It is important that they have access to this information while their parents or family members are still available to pass it on. Young adults with complex health histories may find it useful to keep a summary of their health history, the medications they take, and any particular health issues they have.

Mentors

Given the commonality of many of the difficulties experienced by people who use AAC (Balandin et al., 2007; Buzio et al., 2002; Lo Surdo, 1996), young people may also benefit from interacting with other individuals who use AAC and who have successfully navigated the transition to adult health services. Such interaction may occur over consumer Listservs such as ACOLUG (the Augmentative Communication On-Line Users' Group; Institute on Disabilities at Temple University, 2009), which frequently features lively discussions on medical issues such as obtaining dental services as an adult with cerebral palsy or on personal experiences with specific medical interventions.

On a more personal level, individuals who use AAC may benefit from having a mentor with whom they can discuss strategies for dealing with health providers who may be too busy to listen or who may know little about communicating with someone who uses AAC. The benefits of mentoring for those who are learning to use AAC are recognized by families and service providers (McNaughton et al., 2008; Rackensperger, Krezman, McNaughton, Williams, & D'Silva, 2005); many young people in the process of transitioning find mentoring helpful. Research into web-based mentoring programs in which both mentor and mentee use AAC has demonstrated that such programs are successful (Light et al., 2007). Given that older adults who use AAC have a wealth of experience in managing the health system and recognize this as knowledge that they can share with others we suggest that there is a need for adult mentors who use AAC and who can provide support to young people grappling with the transition to adult health services.

CONCLUSION

Despite recognition of the importance of moving on from pediatric to adult services, young adults may continue to receive health care from children's services for a variety of reasons. These include 1) the complexity of an individual's health condition (Lam et al., 2005), 2) parents' and pediatricians' beliefs that the adult health system will provide inadequate care or inappropriate services for young adults who require care from a multidisciplinary team, and 3) a lack of appropriate transition planning (Reiss & Gibson, 2002).

Reports from older adults and their families (e.g., Balandin et al., 2007; Hemsley, Balandin, & Togher, 2004; Lo Surdo, 1996; Robillard, 1994) have indicated that there is a pressing need to prepare adults who use AAC to deal with adult health care systems and at the same time prepare health systems to provide an appropriate and equitable service for this group (Binks et al., 2007). Some key strategies include supporting the development of needed communication skills and strategies, documenting the individual's medical history, providing access to the individual's medical narratives, supporting the individual in taking a leadership role in medical exchanges, supporting self-determination and self-advocacy in medical (and everyday) decisions, developing and documenting transition plans, and ensuring access to peer collaboration opportunities such as listservs (e.g., ACOLUG) and mentoring. In addition, we would argue that the implementation of health care transition plans requires not only further research and evaluation but also the development of policies to ensure that such plans become a required part of health services.

At the same time, other problems may be even more difficult to overcome. In many countries, health care systems are in crisis, are underfunded, and are coping with having to service an ever increasing number of clients with limited resources (World Health Organization, 2008). Service may be focused on a few highly specialized, expensive, curative interventions so that primary services are not providing optimal health care. Disadvantaged populations, including people with disabilities, may have difficulty accessing available services (World Health Organization, 2008). The World Health Organization (2008) identified the following measures as necessary for improving health care for all: 1) making reforms in terms of the equity of health service provision, 2) making health systems people centered, 3) ensuring that health authorities are more responsible, and 4) developing reforms to protect the health of communities. These measures are keys to ensuring better health for all and will affect not only people who use AAC but also those who support them in their daily lives and in health service provision.

A multifaceted approach will be needed to improve medical transition outcomes for individuals who use AAC. Not only is system change needed to improve access to adult services, but medical professionals require training in how to better interact with individuals with complex communication needs. Families need additional information and supports to help manage the transition from pediatric to adult services. Finally, advocacy and education are important for young people who use AAC—the skills they will require need to be learned long before they transition to adult health services. We would argue that these skills are acquired initially at home and in preschools when young children begin to learn to advocate for themselves. This process continues with the acquisition of literacy skills and with experiences interacting with a range of peers and others in schools and in the general community. Thus, a successful transition for young people who use AAC is facilitated through a lifelong learning process that begins early and continues across the life course. For young people who use AAC to make the transition to adult health services, they and those who support them or who provide such services need to work together to facilitate a smooth transition.

REFERENCES

Adubato, S. (2004). Making the communication connection. *Nursing Management, 35,* 33–35.

American Academy of Pediatrics, American Academy of Family Physicians, & American College of Physicians–American Society of Internal Medicine. (2002). Policy statement. A consensus statement on health care transitions for young adults with special health care needs. *Pediatrics, 110,* 1304–1306.

Andersson, C., & Mattsson, E. (2001). Adults with cerebral palsy: A survey describing problems, needs, and resources, with special emphasis on locomotion. *Developmental Medicine & Child Neurology, 48,* 76–42.

Andrews, G., Henderson, S., & Hall, W. (2001). Prevalence, comorbidity, disability and service utilisation: Overview of the Australian National Mental Health Survey. *British Journal of Psychiatry, 178,* 145–153.

Assistive Technology Law Center. (2006). *SGD funding solutions from Assistive Technology Law Center.* Retrieved September 9, 2009, from http://www.aacfundinghelp.com/

Balandin, S. (2004). "It's hard for them to understand." In S. Millar (Ed.), *Communication matters symposium* (pp. 7–8). Leicester, England: Communication Matters.

Balandin, S., & Armstrong, E. (2001). Teaching with the experts: Lectures in disability and communication. In L. Wilson & S. Hewatt (Eds.), *Speech Pathology Australia national conference* (pp. 251–258). Melbourne, Australia: Speech Pathology Australia.

Balandin, S., & Armstrong, B. (2002, August). *Teachers and learners in AAC: What students think.* Paper presented at the 10th Biennial Conference of the International Society for Augmentative and Alternative Communication, Odense, Denmark.

Balandin, S., Dew, A., Llewellyn, G., & Kendig, H. (2003, March). *Health care experiences of people with cerebral palsy & complex communication needs.* Paper presented at the AGOSCI Something to Say, Sydney, Australia.

Balandin, S., Hemsley, B., Sheppard, J.J., & Hanley, L. (2009). Understanding mealtime changes for adults with cerebral palsy and the implications for support services. *Journal of Intellectual & Developmental Disability, 34,* 197–209.

Balandin, S., Hemsley, B., Sigafoos, J., & Green, V. (2007). Communicating with nurses: The experiences of 10 adults with cerebral palsy and complex communication needs. *Applied Nursing Research, 20,* 56–62.

Balandin, S., & Morgan, J. (1997). Adults with cerebral palsy: What's happening? *Journal of Intellectual and Developmental Disability, 22*(2), 109–124.

Balandin, S., & Morgan, J. (2001). Preparing for the future: Aging and AAC. *Augmentative and Alternative Communication, 17,* 99–108.

Barr, O. (1997). Care of people with learning disabilities in hospital. *Nursing Standard, 12*(8), 49–55.

Berg, N. (2009). *What's it like to live in a nursing home? Exploring the experiences and residential preferences of people under 65, their families and nursing home staff.* Unpublished doctoral dissertation, The University of Sydney, Sydney, Australia.

Bigby, C. (1997a). Later life for adults with intellectual disability: A time of opportunity and vulnerability. *Journal of Intellectual and Developmental Disability, 22*(2), 97–108.

Bigby, C. (1997b). Parental substitutes? The role of siblings in the lives of older people with intellectual disability. *Journal of Gerontological Social Work, 29*(1), 3–21.

Bigby, C. (2000). *Moving on without parents: Planning, transitions and sources of support for older adults with intellectual disabilities.* New South Wales, Australia: Maclennan & Petty.

Binks, J.A., Barden, W., Burke, T., & Young, N.L. (2007). What do we really know about the transition to adult centred health care? A focus on cerebral palsy and spina bifida. *Archives of Physical Medicine and Rehabilitation, 88,* 1064–1073.

Bjornson, K.J., Belza, B., Kartin, D., Logsdon, R.G., & McLaughlin, J. (2008). Self-reported health status and quality of life in youth with cerebral palsy and typically developing youth. *Archives of Physical Medicine and Rehabilitation, 89,* 121–127.

Blackstone, S. (1996). What's standing in the way? *Augmentative Communication News, 9*(4), 1–3.

Bottos, M., Feliciangeli, A., Sciuto, L., Gericke, C., & Vianello, A. (2001). Functional status of adults with cerebral palsy and implications for treatment of children. *Developmental Medicine and Child Neurology, 43,* 516–528.

Bryen, D.N. (2008). Vocabulary to support socially-valued adult roles. *Augmentative and Alternative Communication, 24,* 294–301.

Burtner, A.P., & Dicks, J.L. (1994). Providing oral health care to individuals with severe disabilities residing in the community. *Special Care in Dentistry, 14,* 188–193.

Buzio, A., Morgan, J., & Blount, D. (2002). The experiences of adults with cerebral palsy during periods of hospitalisation. *Australian Journal of Advanced Nursing, 19*(4), 8–14.

Clements, P.T., Focht-New, G., & Faulkner, M.J. (2004). Grief in the shadows: Exploring loss and bereavement in people with developmental disabilities. *Issues in Mental Health Nursing, 25,* 799–808.

Cooper, L., Balandin, S., & Trembath, D. (2009). The loneliness experiences of young adults with cerebral palsy who use alternative and augmentative communication. *Augmentative and Alternative Communication, 23,* 154–164.

Costello, J.M. (2000). AAC intervention in the intensive care unit: The Children's Hospital Boston model. *Augmentative and Alternative Communication, 16,* 137–153.

Dew, A., Balandin, S., & Llewellyn, G. (2007, May). *Exploring transitions of care: Adults with CP and their siblings.* Paper presented at the Sydney Siblings Forum Symposium, Sydney, Australia.

Fitton, P. (1994). *Listen to me—Communicating the needs of people with profound intellectual and multiple disabilities.* London: Jessica Kingsley.

Galambos, N.L., Darrah, J., & Magill-Evans, J. (2007). Subjective age in the transition to adulthood for persons with and without motor disabilities. *Journal of Youth and Adolescence, 36,* 825–834.

Gething, L. (1994). The Interaction with Disabled Persons Scale. *Journal of Social Behavior and Personality, 9*(5), 23–42.

Hemsley, B. (2008). *The experiences and needs of carers of people with cerebral palsy and severe communication impairment in hospital.* Unpublished doctoral dissertation, The University of Sydney, Sydney, Australia.

Hemsley, B., Balandin, S., & Togher, L. (2004). Without AAC: The stories of unpaid carers of adults with cerebral palsy and complex communication needs in hospital. *Augmentative and Alternative Communication, 20,* 243–258.

Hemsley, B., Balandin, S., & Togher, L. (2007). Older unpaid carers' experiences supporting adults with cerebral palsy and complex communication needs in hospital. *Journal of Developmental and Physical Disabilities, 19,* 115–124.

Hemsley, B., Balandin, S., & Togher, L. (2008a). Family caregivers discuss roles and needs in supporting adults with cerebral palsy and complex communication needs in the hospital setting. *Journal of Developmental and Physical Disabilities, 20,* 257–274.

Hemsley, B., Balandin, S., & Togher, L. (2008b). "I've got something to say": Interaction in a focus group of adults with cerebral palsy and complex communication needs. *Augmentative and Alternative Communication, 24,* 1–13.

Hemsley, B., Balandin, S., & Togher, L. (2008c). Professionals' views on the roles and needs of family carers of adults with cerebral palsy and complex communication needs in hospital. *Journal of Intellectual & Developmental Disability, 33,* 127–136.

Hemsley, B., Sigafoos, J., Balandin, S., Forbes, R., Taylor, C., Green, V.A., et al. (2001). Nursing the patient with severe communication impairment. *Journal of Advanced Nursing, 35,* 827–835.

Hines, M. (2009). *Living with autism: A narrative analysis of older parents' experiences.* Unpublished doctoral dissertation, The University of Sydney, Sydney, Australia.

Hudson, B. (2003). From adolescence to young adulthood: The partnership challenge for learning disability services in England. *Disability & Society, 18,* 259–276.

Iacono, T., Balandin, S., & Cupples, L. (2001). Focus group discussions of literacy assessments and web-based reading interventions. *Augmentative and Alternative Communication, 17,* 27–36.

Iacono, T., Cupples, L., Balandin, S., & Cassidy, S. (2001). Access to web-based reading materials for individuals with disability. *ACQuiring Knowledge in Speech, Language and Hearing, 3,* 117–119.

Iacono, T., & Davis, R. (2003). The experiences of people with developmental disability in emergency departments and hospital wards. *Research in Developmental Disabilities, 24,* 247–264.

Institute on Disabilities at Temple University. (2009). Augmentative Communication On-Line Users' Group. Retrieved September 8, 2009, from http://disabilities.temple.edu/programs/aac/acolug/

Juleff, B., & Fox, M. (2003, November). *Something to say about care and communication in hospital.* Paper presented at the Perspectives on Health in Developmental Disability Conference, Sydney, Australia.

Lam, P.-Y., Fitzgerald, B.B., & Sawyer, S. (2005). Young adults in children's hospitals: Why are they there? *Medical Journal of Australia, 182,* 381–384.

Lennox, N., & Diggens, J. (1999). Knowledge, skills and attitudes: Medical schools' coverage of an ideal curriculum on intellectual disability. *Journal of Intellectual and Developmental Disability, 24,* 341–347.

Light, J., McNaughton, D., Krezman, C., Williams, M., Gulens, M., Galskoy, A., et al. (2007). The AAC Mentor Project: Web-based instruction in sociorelational skills and collaborative problem solving for adults who use augmentative and alternative communication. *Augmentative and Alternative Communication, 23,* 56–75.

Light, J.C., Roberts, B., Dimarco, R., & Greiner, N. (1998). Augmentative and alternative communication to support receptive and expressive communication for people with autism. *Journal of Communication Disorders, 31,* 153–180.

Liptak, G. (2008). Health and well being of adults with cerebral palsy. *Current Opinion in Neurology, 21,* 136–142.

Lo Surdo, P. (1996, April). *A brush with death: My hospital experience.* Paper presented at the Ageing and Cerebral Palsy "They Said We'd Never Make It" Conference, Sydney, Australia.

Mann, S., Sripathy, K., Siegler, E.L., Davidow, A., Lipkin, M., & Roter, D.L. (2001). The medical interview: Differences between adult and geriatric outpatients. *Geriatrics, 49,* 65–71.

Marvel, M.K., Epstein, R.M., Flowers, K., & Beckman, H.B. (1999). Soliciting the patient's agenda: Have we improved? *JAMA, 281,* 283–287.

McNaughton, D., & Light, J.C. (1989). Teaching facilitators to support the communication skills of an adult with severe cognitive disabilities: A case study. *Augmentative and Alternative Communication, 5,* 35–41.

McNaughton, D., Rackensperger, T., Benedek-Wood, E., Krezman, C., Williams, M.B., & Light, J.C. (2008). "A child needs to be given a chance to succeed": Parents of individuals who use AAC describe the benefits and challenges of learning AAC technologies. *Augmentative and Alternative Communication, 24,* 43–55.

Merchen, M.A. (1990). Some reasons for being passive from a personal perspective. *Communication Outlook, 12*(1), 10–11.

Murphy, K.P., Molnar, G.E., & Lankasky, K. (1995). Medical and functional status of adults with cerebral palsy. *Developmental Medicine and Child Neurology, 37,* 1075–1084.

Newell, C. (1999). Disabling health systems. *Interaction, 12,* 13–51.

Nieuwenhuijsen, C., van der Laar, Y., Donkervoort, M., Nieuwstraten, W., Roebroek, M.J., & Stam, H. (2008). Unmet needs and health care utilization in young adults with cerebral palsy. *Disability and Rehabilitation, 30,* 1254–1262.

Owens, P.L., Kerker, B.D., Zigler, E., & Horwitz, S.M.(2006). Vision and oral health needs of individuals with intellectual disability. *Mental Retardation and Developmental Disability Research Review, 12,* 28–40.

Pellegrino, L. (1995). Cerebral palsy: A paradigm for developmental disabilities. *Developmental Medicine and Child Neurology, 37,* 834–839.

Poulos, A., Balandin, S., & Llewellyn, G. (2006). Women with cerebral palsy and breast screening by mammography. *Archives of Physical Medicine and Rehabilitation, 87,* 304–307.

Poulos, A.E., Llewellyn, G., & Balandin, S. (2006). What's the point of it? Radiographers, women with disability and mammography screening. *Breast Cancer Research, 8,* S16–S17.

Prior, S., Cummins, K., Waller, A., Kroll, T., & Balandin, S. (2009, June). *Facilitating communication of people with complex communication needs in hospital: A review of the literature.* Poster presented at NHS Scotland Event, Glasgow, Scotland.

Rackensperger, T., Krezman, C., McNaughton, D., Williams, M.B., & D'Silva, K. (2005). "When I first got it, I wanted to throw it off a cliff": The challenges and benefits of learning AAC technologies as described by adults who use AAC. *Augmentative and Alternative Communication, 21,* 165–186.

Regnard, C., Mathews, D., Gibson, L., & Clarke, C. (2003). Difficulties in identifying distress and its causes in people with severe communication problems. *International Journal of Palliative Nursing, 9*(4), 173–176.

Reiss, J., & Gibson, R. (2002). Health care transition: Destination unknown. *Pediatrics, 110,* 1304–1306.

Robey, K.L., Gwiazda, J., & Morse, J. (2001). Nursing students' self attributions of skill, comfort, and approach when imagining themselves caring for persons with physical impairments due to developmental disability. *Journal of Developmental and Physical Disabilities, 13,* 361–371.

Robillard, A.B. (1994). Communication problems in the intensive care unit. *Qualitative Sociology, 17,* 383–395.

Scal, P., & Ireland, M. (2005). Addressing transitions to adult health care for adolescents with special health care needs. *Pediatrics, 115,* 1607–1612.

Sheppard, J.J. (1991). Managing dysphagia in mentally retarded adults. *Dysphagia, 6,* 83–87.

Sheppard, J.J. (2002). Swallowing and feeding in older people with lifelong disability. *Advances in Speech Language Pathology, 4,* 119–121.

Strauss, D., Brooks, J., Rosenbloom, L., & Shavelle, R. (2008). Life expectancy in cerebral palsy: An update. *Developmental Medicine & Child Neurology, 50,* 487–493.

Strauss, D., Cable, W., & Shavelle, R. (1999). Causes of excess mortality in cerebral palsy. *Developmental Medicine and Child Neurology, 41,* 580–585.

Talen, M.R., Grampp, K., Tucker, A., & Schultz, J. (2008). What physicians want from their patients: Identifying what makes good patient communication. *Families Systems and Health, 26,* 58–66.

Tracy, J., & Iacono, T. (2008). People with developmental disabilities teaching medical students—Does it make a difference? *Journal of Intellectual and Developmental Disabilities, 33,* 345–348.

Tuffrey, A., & Pearce, A. (2003). Transition from paediatric to adult medical services for young people with chronic neurological problems. *Journal of Neurology, Neurosurgery & Psychiatry, 78,* 1011–1013.

Tuffrey-Wijne, I., Bernal, J., Jones, A., Butler, G., & Hollins, S. (2006). People with intellectual disabilities and their need for cancer information. *European Journal of Oncology Nursing, 10,* 106–116.

Waller, A. (2006). Communication access to conversational narrative. *Topics in Language Disorders, 26*(3), 221–239.

Whitehouse, S., & Paone, M. (1998). Patients in transition: Bridging the gap from youth to adulthood. *Contemporary Pediatrics, 13,* 15–16.

Williams, M.B. (1993). Getting older. *The UCPA Networker, 7*(1), 13.

Williams, M.B., Krezman, C., & McNaughton, D. (2008). "Reach for the stars": Five principles for the next 25 years of AAC. *Augmentative and Alternative Communication, 24,* 194–206.

Willner, L., & Dunning, D. (1993). *Ageing with cerebral palsy.* London: SCOPE.

World Health Organization. (2000). *Ageing and intellectual disabilities: Improving longevity and promoting healthy ageing.* Geneva: Author.

World Health Organization. (2008). *The world health report 2008: Primary health care now more than ever.* Geneva: Author.

Young, N.L. (2007). The transition to adulthood for children with cerebral palsy: What do we know about their health care needs? *Journal of Pediatric Orthopedics, 27,* 476–478.

Young, N.L., Gilbert, T.K., McCormick, A., Ayling-Campos, A., Boydell, K., Law, M., et al. (2007). Youth and young adults with cerebral palsy: Their use of physician and hospital services. *Archives of Physical Medicine and Rehabilitation, 88,* 696–702.

Zandbelt, L.C., Smets, E.M.A., Oort, F.J., Godfried, M.H., & de Haes, H. (2004). Satisfaction with the outpatient encounter. *Journal of General Internal Medicine, 19,* 1088–1095.

VI

Assessment and Intervention with Teens and Adults

11

AAC Considerations During the Transition to Adult Life

Laura J. Ball, Korey Stading, and Denise Hazelrigg

The term *communication* in its broadest sense can be defined as "any act by which one person gives to or receives from another person information about that person's needs, desires, perceptions, knowledge, or affective states" (National Joint Committee for the Communication Needs of Persons with Severe Disabilities, 1992, p. 2). Communication is the "essence of human life and . . . all people have the right to communicate to the fullest extent possible" (American Speech-Language-Hearing Association, 2005, p. 1). Any individual for whom speech and/or written communication is inadequate to meet various communication needs is likely to benefit from augmentative and alternative communication (AAC). AAC interventions can include the use of both aided (e.g., electronic devices, alphabet boards and wordboards) and unaided (e.g., sign, gestures, pointing) approaches to communication (Beukelman & Mirenda, 2005).

AAC assessment and intervention activities typically focus on teaching communication techniques and strategies to the individual with a disability. However, communication is an interactive process in which each participant adapts to the skills and weaknesses of his or her partner. Therefore, it may be necessary to consider interventions to address not only an individual's use of AAC but also ways to increase opportunities for the individual to successfully communicate with others (Blackstone, Williams, & Wilkins, 2007). More specifically, although the individual with complex communication needs may benefit from the use of AAC techniques, the communication partner may also benefit from instruction in ways to successfully support communicative interaction (Kent-Walsh & McNaughton, 2005).

Complex communication needs may result from a wide range of developmental, physical, cognitive, or social impairments. For many, these disabilities are chronic, requiring AAC support across the life span and, therefore, through numerous life transitions (Lilienfeld & Alant, 2005; Mirenda, 2003). For others, the communication disability is transient, and AAC support for functional communication is required only during a period of recovery from an accident or illness or pending the development of functional spoken communication (Light, Beesley, & Collier, 1988).

When people experience such severe impairments of natural speech or language that they cannot meet their daily communication needs, participation in educational, vocational, and social activities is typically severely restricted, and AAC is required to supplement whatever natural speech they can produce (Beukelman & Mirenda, 2005). Communication limitations often become acutely problematic during important life transitions because the AAC strategies and approaches that have been effective in one set of environments may be less effective in new communication environments (Hamm & Mirenda, 2006; Lund & Light, 2006). In terms of transition planning, the assessment and intervention process for those who use AAC systems requires a focus on functional communication in both current and future contexts (Beukelman & Mirenda, 2005).

In this chapter we provide a brief overview of the AAC assessment and intervention process for transition-age youth and the importance of considering an individual's communication performance and needs in both current and future environments. Individuals interested in a more detailed explanation of the AAC assessment and intervention process are referred to Beukelman and Mirenda (2005).

DEVELOPING THE AAC ASSESSMENT AND INTERVENTION TEAM

As in any assessment activity, the first step is identifying and bringing together the members of the assessment and intervention team. For the young adolescent approaching adulthood, there are many important transitions: from school to work force, postsecondary education, or community activities (Atanasoff, McNaughton, Wolfe, & Light, 1998; Lund & Light, 2006; McNaughton & Bryen, 2007); from home to independent or group home living (see Chapter 9); from an emphasis on family relationships to peer interactions and adult relationships (Smith, 2005; see also Chapter 8). The many changes that occur during the transition from adolescence to adulthood mean that many individuals will be involved in the AAC assessment and intervention activities.

Effective AAC assessment and intervention occur when all stakeholders are well informed and working toward the identification and realization of shared goals. It is often necessary for collaborative teams to coordinate services and support individuals who use AAC in various contexts (Beukelman, Hanson, Hiatt, Fager, & Bilyeu, 2005). Beukelman et al. described the assessment team composition and noted that it "may vary, depending upon the impairment profile, communication needs, and social contexts" (p. 187) of the person who relies on AAC. They also described three general categories of AAC team members: 1) regular, 2) occasional, and 3) specific. Regular team members include individuals who serve regularly on a variety of AAC intervention teams—this typically includes AAC specialists, rehabilitation engineers, and assistive technology specialists. Occasional team members include people who occasionally serve on an AAC team when they are associated in some way with a person who relies on AAC—this may include special education teachers, nurses, and vocational counselors. Specific team members are people who support a specific person but who are not likely to be involved with other AAC teams—for example, the person who uses AAC, family members, general education teachers, and caregivers (Beukelman et al., 2005). There will likely be considerable overlap between the AAC assessment and intervention team (AAC team) and the person's educational transition team. The focus of the AAC team is on maximizing communication in a variety of environments, whereas the transition team addresses a wide range of needs (e.g., living arrangements, employment, recreation).

It is critical that all personnel understand their roles and responsibilities in the assessment and intervention process, including both the outgoing and incoming situations/placements, so that they can meet the needs of the people they serve. Soto, Muller, Hunt, and Goetz (2001) identified five major skills for members of AAC teams: the ability to 1) work collaboratively in a team; 2) use the AAC system to access core curricula or activities; 3) facilitate social interactions; 4) operate, maintain, and integrate the AAC system elements; and 5) create structures that support learning.

The person who will be using the AAC system to communicate is an indispensable member of the AAC team. His or her input and feedback is of critical importance at each stage of the assessment process, because he or she will use the AAC system every day. The AAC team may also use the role of team member participant as a way to teach self-advocacy skills that will become increasingly important with each successive transition. A study by Cameron and Murphy (2002) showed that people of varying ability levels and communication impairments were able to use AAC to express their likes and dislikes about different transition-related topics. When they provided the opportunity for the person who uses AAC to express his or her preferences, care providers learned new information about that person's likes and dislikes that was helpful for providing needed vocabulary (Cameron & Murphy, 2002). An individual who uses AAC encounters many changes with teachers, caregivers, or coworkers throughout the day, and these changes will occur many times over the teen and adult lifetime. Allowing for and supporting the development of self-advocacy skills is essential for enabling people who use AAC to learn to effectively address these challenges.

One AAC team member from the group is assigned the role of advocate. This is a team member who will be consistent across the transition process. The advocate need not have any particular expertise but rather must have a strong vested interest in the ultimate success of the individual's functional communication. Often this advocate is a parent or sibling, but it may also be an AAC specialist, teacher, occupational therapist, or other transition team member. The advocate's role is to ensure communication success throughout the transition process and ultimately across multiple transitions. This person is familiar with the individual's current communication strategies and AAC systems and so can serve as an excellent reference in terms of interpreting behavior and identifying possible strategies that may work in different communication situations. If new strategies or modifications to current systems are needed, the advocate is also helpful because he or she knows what systems have and have not worked for the person in the past. As an individual who communicates with AAC exits the educational system and enters the work force, it is likely that members of the AAC team will change extensively. The presence of a consistent AAC advocate who can communicate and monitor communication goals and objectives makes a critical difference in the potential for successful outcomes in the community.

At this point, it is noteworthy to mention that there may be some differences of opinion among AAC team members in terms of communication needs. It is important to listen to all members' ideas and work to come to a consensus on priorities, keeping in mind that the person using the AAC system will be the ultimate decision maker, either with support or independently. Likewise, if the facilitators' (e.g., parents, educators, coworkers, spouse) needs are not considered or met, the outcome may be poor because these people will work with the individual on a regular basis (Parette & Angelo, 1996).

In the community, family members, friends, and employers may fulfill the advocate role. Family members have a very important role in this process, as they are often the most important communication partners in the individual's life, and their acceptance of AAC influences the use of the recommended communication system (Parette & Angelo, 1996). Not only is the development of family partnerships important in terms of gathering information about the individual, but such partnerships have been shown to affect the carryover of skills addressed in intervention, the maintenance of skills over time in other contexts, and school/caregiver knowledge for setting appropriate expectations (Myers, 2007).

The AAC specialist can provide or help with assessment team preparation. It is important to note that the AAC specialist provides ideas and suggestions for when and how the different AAC techniques may be optimally used with the individual. For example, an AAC specialist may assist the team in identifying AAC options and help with decision making but may not be present at all system trials. Because of this, it is imperative that the transition team identify an AAC coordinator who spends time with the individual on a regular basis. Other team members may then report to the AAC coordinator when successes or problems arise with a particular device. The AAC coordinator contacts the AAC specialist for help with problems or to communicate successes and facilitate subsequent activities.

People who are not on the AAC team but who interact with the individual may require practical demonstrations of the device effectiveness and are therefore provided with specific suggestions for supporting its use. To match features of the AAC system and to accommodate the person's needs while maximizing his or her skills, the AAC team must include members from all communication contexts (e.g., home, school, employment). Members from each of these contexts have expertise in their knowledge of the person and the specific communication needs at their respective sites. The communication needs in all transition settings must be targeted with AAC goals when various devices and/or systems are evaluated. In this way, the team compares and identifies which features are necessary, which features are secondary, and which features may prove distracting or detrimental to functional communication.

ASSESSING CURRENT COMMUNICATION STRATEGIES

When preparing for transitions, it is often useful to begin the process by reviewing or assessing current communication strategies to determine if communication needs are being effectively addressed and capabilities effectively used and to begin to consider whether the current strategies will be successful in the new communication environments. Much of this information may be readily available, and the AAC team can move quickly to the consideration of new goals. However, it should not be assumed that all people who rely on AAC are currently meeting their communication needs and that all planning and intervention should focus on the new transition environments. For some, the assessment will confirm effective communication with current strategies and technologies. However, for others such an assessment will highlight unmet communication needs; inefficient use of communication strategies; or overdependence on trained, familiar communication partners (e.g., family members, classroom aides) who may not be available in new environments.

The first step in such an assessment is to document the individual's communication performance in a variety of contexts and with multiple partners and to consider his or her communication strengths and needs. Most individuals use multiple communication modalities that may include some combination of residual speech, high-tech AAC devices (e.g., computer-based devices that may provide speech synthesis), and low-tech approaches (e.g., alphabet boards and wordboards, symbol displays, sign language, pointing, gestures). With any *AAC system* (i.e., a collection of AAC techniques that are used by an individual to support communication), the individual will not rely on a single component for every interaction. For example, some gesturing and other low-tech options may have been very successful in the past and likely will continue to be functional in the individual's future communication repertoire, especially during predictable activities such as personal care routines. If the individual communicates intentions effectively, efficiently, and appropriately with an existing mode, there may be no reason to consider a new AAC strategy for that activity. However, when a particular communication technique will not be successful in the new setting, an alternative approach should be considered. *Social Networks: A Communication Inventory for Individuals with Complex Communication Needs and Their Communication Partners* (Blackstone & Hunt-Berg, 2003) is widely used by AAC intervention specialists to document communication patterns by those who rely on AAC.

Input should be obtained not only from the members of the AAC assessment team but also from communication partners who interact directly, frequently, and in varied contexts with the person who relies on AAC (e.g., peers, siblings, teachers). These communication partners are in a position to provide rich, comprehensive information related to communication performance and needs within a specific context; any single AAC intervention specialist cannot assume to know or fully understand context-specific details about communication patterns and effectiveness. It is particularly useful to document the extent of support needed from communication partners, as new contexts (e.g., a college dormitory) might not include partners with appropriate training to support communication interaction, and different communication modes may need to be used to replace or support current strategies.

An AAC assessment can be a wide-ranging process, as a number of interrelated factors can influence communication performance. For example, many individuals with severe physical disabilities need specialized seating and positioning support in order to make effective use of AAC technology. In addition, many individuals with disabilities need supports to make full use of their vision and hearing skills. These and other issues may be a part of an AAC assessment—each of these issues does not always need to be investigated exhaustively for each individual, but each is a potential area of concern within an AAC assessment and may need attention.

Many of these assessment domains are interrelated; the order in which they are listed here is not meant to suggest a priority. For example, it may be necessary to ensure that seating and positioning needs have been appropriately addressed before a clear picture of an individual's accessing skills can be obtained, and information on an individual's visual skills will influence the assessment and design of symbol and word displays.

Seating and Positioning

For individuals with physical disabilities, appropriate seating and positioning will determine their ability to control their movements and make accurate and efficient use of low-tech and high-tech AAC systems (Higginbotham, Shane, Russell, & Caves, 2007; McEwen & Karlan, 1989). Occupational therapists and seating specialists play a key role in ensuring that an individual has comfortable seating that provides appropriate support for movement. The assessment team may need to consider the individual's use of an AAC system in a variety of positions (e.g., seated in a power wheelchair, reclining on a sofa, upright in a stander).

Accessing

An *access assessment* involves determining the person's general range of motion, his or her control over movements, and the most economical movements for accessing AAC devices (Beukelman & Mirenda, 2005). Traditionally, assessment activities focused on determining whether a person would access the AAC device *directly* (e.g., using a finger, knuckle, eye gaze, mouth stick, head pointer) or *indirectly* (e.g., scanning with a switch, partner-assisted scanning). Technological developments in tracking eye and head movement now enable people with minimal movement to use computer-based communication and workstation technology (Higginbotham et al., 2007), and assessment teams should regularly review the potential impact of newly developed access technologies for individuals with physical disabilities.

Vision and Hearing

Sensory skills, such as vision and hearing, directly influence the development and use of an individual's AAC system. Many individuals with developmental and acquired disabilities experience significant visual and hearing difficulties (Beckung & Hagberg, 2002; da Costa, Salomao, Berezovsky, de Haro, & Ventura, 2004). An ophthalmologist can contribute important information on how an individual's visual skills can be maximized (e.g., size and location of graphics, use of color). Although speech-language pathologists have some training in enhancing listening performance, it may be useful to consult an audiologist for additional strategies to maximize the individual's participation.

Cognitive-Linguistic Skills

Knowledge of an individual's cognitive and linguistic abilities helps guide the selection of appropriate AAC system components. At times, testing instruments such as standardized norm-referenced measures of intelligence or receptive language can contribute to the cognitive-linguistic assessment process, but these results should always be interpreted with extreme caution (Beukelman &

Mirenda, 2005). Individuals with severe speech disabilities were not included in the validation process for many of the most commonly used standardized language and intelligence assessments, and these individuals typically have had vastly different life experiences than the individuals for whom norms were obtained (Salvia, Ysseldyke, & Bolt, 2009). In addition, these tests may require response modes (e.g., speech) or impose time restrictions that are not appropriate for individuals with physical disabilities (Beukelman & Mirenda, 2005). Standardized test results, therefore, may not provide an accurate picture of an individual's current skills or potential to benefit from educational activities. Informal assessment procedures are often used to provide a broad understanding of cognitive and language abilities. An appropriate AAC system will both be immediately useful to the individual and contain supports for future growth. For example, if an individual demonstrates limited reading and spelling skills, vocabulary may be represented with pictures and photographs. All of these vocabulary items, however, should be clearly labeled with text, and an alphabet line should be included, so that the individual has a means to develop and practice spelling skills.

Natural Speech Skills

Careful assessment of residual, natural speech is particularly important, as some individuals may have relied for years on family or school personnel who are familiar with them and with typical conversational topics to interpret their speech. These supports may not be available in the new living situation, for example, a college dormitory or a group home setting. When assessing people who use some (i.e., residual) natural speech, it is vital to *measure* speech intelligibility or understandability. The word and sentence versions of the Speech Intelligibility Test (Yorkston, Beukelman, Hakel, & Dorsey, 2007) can be used to measure the understandability of teenagers' and adults' speech and provide a useful objective measure of anticipated intelligibility in a variety of environments.

Subjective estimations of intelligibility should be avoided because of inconsistent and often inaccurate results. Commonly, those listeners who are very familiar with the speaker tend to overestimate his or her speech intelligibility because they are familiar with frequent communication topics and with the individual's speech patterns.

· · · · · · · · · · · During his college years, Sam, a student with dysarthric speech due to cerebral palsy, was unwilling to use electronic AAC technology. Rather, he communicated with his residual speech, an alphabet board to resolve communication breakdowns, and occasional writing. As Sam attempted to make the transition to employment, his reduced speech intelligibility interfered with successful interviewing experiences. Follow-up interviews with potential employers revealed that the understandability of his speech was of concern to them. During a transition-related assessment, it became apparent that Sam's speech intelligibility for sentences was approximately 40% when the listener was a stranger and was unfamiliar with the general content of the messages. As part of the assessment, Sam and his parents were asked to estimate his speech intelligibility. His father and mother estimated that Sam was more than 80% intelligible. In a series of counseling sessions, Sam's speech-language pathologist shared information on his scored intelligibility with unfamiliar partners. Following these counseling sessions, Sam decided to supplement his natural speech with an AAC device that provided speech synthesis output.

In time, Sam was hired by an organization that supported children with disabilities. Ten years later, he still speaks and uses his AAC device both as an alternative to speech (with unfamiliar partners) and to augment his speech (with familiar partners). Sam has become very good at predicting which listeners will be able to understand his speech and which listeners will benefit from the use of his AAC device. · · · · · · · · · · · ·

Communication Contexts and Communication Partners

One step in the assessment process is to identify the contexts in which an individual currently participates and communicates and to give careful thought to the unique demands of particular situations with respect to needed vocabulary, typical communication partners, and the need for special strategies. For example, in a high school classroom, an individual will need access to a large vocabulary; however, most communication partners will be familiar with the individual and the AAC system and will understand that time is needed to prepare an appropriate answer to a classroom discussion. If that individual makes use of public transportation to travel to a job site, he or she is more likely to interact with individuals who will have little awareness of AAC, and it will be important that the individual be able to quickly communicate needed information (e.g., WHERE DO I GO FOR THE DOWNTOWN BUS?).

For transition-age youth, the assessment team will need to begin to consider not only current communication contexts but the impact of future contexts. For example, how will the demands of a group home—and communicating personal care needs to group home staff—differ from communicating with a family member who provides care at home? How will the demands of communicating with the public as part of a new job differ from communicating with peers at high school?

Light et al. (1988) provided a description of an AAC intervention for an adolescent girl who had suffered a brain injury. The intervention addressed not only her communication needs while in an acute care rehabilitation setting but also the challenges of communicating once the girl returned to her home community.

Use of AAC

Given the many contexts and communication partners that are typically identified in the assessment process, it is inappropriate to think that one AAC device will fulfill all academic or vocational communication needs. Many AAC devices can provide quick access to large preprogrammed vocabularies and can be used to answer questions in classes and meetings, converse with peers and coworkers, and participate in many group activities. In addition, some can be used to produce written work and complete other academic tasks. However, some individuals may prefer to use an alphabet board for quick one-to-one conversations with familiar partners but use a device to speak with larger groups. They may fingerspell letters with familiar partners but prepare an entire sentence to be spoken aloud with unfamiliar partners. Although these low-tech approaches are typically not sufficient to meet all communication needs, effective low-tech strategies are likely to remain important in specific contexts and should always be available both as a recognized component of the AAC system and as a backup for the high-tech system (Williams, Krezman, & McNaughton, 2008).

IDENTIFYING NEW COMMUNICATION NEEDS

In addition to documenting current performance, the AAC team works to anticipate future changes to the person's communication needs and skills. Some of these anticipated changes involve communication environments, communication partners, and vocabulary.

Communication Environments

The transition from adolescence to adulthood may bring with it changes in living arrangements (e.g., moving from the family home to independent living or a group home), daily activities (e.g., transitioning from high school to postsecondary school, work, or volunteer activities), and social activities (e.g., developing stronger relationships with peers). Many of these new environments will have new but predictable routines, such as getting ready (for school or work), negotiating public transportation, and interacting socially during leisure time. Depending upon the new environments, the individual may have new or changed communication needs, including the following:

- Dealing with a range of settings (e.g., using the communication system in a noisy cafeteria, a quiet café, a lecture hall class)

- Using the AAC device to connect to mainstream technology, such as a cell phone or social networking web sites (e.g., Facebook, MySpace, Twitter)

- Being able to independently maintain and charge a device.

Individuals who will be attending postsecondary programs may have access to an office for students with disabilities to assist in the transition from high school to college (see Chapter 5 for additional information). For all individuals, it will be important that the AAC system be familiar to a wide variety of communication partners so that support can be provided as needed (Hamm & Mirenda, 2006).

Communication Partners

As individuals transition to new environments, they will meet new communication partners. In many situations, a person may need to make use of new communication strategies to meet the demands of the new setting. For example, if transitioning from a school to a work setting, a person may require more formal vocabulary or phrasing. Instead of WHAT'S UP?, the speaker may need to say HOW ARE YOU TODAY? Similarly, if the person transitions from living at home with family to living independently, he or she may require socialization skills never previously considered.

.... Keaton is an 18-year-old with cerebral palsy who graduated from high school and was admitted to a university. Like many college freshmen, he moved into the dormitory. Although his transition team had worked hard to anticipate his academic needs at the university, the social component was not covered comprehensively. As a result, when he met new students, attended sporting events, went to fraternity rush activities, and so forth, he did not have appropriate communication messages stored in his device. Transition teams should consider potential academic, vocational, and social interactions and work to provide comprehensive coverage of communication needs.............

The AAC team also needs to consider whether individuals will need new communication strategies to introduce themselves and their AAC system to others and whether communication partners will need training to support successful communicative interactions.

Changes in Vocabulary

New communication environments and new communication partners bring demands for new vocabulary. An important first step is the completion of a *contextual inventory* in order to identify key words and phrases that will allow the person to successfully communicate in each context. Table 11.1 shows a sample contextual inventory. The transition team lists each of the person's contexts and then scrutinizes them, breaking them into smaller environments or tasks. For example, in postsecondary contexts, students will likely communicate different messages in biology than in art and may have different communication needs in classrooms than in group discussions or laboratory

Table 11.1.   Sample contextual inventory

Place	Conversational topic	What other people are saying	Vocabulary
Work	Work tasks	"I need more supplies."	Supplies
		"How many boxes do we need?"	Boxes
	Lunch	"What's for lunch today?"	Food choices
		"Does anyone have change for a dollar?"	Money
	Break time	"Anybody want to get coffee?"	Snacks
			Drinks
	TV last night	"Did you watch *American Idol* last night?"	TV shows
			Likes/dislikes
Bus	Bus ride	"I need a transfer."	Money
			Tickets
			Places
			Times

contexts. The inventory establishes a list of probable vocabulary for each context, much of which is gleaned from listening to peers in the same contexts. In addition to this specific vocabulary, the person also needs generic vocabulary to have the opportunity to regulate conversations (e.g., directions on how to interact with the person using AAC, CAN YOU COME OVER HERE) and the ability to quickly maintain conversational interactions (e.g., HANG ON A SECOND, BUT . . .). Many daily conversations require nonspecific generic vocabulary consisting of rote social interactive phrases (e.g., "uh-huh," "yeah," "thanks," "how are you?"). Having access to this vocabulary in every context is critical to ensuring successful social communicative development and ongoing interactions (Beukelman & Mirenda, 2005).

For individuals who are not able to spell, the team should also identify the individual(s) who will monitor and update the vocabulary available on the AAC system. In the case of a transition, numerous and exciting new topics for discussion can be included (e.g., a new school, new teachers, new classmates, a new job, new friends). Ensuring that an individual has access to motivating and relevant content will help to ensure that he or she is a meaningful participant in interactions.

Changes in the AAC Assessment Team

The lead professional on the AAC team is often a speech-language pathologist who is typically funded by an age-specific service provider (e.g., the school district, adult services). In these situations, there is a danger that there will be a break or discontinuity in services as the individual who uses AAC moves from high school (and school-based services) to the adult world (and adult services). During a transition, the assessment team should include individuals from both the old as well as the new or anticipated environments. It is often useful to identify a facilitator or advocate who will, in effect, transition with the person and ensure that there is continuity of services from the old to the new environment. This transition team member serves the dual purpose of assisting in the transition and serving as an advocate for the person. The advocate does not necessarily have to be a speech-language pathologist but should be someone with a strong knowledge of the person's skills and needs. Moreover, the advocate must have a strong vested interest in the ultimate success of the individual's functional communication and participation in the new context.

ADDRESSING NEW AND ANTICIPATED COMMUNICATION NEEDS

Assessment includes the determination of specific components that comprise the AAC system. In this respect, individual aspects must be evaluated separately and then assembled to arrive at the optimal match of system features to the person's communication needs. Typically, aspects of systems that are evaluated include 1) effectiveness, 2) efficiency, 3) portability, 4) durability, 5) programming, 6) dependability, and 7) ability to support the development of new skills. In addition, system trials should be performed to ensure that the new approach has the intended impact. Appendix 11.1 provides a form that can be used to gather information during the system trial.

Effectiveness

Although it is difficult to quantify effectiveness, the basic question is whether the AAC system supports the individual in meeting his or her communication goals. In some cases this may be an issue of whether the device has the desired input features (e.g., can a literate individual easily enter the desired text?). Specific output features may be important in some environments (e.g., can the device provide speech output that is loud enough to be heard in a classroom?).

Efficiency

The need for efficient communication in a given situation is influenced by a wide variety of factors. In some contexts or situations (e.g., a classroom discussion), quick communication is necessary, whereas in other situations (e.g., a relaxed conversation with a friend), more time is available to compose messages.

     A variety of techniques can be used to increase efficiency. Most AAC devices provide the ability to store words and phrases for rapid retrieval of predictable vocabulary items. Stored vocabulary can be organized and retrieved using "paging" systems, icons with multiple meanings, and alphabetical organization schemes such as word prediction and abbreviation expansion (i.e., when the person spells an abbreviation, the system is programmed to speak or spell a longer utterance that is represented by the abbreviation, e.g., typing HH might elicit HI, HOW ARE YOU DOING TODAY?). Almost everyone will want to supplement preformulated messages with independently produced vocabulary items, thereby formulating sentences and generating novel messages (Beukelman & Mirenda, 2005).

     Individuals with emerging literacy skills and/or those who communicate with pictures may not be able to spell to communicate unique vocabulary items. The assessment team will need to consider ways both to regularly update the vocabulary available to the individual and to teach the individual strategies that he or she can use with communication partners to support successful interactions (e.g., providing a picture to represent THE WORD IS NOT ON MY BOARD, PLEASE GUESS).

Portability

Considering a person's ability to independently transport the AAC system is particularly important because new transportation challenges are very likely to occur as part of the transition process. If an individual walks under his or her own power, then a portable (e.g., lightweight, small) AAC device that can be carried to various places is essential. When a wheelchair is used for mobility, a less portable device may be feasible. Comparatively large, heavier AAC devices can be mounted to a wheelchair, however this may mean that the person has access to the device only when seated in that particular chair. The AAC team should consider the different contexts (e.g., home, work, riding the bus) and positions (e.g., in bed, in a wheelchair) in which the individual will communicate to ensure that he or she has some method of communicating at all times.

Programming

Many individuals find that communication efficiency can be improved by preprogramming messages for later retrieval. Environments and partners help to determine the messages an individual needs to communicate. Many devices come preprogrammed with high-frequency vocabulary (e.g., common verbs). This vocabulary needs to be individualized with items of special interest to that particular person (e.g., names of family members, vocabulary for participation in an American history class).

On the transition team, AAC staff and caregivers are often responsible for programming a communication device either entirely (i.e., the individual is unable to independently enter vocabulary) or partially (i.e., the individual and team members share in the programming). In the AAC planning meetings, the team creates a schedule for each team member's contribution to AAC system programming and maintenance so that each member has a clear plan for his or her role and the tasks required. In cases in which the person cannot independently manage the maintenance and charging of the device, it is vital to identify a reliable advocate to ensure that the AAC system is set up each morning and closed down for recharging each evening. The person in this role may be the first to become aware of any technical problems that arise so that early reporting and repairs can be arranged.

Dependability

AAC device quality and manufacturer support is particularly important when the person is active in the community. The team must consider all of the contexts in which the individual uses or travels with the device (e.g., working in a factory, traveling on public transit) that may result in damage and require frequent repairs. Both the manufacturer's reputation for completing timely repairs and the availability of technical support for questions regarding day-to-day use are important considerations. The team should consider device durability, system technical support, and manufacturer warranty as well as any other services available for support, such as whether the manufacturer offers a loan or rental system in cases of lengthy repair. The degree to which the manufacturer or vendor provides other customer services, such as training for team members, online tutorials, and local customer support, can also be an important consideration when selecting an AAC device.

Ability to Support the Development of New Skills

For all individuals, especially people with developing cognitive and linguistic skills, assessment ensures that the AAC system supports current communication but also supports the growth of new skills. Obtaining a system that provides for "growth adaptations," such as increases in the number of symbols displayed or the amount of vocabulary that can be stored, will increase the amount of time the person can maximize operational competence without being required to learn a new system to support his or her expanding cognitive-linguistic skills. Likewise, adaptations may be necessary to accommodate for changes in a person experiencing a degenerative disorder. For example, the person may require decreases in the number of symbols or vocabulary to accommodate decreased cognitive-linguistic skills or increased distractibility, alternative options for access to accommodate for progressive paralysis or fatigue, and so forth.

Another important issue to consider when selecting or developing an AAC device is the ways in which the device can be used for a wide variety of applications. As more AAC devices take advantage of computer-based technology, it is possible for them to include additional features. If the AAC team determines that the inclusion of other features on the device is desired, communication and social interaction goals should always remain the first priority. For example, a system with options for environmental control potentially increases independence for activating the television or lights; however, if the extra features interfere with the person's ability to locate communicative utterances in a timely manner, a decision must be made about the relative importance of the trade-off. After determining that communication goals are met, the team must decide which additional features are needed and whether they can be added without negatively affecting the effectiveness of the individual's communication abilities.

AAC System Trials

Trials with new AAC strategies should occur in the various transitional contexts and with the new communication partners and should specifically address the new communication needs. This component of assessment is time consuming; however, real-world assessment during planned visits to the transitional settings is critical to the successful implementation and integration of the AAC system in daily interactions. At these times, the team works to obtain a realistic picture of the device and requests formative feedback regarding the successes and problems of each AAC device from the individual who uses AAC, parents, teachers, and other communication partners. This activity facilitates acceptance of the AAC system by the people who will have the most profound impact on its final success (Parette & Angelo, 1996).

People who rely on AAC for communication require "flexible, individualized assessment approaches to yield accurate results and intervention guidelines" (Snell, 2002, p. 163). It is strongly recommended that structured trials of different AAC systems be completed in each context to ensure that the best outcome is achieved. Considerations include the same features addressed during assessment: effectiveness, efficiency, portability, dependability, programming, and so forth. Questions to be addressed in the trial include the following:

- Is the proposed system effective in facilitating communication on a variety of topics in a variety of environments?

- Does the individual (and/or the support team) have the skills and information needed to maintain the device?

- Have any task-related demands not been addressed?

- Do typical communication partners know how to support effective communication with the individual?

In addition, within any system trial of a high-tech device, the AAC team must also plan a back-up technique in case a device breakdown occurs. The need for a back-up system cannot be underestimated: AAC devices need to be repaired, batteries must be charged, power outages occur. A back-up system is essential for maintaining communication.

PROVIDING SUPPORT FOR EFFECTIVE USE

Once the transition AAC system is chosen, it is implemented. Like assessment, the intervention process is dynamic and is often perceived by team members as a continuation of the assessment process. The unstructured, dynamic nature of AAC intervention may seem like a moving target for many; however, the team must continue to design specific strategies for implementation, modification, support, and follow-up. An AAC device can be well chosen to fit all of an individual's communication needs and still fail solely because of poor implementation. Although some team members will have a larger role than others, the intervention component continues to involve appropriate team members to ensure success.

AAC System Training

The transition team prepares a schedule and evaluation metric to ensure that upon receipt of the AAC device, the individual receives instruction directed at maximizing independence in the use of the complete AAC system. The individual, educators, speech-language pathologists, family, peers, and/or coworkers are trained to operate and support the AAC system at the levels necessary for each of their assigned roles on the team. Some of the roles include troubleshooting, programming messages, setup, and daily maintenance. Specified team members will create communicative messages and vocabulary so that it is readily available. They are aware of and use motivating topics or items to promote the development of communication skills. Such motivators are integrated into messages to create novel interactions, introduce standard communication, or expand existing functional communication using different AAC devices or strategies. For some (e.g., literate people experienced with using AAC devices), initial instruction is sufficient to provide the skills necessary for independent use. Other individuals will benefit from ongoing support from various team members and/or manufacturers.

Communication Opportunities

An individual learning to use an AAC system requires multiple communication opportunities to develop functional communication skills. The extent to which a person has the opportunity to make use of AAC in purposeful ways will ultimately determine the extent to which communication is maintained and generalized across a variety of settings and partners. Team members are responsible for ensuring that people in the transition contexts (e.g., school, home, work, recreation) are aware of their responsibilities to provide communication opportunities (e.g., by asking questions, waiting for the individual to respond, providing choices, expecting use of the AAC device or strategies) and must provide training and support so that opportunities are provided and developed appropriately.

When teaching a new skill, educators must provide repeated opportunities for practice to increase accurate performance and to speed learning. Practice is essential both for individuals who have beginning skills as well as for those who are experiencing new communication demands as a result of transition. Practicing communication in the actual contexts provides the opportunity to rapidly learn the most essential skills. Communication itself is motivating to the majority of people, so simply incorporating its use into daily activities and routines will facilitate learning and use. For individuals with developing communication skills, the AAC technique is directly implemented into functional activities while simultaneously providing motivating consequences to messages. For example, during a group activity, the person uses AAC to produce the message IS IT MY TURN? and the communication partner(s) responds appropriately "Yes!" while placing a ball in position to be kicked. The team supports these people by identifying motivating communication opportunities that are essential to rapidly learning new communication skills.

Given the increased participation of children with severe disabilities in general education classrooms (Wagner et al., 2003), special attention should be given to the support of communication in classroom environments. In academic contexts, communication and social skills should not be excluded from the educational process but instead should be intertwined with educational goals and tasks. Many individuals who rely on AAC require extensive effort to complete academic tasks, leaving little time to address social interactions (Creech, 1992). In other cases, programming devices only with vocabulary for academic tasks leaves little opportunity for teaching social interaction.

Social communication is accepted as an important component in many academic settings (Hunt & Goetz, 1997); thus, assessment for transition must address full participation in all activities, including opportunities to learn social interaction. The AAC team must advocate for these opportunities even if such social interactions are not typically considered a goal in a particular classroom setting. Individuals who use AAC can be supported in increasing their participation in communicative interaction through their partner's use of a least-to-most prompting strategy including wait time and modeling.

With this approach, the partner provides the lowest level of cuing or prompting required to support appropriate participation by the individual who uses AAC. For example, the communication partner would provide *wait time:* pausing during an interaction to provide extra time for the individual to respond. This essential AAC communicative strategy may result in longer overall messages. Some individuals require a pause interval to understand what is said or asked (i.e., comprehension), and, as a result, wait time aids in their processing of the utterance and their responding. Other individuals require extended time to formulate a message because of language delays or impaired physical access to the AAC device. In this case, wait time provides the individual with an opportunity to independently generate a communicative utterance. If communication partners become involved too quickly and interrupt the independent construction of an utterance (e.g., under the impression that they must provide help to prevent the person from struggling), then the individual may become dependent on this assistance and not a functional, independent communicator.

If wait time does not produce the desired results, the communication partner might *model* how the device could be used to participate. Modeling is an effective strategy when teaching vocabulary or sentence formulation. A study by Myers (2007) showed that modeling AAC device interactions had a positive impact on symbol recognition, printed word recognition, awareness of correct word order, and the speed at which new overlays could be introduced. In modeling, a communication partner uses the person's AAC device side-by-side with them while simultaneously speaking. This method provides a model of appropriate vocabulary use during the communication turn and is an excellent example of message formulation to the individual who is learning to use the new AAC device. This strategy may also provide an AAC team member the added bonus of identifying missing vocabulary on the system through personal experience (Myers, 2007).

Over time, team members determine the cues necessary to support functional communication and regularly implement those cues. The team shares these cuing strategies with the individual's communication partners in order to facilitate generalized use. The goal is to gradually eliminate these cues by providing multiple opportunities for new learning, and by always first providing the least amount of cues necessary to support participation.

Follow-Up

Across transitions, an important component of intervention is to ascertain progress toward communication goals. The transition team develops measurable goals for each context, concept, educational/vocational need, and so forth. Initially, these are created from the lists of communication needs created by each team member, which are likely prioritized differently for each person (e.g., communication partner, individual). To determine the outcome of AAC recommendations, it is best to examine the original communication goals outlined for the individual prior to AAC assessment.

When addressing specific communication objectives, transition team members determine the changes expected as a result of AAC introduction (e.g., increased interaction, increased social engagement, progress in academic performance or work productivity, personal autonomy) and collect data that reflect the targeted items. These data may be collected to identify extent of change achieved in specific communication contexts, with specific partners, or in specific interactions. In some cases, the team may discover that strategies that facilitate one goal may impede another. This information is catalogued carefully, and strategies are customized for the success of communication in all transition contexts. In this manner, the team continues to develop goals and measure outcomes across multiple transitions, thereby optimizing independent and comprehensive functional communication.

CONCLUSION

·········· During high school, Larry's AAC team realized that a coordinated effort would be needed to ensure that his transition from high school to adult life would be a success. Larry was a young man with autism who had many community interests but very limited communication skills. Working with Larry, his family, and vocational rehabilitation personnel, the AAC team helped to identify both Larry's communication strengths and his communication needs. Following a series of device trials, the AAC team identified a device that would provide Larry with easy access to highly intelligible synthesized speech in the workplace and would also be highly portable and durable. Using the device, Larry has been an active participant in the workplace and in community recreational activities. (P. Politano, personal communication, May 12, 1999) ··········

Supporting effective communication for an individual with complex communication needs requires the commitment and involvement of the entire AAC team: the individual who uses AAC; family members and friends; and education, communication, and assistive technology professionals. However, if one truly believes that communication is the "essence of human life" (American Speech-Language-Hearing Association, 2005, p. 1), then providing access to effective, efficient, and appropriate communication must be identified as the most important goal in the transition planning process.

REFERENCES

American Speech-Language-Hearing Association. (2005). *Roles and responsibilities of speech-language pathologists with respect to augmentative and alternative communication: Position statement.* Retrieved September 17, 2009, from http://www.asha.org/docs/html/PS2005-00113.html

Atanasoff, L.M., McNaughton, D., Wolfe, P.S., & Light, J. (1998). Communication demands of university settings for students using augmentative and alternative communication (AAC). *Journal of Postsecondary Education and Disability, 13*(3), 32–47.

Beckung, E., & Hagberg, G. (2002). Neuro-impairments, activity limitations, and participation restrictions in children with cerebral palsy. *Developmental Medicine and Child Neurology, 44,* 309–316.

Beukelman, D.R., Hanson, E.K., Hiatt, E., Fager, S., & Bilyeu, D.V. (2005). AAC technology learning part 3: Regular AAC team members. *Augmentative and Alternative Communication, 21,* 187–194.

Beukelman, D.R., & Mirenda, P. (2005). *Augmentative and alternative communication: Supporting children and adults with complex communication needs* (3rd ed.). Baltimore: Paul H. Brookes Publishing Co.

Blackstone, S., & Hunt-Berg, M. (2003). *Social networks: A communication inventory for individuals with complex communication needs and their communication partners.* Monterey, CA: Augmentative Communication.

Blackstone, S.W., Williams, M.B., & Wilkins, D.P. (2007). Key principles underlying research and practice in AAC. *Augmentative and Alternative Communication, 23,* 191–203.

Cameron, L., & Murphy, J. (2002). Enabling young people with a learning disability to make choices at a time of transition. *British Journal of Learning Disabilities, 30,* 105–112.

Creech, R.D. (1992). *Reflections from a unicorn.* Greenville, NC: R.C. Publishing.

da Costa, M.F., Salomao, S.R., Berezovsky, A., de Haro, F.M., & Ventura, D.F. (2004). Relationship between vision and motor impairment in children with spastic cerebral palsy: New evidence from electrophysiology. *Behavioural Brain Research, 149,* 145–150.

Hamm, B., & Mirenda, P. (2006). Post-school quality of life for individuals with developmental disabilities who use AAC. *Augmentative and Alternative Communication, 22,* 134–147.

Higginbotham, D.J., Shane, H., Russell, S., & Caves, K. (2007). Access to AAC: Present, past, and future. *Augmentative and Alternative Communication, 23,* 243–257.

Hunt, P., & Goetz, L. (1997). Research on inclusive educational programs, practices, and outcomes for students with severe disabilities. *Journal of Special Education, 31,* 3–29.

Kent-Walsh, J., & McNaughton, D. (2005). Communication partner instruction in AAC: Present practices and future directions. *Augmentative and Alternative Communication, 21,* 195–204.

Light, J., Beesley, M., & Collier, B. (1988). Transition through multiple augmentative and alternative communication systems: A three-year case study of a head injured adolescent. *Augmentative and Alternative Communication, 4,* 2–14.

Lilienfeld, M., & Alant, E. (2005). The social interaction of an adolescent who uses AAC: The evaluation of a peer-training program. *Augmentative and Alternative Communication, 21,* 278–294.

Lund, S.K., & Light, J. (2006). Long-term outcomes for individuals who use augmentative and alternative communication: Part I—What is a "good" outcome? *Augmentative and Alternative Communication, 22,* 284–299.

McEwen, I.R., & Karlan, G.R. (1989). Assessment of effects of position on communication board access by individuals with cerebral palsy. *Augmentative and Alternative Communication, 5,* 235–242.

McNaughton, D., & Bryen, D.N. (2007). AAC technologies to enhance participation and access to meaningful societal roles for adolescents and adults with developmental disabilities who require AAC. *Augmentative and Alternative Communication, 23,* 217–229.

Mirenda, P. (2003). Toward functional augmentative and alternative communication for students with autism manual signs, graphic symbols, and voice output communication aids. *Language, Speech, and Hearing Services in the Schools, 34,* 203–216.

Myers, C. (2007). "Please listen, it's my turn": Instructional approaches, curricula and contexts for supporting communication and increasing access to inclusion. *Journal of Intellectual & Developmental Disability, 32,* 263–278.

National Joint Committee for the Communication Needs of Persons with Severe Disabilities. (1992). Guidelines for meeting the communication needs of persons with severe disabilities. *ASHA, 33*(Suppl. 5), 1–8.

Parette, H.P., & Angelo, D.H. (1996). Augmentative and alternative communication impact on families: Trends and future directions. *Journal of Special Education, 30,* 77–98.

Salvia, J., Ysseldyke, J.E., & Bolt, S. (2009). *Assessment in special and inclusive education* (11th ed.). Boston: Houghton Mifflin.

Smith, M.M. (2005). The dual challenges of aided communication and adolescence. *Augmentative and Alternative Communication, 21,* 67–79.

Snell, M.E. (2002). Using dynamic assessment with learners who communicate nonsymbolically. *Augmentative and Alternative Communication, 18,* 163–176.

Soto, G., Muller, E., Hunt, P., & Goetz, L. (2001). Professional skills for serving students who use AAC in general education classrooms: A team perspective. *Language, Speech, and Hearing Services in Schools, 32,* 51–56.

Wagner, M., Marder, C., Blackorby, J., Cameto, R., Newman, L., Levine, P., et al. (2003). *The achievements of youth with disabilities during secondary school: A report from the National Longitudinal Transition Study-2.* Menlo Park: CA: SRI International.

Williams, M.B., Krezman, C., & McNaughton, D. (2008). "Reach for the stars": Five principles for the next 25 years of AAC. *Augmentative and Alternative Communication, 24,* 194–206.

Yorkston, K., Beukelman, D., Hakel, M., & Dorsey, M. (2007). *Speech Intelligibility Test.* Lincoln, NE: Madonna Rehabilitation Hospital.

APPENDIX 11.1. Device Trial Worksheet

This device trial was completed at/with (context, communication partners): _____

_____

_____

The following devices were used:

1: _____

2: _____

3: _____

Device	1	2	3	4	5
In this setting and with the people in it, the person . . .					
1. achieves access to the device					
2. has accidental activations on the device					
3. easily uses the device					
4. is effective communicating with device					
5. is accurate communicating with the device					
6. utilizes features of the device					
7. navigates to various messages on the device					
8. likes the device					
9. increases fast, efficient communication with the device					
In this setting and with the people in it, the device . . .					
10. displays text, symbols, photos needed					
11. allows for the person's growth in skills					
12. allows for change in the person's physical skills					
13. provides needed features					
14. has durability suitable to this setting					
15. may be mounted, so the person maintains access					
16. has appropriate manufacturer-provided customer service and technical support					
17 has an accessible cost					
In this setting and with the people in it, communication partners . . .					
18. like the device and enjoy interacting with the person					
19. communicate more readily with the person using the device					
20. achieve successful interactions with the person using the device					

Index

Page references to boxes, figures, and tables are indicated by *b, f,* and *t,* respectively.